D1343396

OXFORD MEDICAL PUBLICATIONS

Paediatric Haematology and Oncology

Oxford Specialists Handbooks published and forthcoming

www.oup.co.uk/academic/medicine/osh/

Oxford Specialist Handbooks in Paediatrics

Paediatric Haematology and Oncology

Edited by

Simon Bailey

Consultant Paediatric Oncologist,
and Honorary Clinical Senior Lecturer
Newcastle upon Tyne Hospitals NHS Foundation Trust

and

Rod Skinner

Consultant and Honorary Clinical Senior Lecturer in
Paediatric Oncology/Bone Marrow Transplantation,
Newcastle upon Tyne Hospitals NHS Foundation Trust

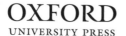

OXFORD
UNIVERSITY PRESS

OXFORD
UNIVERSITY PRESS

Great Clarendon Street, Oxford OX2 6DP

Oxford University Press is a department of the University of Oxford.
It furthers the University's objective of excellence in research, scholarship,
and education by publishing worldwide in

Oxford New York

Auckland Cape Town Dar es Salaam Hong Kong Karachi
Kuala Lumpur Madrid Melbourne Mexico City Nairobi
New Delhi Shanghai Taipei Toronto

With offices in

Argentina Austria Brazil Chile Czech Republic France Greece
Guatemala Hungary Italy Japan Poland Portugal Singapore
South Korea Switzerland Thailand Turkey Ukraine Vietnam

Oxford is a registered trade mark of Oxford University Press
in the UK and in certain other countries

Published in the United States
by Oxford University Press Inc., New York

British Library Cataloguing in Publication Data
Data available

Library of Congress Cataloging-in-Publication-Data
Paediatric haematology and oncology / edited by Simon Bailey and Rod Skinner.
   p. ; cm.—(Oxford specialist handbooks in paediatrics)
   Includes index.
   ISBN 978-0-19-929967-6 (alk. paper)
   1. Pediatric hematology. 2. Tumors in children. I. Bailey, Simon, 1964–II. Skinner, Rod, 1959–III.
   Series: Oxford specialist handbooks in paediatrics.
   [DNLM: 1. Neoplasms. 2. Child. 3. Hematologic Diseases. QZ 275 P126 2009]
   RJ411.P345 2009
   618.92′15—dc22

                                                                                        2009019006

Typeset by Cepha Imaging Private Ltd., Bangalore, India
Printed in China
on acid-free paper through
Asia Pacific Offset

ISBN 978–0–19–929967–6

10 9 8 7 6 5 4 3 2 1

Haematological and Oncological emergencies

Acknowledgements

Numerous people have helped and supported us during the writing and editing of this Handbook. Several colleagues have contributed helpful material and made excellent suggestions that have improved individual sections and chapters. We would particularly like to thank Denise Blake (Chemotherapy), Dr Steve Pedler (Severe sepsis), Dr Peter Carey (Acute myeloid leukaemia, Myelodysplasia, Myeloproliferative diseases, Bone marrow failure), Professor Josef Vormoor (Acute myeloid leukaemia), Professor Irene Roberts (the Chronic myeloid leukaemia section of Myeloproliferative diseases), and Dr Mario Abinun, Dr Andy Gennery, Dr Rob Wynne, Dr Paul Veys, and Professor Ajay Vora (sections of Haemopoietic stem cell transplantation). Dr Peter Carey has also contributed numerous photographs of blood films and bone marrow smears.

Our particular thanks go to everybody who has contributed so willingly and efficiently to writing chapters for this Handbook.

Finally, we are indebted to our wives and our children who have tolerated us during the last three years of writing and editing!

Contents

Symbols

📖	cross references
→	leading to
↓	decreased
↑	increased
α	alpha
β	beta
γ	gamma
κ	kappa
λ	lambda
σ	sigma
►►	Don't dawdle!
►	Important
−ve	negative
+ve	positive
⚠	warning
Δ	differential diagnosis
1°	primary
2°	secondary
<	less than
>	greater than

Abbreviations

μT	microTesla
ACC	adrenocortical carcinoma
ACTH	adrenocorticotrophic hormone
AD	autosomal dominant
AFP	α-fetoprotein
AIHA	autoimmune haemolytic anaemia
ALAL	acute leukaemia of ambiguous lineage
ALCL	anaplastic large cell lymphoma
ALD	adrenoleucodystrophy
ALG	anti-lymphocyte globulin
ALL	acute lymphoblastic leukaemia
ALP	alkaline phosphatase
AMKL	acute megakaryoblastic leukaemia
AML	acute myeloid leukaemia
ANC	absolute neutrophil count
APC	adenomatous polyposis coli
APL	acute promyelocytic leukaemia
APLS	Advanced Paediatric Life Support
APrC	antigen-presenting cell
APT	AST, ALP, GGT
APTT	activated partial thromboplastin time
AR	autosomal recessive
ARMS	alveolar rhabdomyosarcoma
ASAP	as soon as possible
ASR	age-standardized annual incidence
AST	aspartate transaminase
ATG	anti-thymocyte globulin
ATM	ataxia telangiectasia mutated (gene)
ATRA	all-trans retinoic acid
ATRT	atypical teratoid rhabdoid tumours
AUC	area under the curve
BAL	bronchoalveolar lavage
BCC	basal cell carcinomas
BCG	Bacillus Calmette-Guérin
BCNU	bis-chloronitrosourea (carmustine)
bd	twice daily
BDNF	brain-derived neurotrophic factor
BL	Burkitt's lymphoma
BM	bone marrow
BMA	bone marrow aspiration
BMD	bone mineral density
BMT	bone marrow transplant
BNF	British National Formulary
BP	blood pressure
Bu	busulfan

BWS	Beckwith-Wiedemann syndrome
CAD	coronary artery disease
CAMT	congenital amegakaryocytic thrombocytopenia
CCLG	Children's Cancer and Leukaemia Group
CCNU	chloroethylcyclo-hexylnitrosourea
CDI	central diabetes insipidus
CDK	cyclin-dependant kinase
CEA	carcinoembryonic antigen
CGH	comparative genomic hybridization
CHAD	cold haemaglutinin disease
CI	confidence interval
CIMF	chronic idiopathic myelofibrosis
CINV	chemotherapy-induced nausea and vomiting
CJD	Creutzfeld-Jacob disease
CML	chronic myeloid leukaemia
CMML	chronic myelomonocytic leukaemia
CMV	cytomegalovirus
CNS	central nervous system
CNSHA	congenital non-spherocytic haemolytic anaemia
COG	Clinical Oncology Group
CP	chronic phase
CPC	choroid plexus carcinoma
CPP	choroid plexus papilloma
CR	complete remission
CRABP2	cellular retinoic acid binding protein
CRBP	cellular retinol binding protein
CRP	C-reactive protein
CSF	colony-stimulating factor
CSF	cerebrospinal fluid
CSVT	cavernous sinus venous thrombosis
CT	computed tomography
CTPA	CT pulmonary angiography
CTX	chemotherapy
CTZ	chemoreceptor trigger zone
CVA	cerebrovascular accident
CVAD	central venous access devices
CVC	central venous catheter
CVP	central venous pressure
CXR	chest X-ray
DAT	direct antiglobulin test
DBA	Diamond-Blackfan anaemia
DDAVP	desmopressin acetate
DDS	Denys-Drash syndrome
DHPLC	denaturing high performance liquid chromatography
DIC	disseminated intravascular coagulation
DKC	dyskeratosis congenita
DLCL	diffuse large cell lymphoma
DLI	donor lymphocyte infusion
DLT	dose-limiting toxicity
DNA	deoxyribosenucleic acid
DNET	dysembryoplastic neuroepithelial tumour

DPG	diffuse intrinsic pontine glioma
DS	Down syndrome
DWI	diffusion-weighted imaging
DVT	deep vein thrombosis
E	epithelial
EBV	Epstein-Barr virus
ECG	electrocardiogram
ECP	extracorporeal photopheresis
EFS	event-free survival
EGF	epidermal growth factor
EGIL	European Group on Immunological Classification of Leukemias
EIA	enzyme immunoassay
EM	electron microscopy
EMA	eosin-5-maleamide
emf	electromagnetic fields
ENT	Ear, Nose and Throat
EPO	erythropoietin
ES	Ewing's sarcoma
ESBL	extended spectrum beta-lactamase
ESFT	Ewing's sarcoma family of tumours
ET	essential thrombocythaemia
EUD	European Union Directive
EVD	external ventricular drain
FA	Fanconi anaemia
FEIBA	factor VIII inhibitor by-pass agent
FFP	fresh frozen plasma
FGF	fibroblast growth factor
FH	favourable histology
FISH	fluorescent in-situ hybridization
FNA	fine needle aspiration
FSH	follicle-stimulating hormone
G6PD	glucose-6-phosphate dehydrogenase
GA	general anaesthetic
GBM	glioblastoma multiforme
GCP	Good Clinical Practice
GCT	germ cell tumours
GDNF	glial-derived neurotrophic factor
GFR	glomerular filtration rate
GGT	gamma glutamyl transferase
GH	growth hormone
GI	gastrointestinal
GIST	gastrointestinal stromal tumours
GIT	gastrointestinal tract
GM-CSF	granulocyte macrophage colony-stimulating factor
GN	ganglioneuroma
GNB	ganglioneuroblastoma
GST	glutathione-S-transferase
GTR	gross total resection
GvHD	graft-versus-host disease
GvL	graft versus leukaemia

H&E	haematoxylin & eosin
HA	hypoplastic anaemia
HAS	human albumin solution
Hb	haemaglobin
HB	hepatoblastoma
HbS	sickle cell Hb
HC	*haemorrhagic cystitis*
HCC	hepatocellular carcinoma
HCG	human chorionic gonadotrophin
HD	Hodgkin disease
HDAC	histone deacetylase
HDN	haemorrhagic disease of the newborn
HE	hereditary elliptocytosis
HEPA	high efficiency particulate air
HL	Hodgkins lymphoma
HLA	human leukocyte antigen
HLH	haemophagocytic lymphophistiocytosis
HMPV	human metapneumovirus
HNIG	human normal immunoglobulin
HNPCC	hereditary non-polyposis colon cancer
HPA	hypothalamic-pituitary axis
HPLC	high pressure liquid chromatography
HPP	hereditary pyropoikilocytosis
HR	hormone replacement
HS	hereditary spherocytosis
HSC	haemopoietic stem cells
HSCT	haemopoietic stem cell transplantation
HSV	herpes simplex virus
HTA	Human Tissue Authority
HUS	haemolytic-uraemic syndrome
HVA	homovanillic acid
HVOD	hepatic veno-occlusive disease
HZV	herpes zoster virus
IBMFS	inherited bone marrow failure syndrome
ICH	intracranial haemorrhage
ICP	intracranial pressure
ID	immunodeficiency
IEF	iso-electric focusing
IF	immunofluorescence
IGF	insulin-like growth factors
IM	intramuscular
INR	International Normalized Ratio
INSS	International Neuroblastoma Staging System
IPV	inactivated poliomyelitis virus
IST	immunosuppressive treatment
ITP	immune thrombocytopenic purpura
ITU	intensive care unit
IUT	intrauterine transfusion
IV	intravenous
IVC	inferior vena cava
JIA	juvenile idiopathic arthritis

JLTG	Japanese Liver Tumour Group
JMML	juvenile myelomonocytic leukaemia
JXG	juvenile xanthogranuloma
LAE	late adverse effect
LAF	laminar air flow
LAIP	leukaemia-associated immunophenotype
LBW	low birth weight
LCH	Langerhans cell histiocytosis
LDH	lactate dehydrogenase
LFT	liver function tests
LH	luteinizing hormone
LL	lymphocytic lymphoma
LMWH	low molecular weight heparin
LOH	loss of heterozygosity
LP	lumbar puncture
LPHD	lymphocyte predominant Hodgkin disease
LTFU	long-term follow-up
MAA	moderate aplastic anaemia
MAHA	micro-angiopathic haemolytic anaemia
MAP	mitogen-activated protein
MBEN	medulloblastoma with extensive nodularity
MBL	medulloblastoma
MCV	mean corpuscular volume
MDR	multidrug resistance
MDS	myelodysplasia
MDT	multidisciplinary team
MEN	multiple endocrine neoplasia
MFB	multifocal bone
MGCT	malignant germ cell tumour
MHRA	Medicines and Healthcare Regulatory Agency
MIBG	meta-iodobenzylguanidine
MIC	minimal intensity conditioning
MLPA	multiplex ligation PCR amplification
MMF	mycophenolate mofetil
MMP	matrix metalloproteinase
MMR	measles, mumps, rubella
MMUD	mismatched unrelated donor
MOF	multi-organ failure
MPD	myeloproliferative diseases
MPNST	malignant peripheral nerve sheath tumour
MPV	mean platelet volume
MRA	magnetic resonance angiogram
MRD	minimal residual disease
MRI	magnetic resonance imaging
MRSA	methicillin-resistant *Staphylococcus aureus*
MRV	magnetic resonance venography
MS	multisystem
MSC	mesenchymal stem cells
MST	morphine sulphate tablets
MTD	maximum tolerated dose
MUD	matched unrelated donor

NAI	non-accidental injury
NAITP	neonatal alloimmune thrombocytopaenic purpura
NB	neuroblastoma
NBL	neuroblastoma
NDI	nephrogenic diabetes insipidus
NF1	neurofibromatosis type 1
NG	nasogastric
NGF	nerve growth factor
NHL	non-Hodgkin lymphoma
NICE	National Institute for Health and Clinical Excellence
NPC	nasopharyngeal carcinoma
NPS	nasopharyngeal secretions
NSAA	non-severe aplastic anaemia
NSE	non-specific esterase
NSpE	neurone specific enolase
NT	neurotrophins
NTM	non-tuberculous mycobacterial
OCP	oral contraceptive pill
od	once daily
OR	odds ratio
PA	pernicious anaemia
PARP1	polyADPribosepolymerase 1
PAS	periodic acid-Schiff
PBSC	peripheral blood stem cells
PCA	patient-controlled analgesia
PCH	paroxysmal cold haemoglobinuria
PCP	*Pneumocystis jiroveci* pneumonia
PCR	polymerase chain reaction
PCToma	phaeochromocytoma
PCV	pneumococcal conjugate vaccine
PDGF	platelet derived growth factor
PE	pulmonary embolism
PEG	percutaneous endoscopic gastrostomy
PEM	protein energy malnutrition
PET	positron emission tomography
PFA	platelet function analyser
PFT	pulmonary function tests
PICU	paediatric intensive care unit
PK	pyruvate kinase
PKC	protein kinase C
PML	progressive multifocal leucoencephalopathy
PN	parenteral nutrition
PNET	primitive neuroectodermal tumour
PNH	paroxysmal nocturnal haemoglobinuria
PPB	pleuropulmonary blastoma
pPNET	peripheral primitive neuroectodermal tumour
PPSV	pneumococcal polysaccharide vaccine
PRN	per requirement
PT	prothrombin time
PTC	Principle Treatment Centre
PTH	parathyroid hormone

PTLD	post-transplant lymphoproliferative disorders
PV	polycythaemia vera
qds	four times daily
R&D	research and development
RA	retinoic acid
RAR	retinoic acid receptor
RARE	retinoic acid response element
Rb	retinoblastoma
RBP	retinol binding protein
RC	refractory cytopenia
RD	related donor
RA	refractory anaemia
RAEB	refractory anaemia with excess blasts
RAEB-t	refractory anaemia with excess blasts in transformation
RARS	refractory anaemia with ringed sideroblasts
RIC	reduced intensity conditioning
RMS	rhabdomyosarcoma
RR	relative risk/risk ratio
RRT	regimen-related toxicity
rSBP	raised systolic blood pressure
RSV	respiratory syncytial virus
RT	radiotherapy
RTA	renal tubular acidosis
SAA	severe aplastic anaemia
SaO_2	arterial oxygen saturation
SBP	systolic blood pressure
SC	subcutaneous
SCD	sickle cell disease
SCF	stem cell factor
SCID	severe combined immunodeficiency
SDS	Schwachman-Diamond syndrome
SEGA	sub-ependymal giant cell astrocytoma
SIADH	syndrome of inappropriate antidiuretic hormone secretion
SIOP	International Society of Paediatric Oncology
SIOPEL	International Society of Paediatric Oncology Epithelial Liver Tumour Strategy Group
SLE	systemic lupus erythematosus
SMS	superior mediastinal syndrome
SMR	standardized mortality ratio
SNP	single nucleotide polymorphism
SNS	sympathetic nervous system
SOS	sinusoidal obstruction syndrome
SRSV	small round structured virus
SS	single system
SSCP	single strand conformational polymorphisms
STS	soft tissue sarcoma
SVC	superior vena cava
SVCS	superior vena cava syndrome
T	Tesla
TACE	trans-arterial chemoembolization

TAM	transient abnormal myelopoiesis
TAR	thrombocytopenia absent radii
TBI	total body irradiation
TC^{99} MDP	technetium ^{99m} labelled methylene diphosphonate
TCD	transcranial Doppler
tds	three times daily
TGN	thioguanine nucleotides
TIMP	tissue inhibitors of MMP
TK	tyrosine kinase
TLI	total lymphoid irradiation
TLS	tumour lysis syndrome
TMZ	temozolamide
TNS	transcutaneous electrical nerve stimulation
TOF	tracheo-oesophageal fistula
TPMT	thiopurine methyltransferase
TRALI	transfusion related acute lung injury
TS	tumour suppressor
TSC	tuberous sclerosis
TSH	thyroid stimulating hormone
TT	thrombin time
TV	testicular volume
U&E	urea and electrolytes
UCB	umbilical cord blood
UH	unfavourable histology
URD	unrelated donors
US	ultrasound
UTI	urinary tract infection
UV	ultraviolet
WAGR	Wilms' tumour, aniridia, genitourinary abnormalities, mental retardation
WAS	Wiskott-Aldrich syndrome
WCC	white cell count
VEGF	vascular endothelial growth factor
VEGFR	vascular endothelial growth factor receptor
VHL	Von Hippel-Lindau disease
VIP	vasoactive intestinal peptide
VKDCF	vitamin K-dependent clotting factors
VMA	vanillylmandelic acid
VP	ventriculo-peritoneal
VRE	vancomycin-resistant enterococcus
VSAA	very severe aplastic anaemia
WT	Wilms' tumour
VTE	venous thromboembolism
VWD	von Willebrand disease
VWF	von Willebrand factor
VZIG	varicella zoster immunoglobulin
VZV	varicella-zoster virus
VZV/HZV	varicella/herpes zoster virus
XIAP	X inhibitor of apoptosis protein
XLP	X-linked lymphoproliferative disease
ZPP	zinc protoporphyrin

List of Contributors

Viv Allison
Paediatric Oncology Outreach Nurse Specialist, Royal Victoria Infirmary, Newcastle upon Tyne Hospitals NHS Foundation Trust, UK

Simon Bailey
Consultant and Honorary Clinical Senior Lecturer in Paediatric and Adolescent Oncology, Victoria Royal Infirmary, Newcastle upon Tyne Hospitals NHS Foundation Trust, UK

A. Martin Barrett
Consultant Paediatric Surgeon, Royal Victoria Infirmary, Newcastle upon Tyne Hospitals NHS Foundation Trust, UK

Tina Biss
Specialist Registrar in Haematology, Newcastle upon Tyne Hospitals NHS Foundation Trust, UK

Bernadette Brennan
Consultant Paediatric Oncologist, Royal Manchester Children's Hospital, UK

Penelope Brock
Consultant Paediatric Oncologist and Honorary Senior Lecturer, Great Ormond Street Hospital NHS Trust and Institute of Child Health, London, UK

Quentin D. Campbell-Hewson
Consultant Paediatric and Adolescent Oncologist, Royal Victoria Infirmary, Newcastle upon Tyne Hospitals NHS Foundation Trust, UK

Peter J. Carey
Consultant in Haematology, Royal Victoria Infirmary, Newcastle upon Tyne Hospitals NHS Foundation Trust, UK

G. Chinnaswamy
Northern Institute for Cancer Research, University of Newcastle upon Tyne, UK

Julia Clark
Consultant Paediatric Immunology and Infectious Diseases, Newcastle General Hospital, Newcastle upon Tyne Hospitals NHS Foundation Trust, UK

Anita Devlin
Consultant Paediatric Neurologist, Newcastle General Hospital, Newcastle upon Tyne Hospitals NHS Foundation Trust, UK

Angela Edgar
Consultant Paediatric Oncologist, Royal Hospital For Sick Children, Edinburgh, UK

Amanda Gerrard
Paediatric Oncology Outreach Nurse Specialist, Royal Victoria Infirmary, Newcastle upon Tyne Hospitals NHS Foundation Trust, UK

Juliet Hale
Consultant Paediatric and Adolescent Oncologist, Royal Victoria Infirmary, Newcastle upon Tyne Hospitals NHS Foundation Trust, UK

John Hanley
Consultant Haematologist, Royal Victoria Infirmary, Newcastle upon Tyne Hospitals NHS Foundation Trust, UK

Darren Hargrave
Oak Foundation Consultant Paediatric Oncologist in Drug Development, Royal Marsden Hospital, Surrey, UK

Helen Jenkinson
Consultant Paediatric Oncologist,
Birmingham Children's Hospital, UK

Hina Johnstone
Paediatric Oncology Outreach
Nurse Specialist, Royal Victoria
Infirmary, Newcastle upon Tyne
Hospitals NHS Foundation
Trust, UK

Orla Keating
CLIC Sargent Social Worker,
Newcastle upon Tyne, UK

Rajesh G. Krishnan
Consultant Paediatric
Nephrologist, Children's Kidney
Centre, University Hospital of
Wales, Cardiff, UK

Sheila M. Lane
Consultant Paediatric Oncologist,
Children's Hospital, Oxford, UK

Joanne Lewis
Consultant Clinical Oncologist,
Northern Centre for Cancer Care,
Freeman Hospital, Newcastle upon
Tyne Hospitals NHS Foundation
Trust, UK

Jan McBride
CLIC Sargent Social Worker,
Newcastle upon Tyne, UK

Sharon McGeary
Paediatric Oncology Outreach
Nurse Specialist, Royal Victoria
Infirmary, Newcastle upon Tyne
Hospitals NHS Foundation
Trust, UK

Kieran McHugh
Consultant Paediatric Radiologist,
Great Ormond Street Hospital
NHS Trust, London, UK

Louise Parker
Chair in Population Cancer
Research, Canadian Cancer
Society (Nova Scotia Division)
Dalhousie University, Canada

Anne Parry
Paediatric Oncology Research Sister,
Newcastle upon Tyne Hospitals
NHS Foundation Trust, UK

Bob Phillips
Locum Consultant in Paediatric
Oncology, Leeds Teaching Hospital
Trust, and MRC Research Fellow,
Centre for Reviews and
Dissemination, University of York,
UK

Lisa Price
Paediatric Oncology Research Sister,
Newcastle upon Tyne Hospitals
NHS Foundation Trust, UK

Rod Skinner
Consultant and Honorary Clinical
Senior Lecturer in Paediatric and
Adolescent Oncology/BMT, Royal
Victoria Infirmary and Newcastle
upon Tyne Hospitals NHS
Foundation Trust, UK

Clavin Soh
Consultant Neuroradiologist,
Salford Royal NHS Foundation
Trust, UK

Deborah Tweddle
Clinical Senior Lecturer and
Honorary Consultant in Paediatric
and Adolescent Oncology,
Newcastle University, UK

H. Josef Vormoor
Sir James Spence Chair of Child
Health and Honorary Consultant
in Paediatric and Adolescent
Oncology, Northern Institute for
Cancer Research, Newcastle
University, UK

Kevin P. Windebank
Senior Lecturer in Child Health,
Newcastle University, UK
and Honorary Consultant in
Paediatric and Adolescent
Oncology, Newcastle upon Tyne
Hospitals NHS Foundation Trust

Introduction

Although a few children with solid tumours were treated successfully with surgery and/or radiotherapy in the first half of the 20th century, the overall survival rate of childhood malignancy only increased appreciably after the late 1950s following the introduction of combination chemotherapy, initially in acute lymphoblastic leukaemia and then in solid tumours. Whereas <10% of children with malignancy survived in the 1950s, paediatric haematologists and oncologists in developed countries in 2008 expect that about 75% of children with cancer or leukaemia will survive at least 5 years from diagnosis, and anticipate that most of these will be cured. There are several reasons for this hugely impressive increase in survival, including great advances in the availability and use of chemotherapy, as well as major improvements in surgical and radiotherapeutic techniques and in supportive care. However, the most important factors are probably summarized by the concept of working together. This is seen in many ways:

- The use of multimodality treatment, where several different cytotoxic drugs are used together (combination chemotherapy) in a planned manner, often with additional radiotherapy and/or surgery (Multimodality treatment 📖 p. 130).
- Multidisciplinary teamwork with important contributions from numerous different healthcare, social-care, and scientific professionals, including:
  - doctors (e.g. paediatricians, surgeons, radiotherapists, radiologists, endocrinologists);
  - nurses (including specialist nurses, e.g. palliative care nurses);
  - pharmacists;
  - dieticians;
  - therapists (e.g. physiotherapists, occupational therapists);
  - social workers;
  - psychologists;
  - teachers;
  - laboratory staff (e.g. in microbiology laboratory);
  - research scientists.
- The widespread and extremely successful use of clinical trials to achieve sustained and progressive improvements in treatment and hence survival (Clinical trials 📖 pp. 202–204).

However, paediatric haematologists and oncologists cannot rest on their laurels since this success has come only at a significant price for the patients. Despite efforts to reduce the amount of potentially toxic treatment given to children with malignancy, many still suffer from significant late adverse effects of treatment, which may cause chronic ill-health with considerable impact on the survivor's quality of life (Long-term follow-up 📖 pp. 294–312). Given that children cured of malignancy may expect to live for a further 60–80 years, it is clearly vital to reduce the burden of late toxicity. Therefore, in light of the great improvements in survival of many childhood cancers and leukaemias, coupled with increasing recognition of the potential chronic toxicity of treatment for malignancy, the approach to treatment in many good prognosis malignancies over the last two decades has shifted noticeably to one of 'cure at least cost'. The aim of paediatric oncologists has been to achieve this by appropriate reduction of the intensity and/or duration of treatment in carefully identified good prognosis patients. Such stratification of treatment relies on detailed information about a patient's response to treatment and survival prognosis based on several factors, including:

- **Patient factors:** e.g. age, sex.
- **Disease factors**: e.g. disease burden as judged by haematological indices (e.g. white cell count), disease stage determined by imaging, histological subtypes, biological/molecular genetic characteristics (e.g. *MYCN* in neuroblastoma).

However, in some childhood malignancies survival rates remain very poor. New and more effective treatment strategies are needed urgently in these poor prognosis conditions, where the historically accepted philosophy of 'cure at any cost' remains applicable.

Aim

This handbook aims to provide trainees in paediatric haematology/oncology, as well as staff in related medical or other healthcare disciplines, with an easily accessible source of information about the basic principles of childhood cancer and leukaemia, as well as much of the more detailed specialist knowledge required to care for children with these conditions.

Layout

The book is divided into twelve sections:
- **Introduction to paediatric haematology and oncology**, including a section on the status of paediatric haematology and oncology in the developing world.
- **General approaches to suspected cancer** in the child who may have malignancy.
- **Oncological emergencies** in paediatric haematology and oncology.
- **General principles** of management of a child with malignancy.
- **Supportive care** of children with malignancy.
- **Long-term follow-up** after treatment
- **Benign haematological diseases, Malignant haematological diseases, Solid tumours, Central nervous system tumours,** and **Other conditions,** describing common and rarer paediatric malignancies.
- **New treatment strategies**, describing possible future directions in paediatric oncology.

The book concludes with a general information section, including information about normal values of laboratory tests, and helpful websites.

Introduction to paediatric haematology and oncology

Epidemiology of childhood cancer

What is epidemiology?

Epidemiology is the study of the occurrence and outcome of disease at the population level. This may not sound too exciting, but epidemiology is the tool that provides (or attempts to provide) the answers to the most important and urgent questions that families and doctors ask when a child is diagnosed with cancer:

- Why has my child got this disease?
- Who else gets this disease?
- What is going to be the outcome?

From an epidemiological point of view, the study of childhood cancer presents a real challenge because it is such a rare disease. It can be very difficult to conduct studies of sufficient size to have enough statistical power to answer the questions posed of them in a reliable and robust way. Even missing one or two cases in some instances can bias results, leading the researcher towards an erroneous conclusion. Bias can go in either direction, suggesting a positive association or effect when none exists, or suggesting no relationship between two factors when the truth is that there may well be an association hidden under an unsatisfactory study design. Because the numbers of cases of cancer in children do tend to be small, especially when considering subgroups, such as particular forms of leukaemia or solid tumours, it is very important to be aware of the limitations of all epidemiological studies in this field, and to understand the importance of the 95% confidence interval in indicating uncertainty.

Uncertainty in epidemiology

Uncertainty is unavoidable in epidemiological investigation. Even in calculating something as apparently straightforward as an incidence rate (see Definitions 📖 pp.17–19), which is the ratio of two numbers (the *numerator* being the number of cases observed in a given time period and the *denominator* being the population from which those cases were drawn), there are several potential sources of uncertainty. For example, in the numerator there is the potential for some cases to have been missed altogether and, for some cases, to be counted when, in fact, they are not truly cases of the disease of interest. This can happen for a number of reasons, including clerical coding error and misdiagnosis. So the number of cases identified in a population can be inflated or deflated. The number of cases arising from a given size of population will also vary from time to time and from place to place merely because of chance. The denominator is also uncertain, since in general the census is relied upon to inform about the 'population at risk', but since the census only happens every 10 years, in between censuses an educated guess is made as to what the population is. These uncertainties can have particularly big effects in childhood cancer, where numbers of cases are small and, in some instances, time periods and spatial units of interest are small too.

Much of epidemiological research is about to trying to find associations between past exposures and current disease leading to clues about disease causation. A much used study design for this is the case-control study (see Definitions 📖 pp.17–19), where exposure history is constructed for a group with disease (*cases*) and compared with the exposure history of a group of similar, but disease free individuals (*controls*). The objective is to identify exposures which are associated with having the disease, and the measure of the magnitude of any such association is reported as the odds ratio (OR; see Definitions 📖 pp.17–19). An OR of 1.3, for example, implies a 30% increase in risk of disease in those who had the exposure under study, and an OR of 2 indicates a doubling of risk. Uncertainty is even more of a problem in producing ORs than in producing incidence rate estimates. This is because measuring 'exposure' is always challenging. By definition, in a case-control study, the 'exposure' is in the past and this adds the potential for the introduction of error into the exposure estimate. A further complication is that cases and especially controls included in research studies may not be typical of all potential cases or all potential controls, and this can introduce bias into the study and, again, lead the researcher to the wrong conclusion. Case-control studies of the causes of childhood cancer have included investigation of factors, such as the role of maternal diet, exposures to agrochemicals, X-rays, paternal occupations, etc. In all of these cases, there is uncertainty and error in exposure estimates because of limitations in recording, measurement, or recall.

Confidence intervals

While the assessment of error in exposure estimates is generally not fully addressed in the majority of reports of epidemiological studies, we have a major tool to help us estimate the extent of uncertainty associated with rates or odds ratios – the 95% confidence interval (95% CI). All studies report a point estimate for rates or odds ratios, but not all studies should (nor do) carry the same weight – some studies are better than others, either because of their size (bigger is usually better) or the precision of their exposure assessments. The 95% CI for each estimate tells us the range of likely values that the point estimate could take, given the characteristics of the study. For example, two studies may have investigated the association between *in utero* X-ray exposure and risk of childhood cancer. Both produce the same OR, but one study has a much narrower confidence interval. Therefore, its effect estimate (OR) is more likely to be robust and reliable.

In epidemiology there is a move away from reporting the traditional statistical significance of a finding (e.g. $p = 0.05$) towards reporting the 95% CI of the effect estimate. This is because, for the reasons outlined above, the 95% CI, in addition, gives an indication of the robustness and reliability of the point estimate.

Who gets childhood cancer?

Disease groups

There are about 1400 new cases of childhood cancer in the United Kingdom each year. Around a third of childhood cancers are leukaemias, a quarter are brain tumours and the remainder comprise a number of increasingly rare diseases, including neuroblastoma, bone tumours, sarcomas, and other rare tumours (see Fig. 1.1).

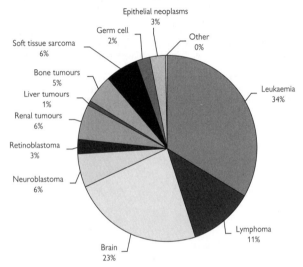

Fig. 1.1 Distribution of types of childhood cancer.

Leukaemias, lymphomas, brain tumours, and soft tissues sarcomas are themselves groups of distinct diseases, the constituents of which are shown in Fig. 1.2.

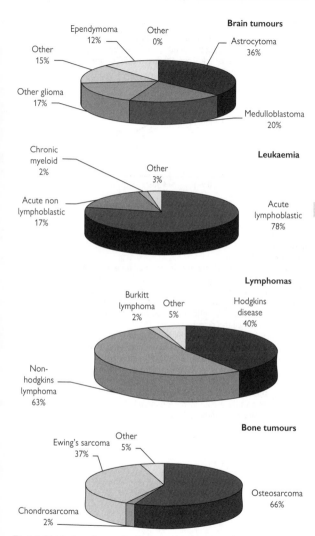

Fig. 1.2 Distribution of types of malignancy within the major subgroups of childhood cancer.

Incidence rates

Overall, childhood cancer is a rare disease and accounts for <1% of all cancer cases. Cancer affects 1 in 600 individuals by the age of 14 years and 1 in 300 by the age of 24. Boys are around 20% more likely to develop cancer than girls (see Fig. 1.3).

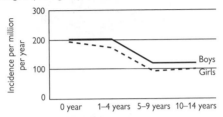

Fig. 1.3 Cancer incidence by age and sex (Europe).

Knowing the overall incidence of childhood cancer and its constituent parts is relevant to the ability to plan and develop the appropriate health and health-related services required to care for these children in both the short- and long-term.

Understanding changes in incidence over time and differences between different populations, e.g. between boys and girls, the affluent and the less affluent, and different populations (e.g. countries, people of different ethnicity) provides essential clues to the aetiology of disease, and in particular the balance between genetic factors vs. environmental and lifestyle factors in the causation of the disease.

The incidence of many childhood cancers, especially leukaemias, melanomas, and brain tumours has been increasing in most Western countries in recent decades (Table 1.1). This implies that environmental factors play a role in the aetiology of these diseases and that changes in environmental exposures result in changing patterns of disease. This does not preclude the potential of gene environment or epigenomic environment interactions to play a role in determining individual risk of cancer in the face of changing environmental risk.

Table 1.1 Temporal trends in childhood cancer rates in Europe 1970–1999

Malignancy	Annual Percentage Increase in Incidence Rate
Leukaemia	1.4%
Lymphoma	1.3%
Hodgkin disease	1.5%
Central nervous system (Eastern Europe)	2.5%
Central nervous system (Western Europe)	0.8%
Neuroblastoma	2.0%
Germ cell tumours	1.8%
Renal tumours	1.1%
Hepatic tumours	1.0%
Bone tumours	0.4%

What happens to children with cancer?

Survival

In the developed world the majority of children diagnosed with cancer will survive for at least 5 years and most of these will probably be cured.

There are big differences in survival for different cancers: death from retinoblastoma for example is uncommon with 5 year survival being in excess of 99% for this disease. Over 85% of children with leukaemia will be cured but for many of the solid tumours survival is lower, e.g. 5-year survival from brain tumours is around 75% and for bone tumours it is 72%. For each disease within the childhood cancer spectrum, there are characteristics of the child and disease at diagnosis, which allows identification of those in lower and higher risk groups, and therapy is tailored not only for each disease, but also for the various risk groups within each disease. Factors such as age, gender, and burden of disease at diagnosis, all influence response to treatment and, hence, whether an individual child is perceived as low or high risk for that particular disease.

Figure 1.4 shows the changes in survival over time for children with a number of different malignant diseases.

The surgical, chemotherapy, radiotherapy, and stem cell transplant regimens used in childhood cancer, and advances in supportive care have been responsible for the tremendous improvements in outcome over recent decades. However, all of these modes of treatment are toxic and cure has come at a cost, one of which is iatrogenic disease, which includes secondary cancer. Children treated with these therapies are at an average risk of a second malignancy at least four times that of the rest of the population. The implications of this are that, while it is important to reduce exposures wherever possible and to protect patients from their consequences, long-term follow-up and education of survivors is a necessary part of care of these patients (Long-term follow-up ▢ pp.294–312).

Survival for specific cancers has not only changed over time, but also varies between countries and, for many (but not all), is consistently poorer in the UK than elsewhere in mainland Europe and North America. The reasons for these differences are complex and may include differences in treatment delay (the interval between onset of symptoms and starting appropriate therapy), as well as differences in therapeutic approach.

Late effects of cancer therapy

The cure of cancer does not come without cost and there are many late effects of cancer therapy (Long-term follow-up ▢ pp.294–312). At least 60–70% of all cancer survivors have a long-term medical condition consequent to their cancer therapy and second malignancy is a major cause of death later than 5 years from diagnosis.

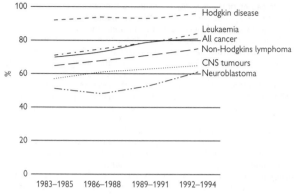

Fig. 1.4 Trends in 5-year survival in childhood cancer (Europe).

Causes of childhood cancer

Childhood cancer is a rare disease, affecting only 1 in 600 children by the age of 14 years. This is in dramatic contrast with adult cancer, the lifetime risk of which is 1 in 2 in men and 1 in 3 in women. Many of the causes of adult cancers are known and most involve long-term exposures over years or decades to exogenous agents, such as the 4000 or so carcinogenic or otherwise noxious constituents of tobacco smoke, high fat and low anti-oxidant diets, or endogenous agents, such as oestrogen. For children, the obvious observation is that they have not yet lived long enough to have had the opportunity to have been exposed to anything for years let alone decades. The pattern of cancers in children reflects this: carcinomas, which make up the majority of adult cancers, are rare in children, whereas two-thirds of cancers comprise leukaemia and brain tumours.

The causes of the majority of childhood cancers are unknown. With a few rare exceptions (such as bilateral retinoblastoma, which accounts for less than 1% of all childhood tumours, and some rare heritable conditions, such as Li Fraumeni syndrome), childhood cancer is not an inherited disease. Overall, the heritable component of childhood cancer is estimated to be around 2–3% at most. That said, the siblings of children with some malignancies, e.g. infantile acute lymphoblastic leukaemia, are at higher risk of developing malignancies, although the increase in risk is small. For children with some constitutional genetic conditions, e.g. Down syndrome and neurofibromatosis, the risk of cancer is increased, specifically Down syndrome confers a 150-fold increased risk of acute myeloid leukaemia (AML). Children with significant congenital anomalies are at higher risk of cancer than other children, e.g. there is an increased risk of Wilms' tumour in children born with Beckwith-Wiedemann syndrome, such that screening is recommended for children with this syndrome. This increased risk of malignant disease in children with congenital anomalies suggests a common cause to these conditions, and that the origins of many childhood cancers may lie in the period preceding birth. It is possible that peri-conceptional or gestational exposures may be important in affecting the genome, the epigenome or the proteome and, hence, increase susceptibility to cancer in childhood.

Although the potential time period for children to experience a carcinogenic exposure is short, because of the tremendous rate of growth and development during the post-conceptional period, there is potential for greatly increased vulnerability. In the transmogrification from fertilized egg to adult human, there are some 42 sequential cell divisions, over 90% of which occur *in utero* and during the first months of life. This period of extensive DNA replication reflects a period of genomic sensitivity and certainly the carcinogenic effect of radiation exposure is greatly enhanced in the foetus and the child.

Leukaemia

Leukaemia, and in particular acute lymphoblastic leukaemia (ALL), has been the most studied childhood malignancy from an epidemiological/aetiological perspective. There are several reasons for this. First, leukaemia is the most common malignancy of childhood, which means that from an epidemiological point of view it is the easiest to study. Secondly, it has a striking age incidence pattern – peaking at the age of around 4–6 years and then declining rapidly. Thirdly, this age peak emerged in the developed world over a period of several decades during the twentieth century, and is continuing to emerge in the developing world, where it was previously absent. This changing epidemiology, with a growing number of cases, has increased awareness and concern about this disease. In addition, the observation in the 1980s of apparent clusters of childhood leukaemia led to intense interest in the possibility of an environmental factor, causing childhood leukaemia, and the search for this factor has been the object of a great deal of research. It should be noted that because many epidemiological studies were retrospective, relying on historical ascertainment of cases, they were not able to necessarily distinguish between the various subtypes of childhood leukaemia and some also included non-Hodgkin lymphoma. In general, however, the leukaemias in this age group are predominantly acute lymphoblastic leukaemia, the main thrust of the hypotheses outlined below.

Radiation

Ionizing radiation

Ionizing radiation has been recognized as a potent carcinogen for over a century and exposure is known to cause leukaemia in adults. A higher rate of leukaemia was observed in the radiation-exposed survivors of the bombs at Nagasaki and Hiroshima. Because of this and because one of the largest and most persistent 'clusters' of childhood leukaemia was reported in the village of Seascale adjacent to the Sellafield nuclear installation in Cumbria, the role of ionizing radiation and electromagnetic fields has been much studied in childhood leukaemia.

There is agreement that *in utero* X-ray exposure increases the risk of all cancer, including leukaemia, in children born subsequently by around 30%. However, it is not an important cause of cancer in children in the UK or elsewhere where X-ray exposure during pregnancy is limited. Exposure to natural background radiation (due predominantly to radon exposure) has not been found to be strongly associated with childhood leukaemia. Studies of the role of paternal exposure to radiation have been equivocal, but since such exposures are now generally low due to vigilant radiation protection regimens, any increased risk they may bring makes a very small contribution to the overall burden of childhood leukaemia in the population.

Non-ionizing radiation

Studies of non-ionizing radiation, such as electromagnetic fields (emf) from electric power lines or appliances suggest that exposures greater than $0.4\mu T$ may increase the risk of childhood leukaemia. However, there are concerns about the reliability of these studies and again, even if this finding was accepted, such high exposures to emf are uncommon, implying that the vast majority of ALL cases are not caused by such exposures.

Other environmental exposures

Studies of other environmental exposures, such as agrochemicals, have had equivocal results, but there is some evidence that exposure to these agents is associated with small increased risks of leukaemia, especially in those who are genetically susceptible.

Clustering and infection

A characteristic of the occurrence of ALL is its tendency to 'cluster', i.e. there are places where, for a period of time, there are more cases than would be expected by chance alone. This has led to the generation of hypotheses around the role of community and individual infection in the aetiology of childhood leukaemia. Kinlen has studied many circumstances where there has been unusual population mixing, such as new towns, commuter towns, and war time evacuation of children from cities to rural communities. He found high rates of childhood leukaemia associated with many of these phenomena, leading to the hypothesis that high levels of circulating infections in circumstances, where herd immunity is low, leads to childhood leukaemia as a rare and unusual response to a common infection. There is some evidence that this explanation could account for more than half of all cases, and it is consistent with many of the current and historical features of the epidemiology of childhood leukaemia.

Solid tumours

In general, solid tumours have not been studied as much as leukaemias from an epidemiological point of view, the major reason being the challenge of studying these very rare diseases.

The causes of most solid tumours remain unknown. Retinoblastoma can arise from an inherited or a new mutation, and it is estimated that slightly less than half of retinoblastoma arising in the UK is inherited. While, as noted above, some characteristic congenital conditions increase the risk of solid tumours (such as Wilms' tumour), the vast majority of solid tumours are not inherited. As for leukaemia, there is evidence that *in utero* exposure to X-rays can increase the risk of solid tumours, but since very few women receive such investigations, this plays almost no causal role at a population level.

Implications for primary prevention and screening

For the vast majority of childhood cancers, the cause or causes remain unknown. This means there is currently little prospect of primary prevention of childhood cancer, although the role of infection and maturation of the immune system in leukaemia may point to a role for vaccination as an immune system maturation device. Breast feeding (exclusive and of long duration) protects against the development of leukaemia, probably by playing a similar role.

Screening for Wilms' tumour is recommended for children with Beckwith-Wiedemann syndrome and a few other rare congenital conditions.

Attempts were made to screen for neuroblastoma using urine catecholamine measurements in infants. While some cases of neuroblastoma were found by this approach, which was implemented throughout Japan for a number of years and investigated in research projects in North America, Germany, France, and the UK, it was eventually concluded that such screening did not reduce mortality and may have increased morbidity from this disease.

Definitions

Incidence

Incidence rate

This is the rate of occurrence of new cases of disease within the population. Generally, for childhood cancer, the incidence is reported as the number of cases per year per million population within a specific group, with respect to age and sex. For example, during 1971–1980 in England and Wales, the incidence rate of childhood cancer in boys aged 0–14 years was 114.1 per million per year.

Age-adjusted incidence rate

Age-adjusted incidence rate takes into account the fact that the age distribution of the population being studied may be different from that of a population with which you may wish to compare it. Commonly, a standard European or World population is used for the adjustment, which then allows direct comparison of rates between countries that may have different proportions of younger and older individuals. For example, during 1971–1980 in England and Wales, the age-adjusted incidence rate of childhood cancer in boys aged 0–14 years was 119.6 per million per year.

Cumulative incidence rate

The cumulative incidence rate is the risk aggregated over several years – typically up to age 14. For example, during 1971–1980 in England and Wales, the cumulative incidence rate of childhood cancer in boys up to age 15 years was 1310 per million or 1.3 per 10000.

Mortality

Mortality rate

The mortality rate is the number of deaths within a specific population during a specific time period – typically a year. Thus, for childhood cancer, the mortality rate would typically be reported as 20 per million per year.

Standardized mortality rate

The standardized mortality rate, like the adjusted incidence rate, takes into account the differences in age and/or sex distribution between populations, and allows direct comparison of mortality rates between different populations.

Standardized mortality ratio

For estimation of the standardized mortality ratio (SMR), the mortality rate in a reference population is considered to be equal to 100 and the SMR of the study population is the ratio of the observed number of deaths to the number that would be expected if the mortality rate was the same as that of the reference population. Populations with mortality rates lower than the reference population will have SMRs less than 100, while populations with rates higher than the reference population will have SMRs higher than 100.

Survival rate

The survival rate is the proportion of those diagnosed with the disease who survive for a given period of time. Typically, for childhood, ALL 5-year survival is around 85%.

Prevalence

The prevalence of disease is a measure of the number of people within a specific population who have the disease at any one time. Prevalence depends on both the incidence of disease and the duration of symptoms. For acute illness, prevalence is less than incidence, but for chronic disease, the prevalence may be higher.

The prevalence of childhood cancer is typically around 400 per million.

Measures of effect

Relative risk/risk ratio

The relative risk (or risk ratio, RR) is a comparison of the risk of disease in an exposed population with the risk of disease in an unexposed population. True relative risk estimates are only available from cohort studies. OR (see below) are used as an approximation to the RR, although they can overestimate the magnitude of the effect in small studies.

Odds ratio

The odds ratio is directly calculable from case-control studies and is the effect estimator from logistic regression analyses. It is the ratio of the odds of exposure in the diseased vs. the disease-free population. It is used as an estimate of the RR, but the two measures are not necessarily the same.

Confidence interval

Confidence intervals are a probabilistic window around a measured rate or point estimate of effect (OR or RR, for example) within which the true point estimate is likely to occur. 95% CI are typically reported; these encompass 95% of all probable values of the point estimate given the dataset scope and limitations. The width of the 95% CI depends on both the size (and statistical power) of the study and the heterogeneity of the exposure measurements. A narrow 95% CI implies a more robust study finding than a wider one.

Study design

Case-control study

Case-control studies capture retrospective data on exposure and compare exposure histories in the diseased group (cases) with a disease-free group (controls). Case control studies are more efficient for the study of rare diseases, such as childhood cancer.

Cohort study

Cohort studies may be retrospective or prospective and involve capturing exposure data on a large population from which the cases will (or have) emerge(d). For rare diseases, such as childhood cancer, cohort studies must capture information on huge populations (typically, several hundred thousands or even millions of person years) for a sufficient number of cases to arise to make the observations robust. Cohort studies are generally more expensive and resource intensive than case-control studies, although they may be less prone to bias.

Clustering analysis/incidence rate heterogeneity studies

There are several different approaches used to determine whether there are differences in the rates of disease between places and between different time periods. Space–time clustering investigated whether cases are closer in space and time than would be expected by chance. This would occur, for example, if an infection agent was involved in the aetiology of the disease. Childhood leukaemia cases tend to demonstrate space–time clustering, especially when place and time of birth (vs. diagnosis) are considered. Other statistical tests compare rates between one place and another, and between one time period and another. This addresses other hypotheses of causation, such as whether there may be more cases in one place due to an environmental factor, such as a source of pollution.

Biology and genetics of childhood cancer

What is cancer?

- Cancer is the uncontrolled proliferation of abnormal cells.
- A malignant tumour invades and destroys the tissue in which it originates, and can spread (metastasize) to distant sites.
- A benign tumour is non-invasive and does not metastasize.
- Cancer is a genetic disease of somatic cells and sometimes germ cells.
- Most cancers originate from a single aberrant cell, i.e. they are clonal.

What causes cancer?

- Good evidence to show that both physicochemical agents and viruses are tumourigenic for human cancers.
- Physicochemical agents modify normal genes to become cancer genes (oncogenes), e.g. via mutation.
- Viruses may trigger oncogenesis [e.g. Epstein-Barr virus (EBV) in endemic Burkitt's lymphoma] and may carry their own oncogenes, e.g. *KIT, MYCC, ABL*.
- For most childhood cancers it is unclear what triggers oncogenesis, but the role of oncogenes and anti-oncogenes (tumour suppressor genes) is well established.

Oncogenes

- These are the 'tumour accelerators'.
- They are normal cellular genes (proto-oncogenes), which have been altered in some way to become constitutively active (gain of function):
  - amplification, e.g. *MYCC, MYCN, Erb-B2*;
  - activating mutation, e.g. c-*KIT*;
  - translocation, e.g. t(9;22) *BCR/ABL*.
- Usually act in a dominant manner at the cellular level.
- There are >100 oncogenes, which code for oncoproteins.
- Can act anywhere in the cell, ranging from external growth stimulus to transcription factor in the nucleus, regulating the transcription of proliferation-related genes.

Growth factors

- Epidermal growth factor (EGF).
- Platelet derived growth factor (PDGF).
- Fibroblast growth factors (FGF1-9).
- Insulin-like growth factors (IGF1,2).
- Vascular endothelial growth factor (VEGF).
- Stem cell factor (SCF).
- Glial-derived neurotrophic factor (GDNF).
- Nerve growth factor (NGF).
- Brain-derived neurotrophic factor (BDNF).
- Neurotrophins 3–5 (NT3-5).

Transmembrane growth factor-receptors = tyrosine kinases

- *ErbB1–4* – EGF receptor.
- PDGF receptor α, β.
- VEGF receptor.
- c-*KIT* – SCF receptor.
- *RET* – GDNF receptor.
- IGF1 receptor α, β.
- *TrkA, NGFR* – NGF receptor.
- *TrkB, TrkC* – BDNF and NT-3 receptors, respectively.

Cytoplasm

- Intracellular tyrosine kinases, e.g. *BCR-ABL*: kinases phosphorylate proteins at serine, threonine and tyrosine residues.
- 2nd messengers:
  - protein kinases, e.g. protein kinase C (PKC);
  - GTPases, e.g. *K-RAS, N-RAS, H-RAS*;
  - phospholipase C, phosphoinositol 3 kinase (PI3 kinase).
- Other intracellular signal transduction pathways: mitogen-activated protein (MAP) kinase.
- Mitochondria: BCL-2 anti-apoptosis.

Nucleus

- Transcription factors, e.g. *MYCC, MYCN FOS, JUN, MDM2*.
- Transcriptional co-factors, e.g. histone deacetylases (HDAC).
- Cyclins and cyclin-dependent kinases, e.g. CCND1, CDK4.

Tumour suppressor genes

- These are the 'tumour brakes'.
- First observed in cell fusion studies when some human tumour cells fused with normal cells produced hybrids that had lost their malignant properties.
- Usually act in a recessive manner at the cellular level.
- Become inactivated (loss of function) by various mechanisms in cancer:
  - gene deletion of one allele (loss of heterozygosity) and deletion, or inactivating mutation of 2nd allele, e.g. *p53, Rb*.
  - epigenetic silencing through methylation, e.g. *p16(CDKN2A)*.
- The heritable form of retinoblastoma (Rb), based on germline mutations in the Rb tumour suppressor (TS) gene and the 2nd hit required for oncogenesis (Knudson's 2 hit hypothesis), supported the concept of the presence of TS genes, which are recessive at the cellular level but dominantly inherited.

TS genes (and their loci) include:
- **Cytoplasm:**
  - *APC* (adenomatous polyposis coli) (5q21) – tyrosine phosphorylation;
  - *PTEN* (phosphatase and tensin homologue deleted on chromosome 10) (10q23) – phosphatase, removes phosphate groups and inhibits PI3kinase and AKT kinases;
  - *Neurofibromin* – (the *NF1* gene product) (17q11), a GTPase activating protein (inhibits RAS);
  - *Merlin* (the *NF2* gene product) (22q12) – cytoskeletal protein;
- **Nuclear transcription factors:**
  - *p53* (17p13) *53kd protein* – transcriptionally regulates G1 to S checkpoint → cell cycle arrest, and apoptosis;
    - guardian of the genome
    - activated in response to stress e.g. DNA damage
  - *WT1* (Wilms' tumour 1)(11p13) – transcriptional activator or repressor for growth factor genes;
  - *PML* (Promyelocytic Leukaemia)(15q22) – transcriptional repression;
  - *VHL* (Von Hippel Lindau)(3p25) – represses hypoxia-induced genes, e.g. VEGF.
- Cell cycle inhibitors:
  - *Rb* (13q14) – inhibits G1 to S checkpoint;
  - *p16^{INK4a}/p14^{ARF}* (9p21) – cyclin-dependent kinase inhibitors.
- **DNA repair genes:**
  - *ATM* (11q23) – ataxia telangiectasia mutated;
  - *BRCA1* (breast cancer 1)(17q21) and *BRCA 2* (Fanconi anaemia);
  - *CHK1* – checkpoint kinase 1, cell cycle checkpoint control;
  - *hMLH1* (3p21), *hMSH2* (2p22) – mismatch repair genes.
- **Cell death inducing genes:**
  - *DCC* (deleted in colon cancer)(18q21) – caspase substrate;
  - *FAS (CD95)* (10q24) – cell death receptor.

DNA repair genes

Types of DNA repair

Nucleotide excision repair
- Used to repair UV irradiation-induced pyrimidine dimers and single stand breaks.
- Involves the enzyme polyADPribosepolymerase 1 (PARP1).

Homologous recombination
- Used to repair double strand breaks, e.g. from ionizing radiation, involves *ATM* to sense the damage, DNA dependent protein kinases (DNA PKs) and *BRCA1/2* to repair it.
- *BRCA2* is one of the Fanconi anaemia genes.

Non homologous end joining
- Also used to repair DNA double strand breaks; more error prone.
- Also involves *ATM*, DNA PKs.

Mismatch repair
- Uses mismatch repair enzymes, e.g. *hMLH1* and *hMSH2* to remove mistakes in DNA that occur more frequently at sites of DNA repeats called microsatellites.
- Mutated in hereditary non-polyposis colon cancer (HNPCC).
- Defective mismatch repair leads to microsatellite instability, but rarely found in paediatric tumours.

In cancers, it is the powerful combination of oncogene activation and tumour suppressor gene inactivation, combined with the inability to repair these genetic hits and the evasion of apoptosis, which enables the tumour cells to divide and eventually conquer.

Apoptosis: programmed, energy-dependent cell death occurring in response to radiotherapy (RT), chemotherapy (CTX), growth factor withdrawal, cytotoxic lymphocyte killing.
- **Characteristic morphology:** nuclear condensation and fragmentation with cell membrane sparing.
- **Biochemical:** DNA fragmentation.
- BCL-2 family includes pro-apoptotic (BAX) and anti-apoptotic (BCL-2) members present in mitochondria.
- **Two mechanisms:**
  - *mitochondrial* – e.g. from CTX via *p53* inducing BAX;
  - → cytochrome C release from mitochondria and caspase 9 cleavage/ activation;
  - *non-mitochondrial* via death receptors (FAS, TNF pathways), e.g. lymphocyte mediated cytolysis, involves caspase 8 cleavage;
  - final common pathway of caspase 3 cleavage → apoptosis.

Tumourigenesis is a multi-step process leading to genetic alterations in:
- Regulation of cell cycle progression.
- Apoptosis.
- Differentiation.
- Angiogenesis and metastasis:
  - the genes and chromosomes involved may occur in cancer cells, normal somatic cells and germ cells;
  - some of these alterations and the methods of detection are outlined below.

Non-random, somatic genetic abnormalities in childhood cancers

Whole chromosome abnormalities

- **Detected by karyotype analysis:** G banding of metaphase chromosome spreads.
- **Ploidy:**
  - this is the total number of chromosomes in a cell;
  - diploid = 46, haploid = 23;
  - aneuploidy = gain or loss of 1 or more whole chromosomes;
  - hyperdiploidy = 47–50:
    - associated with a good prognosis in ALL;
    - triploidy associated with a good prognosis in infants with neuroblastoma (NBL).
- **Monosomy:**
  - instead of two copies of a chromosome present in somatic cells there is only one copy;
  - monosomy 5 or 7 is associated with a poor prognosis in AML.
- **Trisomy:** acquired trisomy 21 is frequently found in ALL and AML.

Partial chromosome abnormalities

Can be detected from karyotype, but more refined mapping is possible using:

- Fluorescent *in-situ* hybridization (FISH).
- Southern blot.
- Multiplex ligation PCR amplification (MLPA).
- Comparative genomic hybridization (CGH).
- Array CGH.
- Single nucleotide polymorphism (SNP) chips.
- **NB:** All except FISH are DNA averaging techniques, a normal result does not exclude abnormalities if tumour cell content <60%.
- FISH is the most sensitive and can be performed on single cells.

Deletions

- Loss of either short (p = petite) or long (q) arm of one chromosome.
- Leads to loss of heterozygosity (LOH).
- 1p loss, 11q loss, 3p loss all occur frequently in NBL and are associated with a poor prognosis.
- 17p loss in medulloblastoma is associated with a poor prognosis.

Other

Inversion of chromosome 16 in AML M4Eo is associated with good risk disease.

Gains

- Gain of p or q arm of chromosome.
- Unbalanced 17q gain or 2p gain in NBL.

Translocations

- Detectable by karyotypic analysis, break-apart FISH probes or reverse transcription-PCR for fusion transcripts.
- Not detectable by other methods.
- Frequent in haematological malignancies.
- Also found in some solid tumours but rare in NBL.

Transcriptional control chimeric genes

- **t(8;14)(q24;q32), Burkitt's lymphoma:**
  - translocation of *MYCC* including promoter to control of immunoglobulin heavy chain (chromosome 14), or light chain κ or λ (chromosomes 2, 22) enhancers;
  - leads to overactive *MYCC*;
  - not of prognostic significance.
- **t(15;17)(q21;q21), acute promyelocytic leukaemia (M3):**
  - fusion of *PML* gene (chromosome 15) with the retinoic acid receptor – α (*RARA*) (chromosome 17);
  - associated with good risk disease;
  - associated with response to ATRA (see Targeted treatments for molecular defects in childhood cancers, Differentiation, 📖 p.36).
- **t(X;18)(p11;q11), synovial sarcoma:**
  - chimeric transcriptional control genes;
  - *SYT-SSX1* – occurs in 65% of synovial sarcomas;
  - *SYT-SX2* – occurs in 35% of synovial sarcomas.
- **t(11;22)(q24;q12), Ewing's sarcoma (ES)/PNET:**
  - chimeric Ewing's sarcoma *EWS/Fli1* transcript present in >85% ES;
  - also t(21;22) – 10% ES;
  - *others* – t(7;22), t(17;22), t(2;22) – all rare;
  - uncertain prognostic significance.
- **t(2;13)(q35;q14), alveolar rhabdomyosarcoma (RMS):**
  - *PAX 3*/Forkhead(*FKHR*) fusion transcript;
  - occurs in 60% alveolar RMS;
  - associated with a worse prognosis in metastatic disease;
  - also t(1;13)(p36;q14) – 15–20% alveolar ARMS;
  - PAX7/Forkhead(FKHR) fusion transcript;
  - associated with a better prognosis in metastatic disease.

Tyrosine kinase chimeric genes

- **t(9;22)(q34;q11), *BCR/ABL* in CML (= Philadelphia chromosome):**
  - also found in 3–5% ALL, where it is a poor prognostic marker;
  - leads to fusion transcript and chimeric oncoprotein;
  - constitutively active tyrosine kinase;
  - targeted by kinase inhibitors e.g. imatinib (Targeted treatments for molecular defects in childhood cancers 📖 p.34).
- **t(2;5)(p23;q35), anaplastic large cell non-Hodgkin lymphoma:**
  - anaplastic lymphoma kinase (*ALK*)/nucleophosmin (*NPM*) fusion transcript.
  - not prognostic.

Single gene defects
- **Deletions:**
  - may be homozygous or heterozygous (LOH);
  - *p16 +/– p14 (CDKN2A)* – melanoma, glioblastoma, T-cell ALL, NBL, ES;
  - *Rb* – retinoblastoma, sarcoma;
  - *p53* – osteosarcoma, mouse knockouts develop tumours, but viable;
  - *WT1* – LOH in 20% Wilms' tumour, mouse knockouts lethal as WT1 needed for kidney and gonad development.

NB. Epigenetic silencing through methylation, e.g. for *p16*, *WT1*, and caspase 8, can occur as an alternative mechanism of loss of function in TS genes.

- **Amplification:**
  - present cytogenetically as extrachromsomal double minutes and homogenously staining regions;
  - most easily detected by FISH;
  - *MYCN:*
    - transcription factor controlling cell cycle related genes and apoptosis;
    - amplified 10–300-fold in 20–25% of NBL and alveolar RMS;
    - poor prognostic marker.
  - *MDM2:*
    - negatively regulates *p53*;
    - amplified in osteosarcomas and rarely NBL;
    - often co-amplified with *Gli* and *CDK4*.

- **Mutations:**
  - can screen by denaturing high performance liquid chromatography (DHPLC) or single strand conformational polymorphisms (SSCP);
  - best detected by direct sequencing of DNA;
  - may be homozygous (mutation of one allele and deletion of 2nd allele) or heterozygous (2nd allele normal);
  - *p53*:
    - mis-sense mutations most common;
    - rare in embryonal paediatric tumours;
    - present in sarcomas;
    - more frequent at relapse, e.g. leukaemia, Wilms' tumour, NBL
  - *Ras* – activating mutations in codons 13 or 61 of *N-ras* in 20% of AML patients;
  - *Rb*:
    - point mutations affecting mRNA splicing, frameshift mutations → truncated protein;
    - occur in osteosarcoma, Burkitt's lymphoma, and glioblastoma;
  - *ATM*:
    - bi-allelic point mutation;
    - leukaemia/lymphoma;
  - *PTCH*:
    - homologue of *Drosophila* segment polarity gene;
    - sonic hedgehog receptor;
    - mutated in 10% medulloblastoma;
  - *c-kit*:
    - activating mutations in gastrointestinal stromal tumours (GIST);
    - if present, sensitive to imatinib therapy;
    - rarely involved in childhood tumours.

Heritable genetic abnormalities associated with childhood cancers

4–10% childhood cancer results from inherited genetic mutations.

Constitutional chromosomal abnormalities

Down syndrome (DS, trisomy 21)
- 2–3% risk of acute leukaemia: ALL (60%) or AML (40%).
- Most of the ↑ risk of AML occurs <4 years age.
- Up to 70% of DS-associated AML is M7 (Acute myeloid leukaemia, Treatment, Down Syndrome–acute myeloid leukaemia ☐ pp.416–417).

Cancer predisposition syndromes

Features of an autosomal dominant (AD) cancer family syndrome
- Multiple generations affected with cancer.
- Transmission may occur through either parent.
- Earlier age of onset compared with sporadic cases.
- ↑ Multiple and/or bilateral tumours.
- Also metachronous tumours.
- ↑ Risk of only a few cancer types.
- Variable penetrance, so carriers don't necessarily develop cancer.

NF1 (AD) Von Recklinghausen's disease
- Commonest AD disorder 1 in 2500.
- Accounts for 50% of all optic gliomas, usually by age 6 years.
- **Plexiform neurofibromas:** congenital, develop in early life, may be disabling.
- Benign neurofibromas.
- ↑ Risk of phaeochromocytoma (PCToma), JMML, other CNS gliomas, malignant peripheral nerve sheath tumour (MPNST, 50% have NF1), sarcomas.
- Germline *Neurofibromin* mutations with loss of 2nd copy.

NF2 (AD)
- Bilateral acoustic neuromas.
- Astrocytomas, meningiomas, melanomas.

Multiple endocrine neoplasia (MEN) (AD)
- **MEN1:** parathyroid, islet cell, and pituitary tumours.
- *MEN1* gene on chromosome 11.
- **MEN2a:** medullary thyroid carcinoma, parathyroid adenoma, PCToma.
- **MEN2b:** as for 2a, also including gastrointestinal (GI) ganglioneuromas, skeletal abnormalities, onset in infancy.
- Activating *RET* mutation (10q11) in MEN2a and b.
- Inactivating *RET* mutation → Hirschsprung disease.

Li-Fraumeni (AD):

- Germline heterozygous mutations in *p53* gene or occasionally checkpoint kinase 2 (*chk2*).
- Classic: proband with sarcoma <45 years *plus* 1st degree relative with any cancer <45 years *plus* 1st degree relative with any cancer <45 years or sarcoma at any age.
- RMS, other soft tissue sarcoma, pre-menopausal breast cancer, brain tumours, adrenocortical carcinoma, acute leukaemia, choroid plexus carcinoma.
- ↑ Risk of 2nd cancer (cumulative probability 57%).

Turcot syndrome (AD)

- Brain tumours (gliomas, ependymomas, medulloblastoma) with polyposis and colon cancer:
  - *APC* mutation (medulloblastoma); or
  - HNPCC loci (*hMLH1, hMSH2*; glioblastoma multiforme).

Tuberous sclerosis (TSC) (AD)

- Seizures, developmental delay, adenoma sebaceum.
- Two-thirds of cases are new mutations.
- At least 2 genes are involved:
  - *TSC1* (9q34) Hamartin;
  - *TSC2* (16p13) Tuberin.
- Cardiac rhabdomyosarcomas develop *in utero* and often regress postnatally.
- Retinal hamartomatas, giant cell astrocytoma, renal angiomyolipomas.

von Hippel-Lindau disease (AD)

- Multiple cerebellar haemangioblastoma, retinal angioma (usually in 2nd or 3rd decade of life), renal cell carcinoma (+ cysts), PCToma.
- Surveillance required if VHL mutations present.

Gorlin syndrome (AD)

- Multiple naevoid basal cell carcinomas (BCC): 30% of <20-year-olds with BCC have Gorlin's.
- Odontogenic jaw cysts, bifid ribs, palmar/plantar pits, facial dysmorphism, short 4th metacarpal.
- Medulloblastoma (MBL): 10% of <2-year-olds with MBL have Gorlin's.
- RT → multiple naevi in RT field + ↑ risk of meningioma and ependymoma.
- Mutations in *PTCH*.

Familial adenomatous polyposis (AD)

- Extensive polyposis in 2nd and 3rd decade of life, with colorectal cancer, dermoid cysts, mandibular cysts, and osteomas.
- Carriers have increased risk of upper GI cancer, thyroid cancer (1%), and hepatoblastoma (1 in 250 lifetime risk).
- Surveillance sigmoidoscopies recommended from 8 years of age.

Familial retinoblastoma (AD)
- Accounts for 40% retinoblastoma.
- 85% are *de novo* germline mutations.
- Age of onset earlier than sporadic (usually <1 year).
- Bilateral tumours frequent.
- ↑ Risk of other tumours, e.g. osteosarcoma, soft tissue sarcoma, melanoma.

Constitutional abnormalities → ↑ risk of Wilms' tumour

3–5% Wilms' tumour cases are hereditary.

WAGR
- <u>W</u>ilms' tumour, <u>A</u>niridia, <u>g</u>enitourinary abnormalities, mental <u>r</u>etardation.
- Interstitial deletion of *WT1* allele and mutated 2nd allele.

Beckwith-Wiedemann syndrome:
- Macroglossia, unusual ear creases, somatic gigantism, visceromegaly, neonatal hypoglycaemia, abdominal wall defects.
- May include hemihypertrophy, but this can also occur in isolation.
- ↑ Risk of WT.
- Duplication of 11p15 with genomic imprinting (paternal).
- Leads to LOH without copy number change = uniparental disomy.
- Includes *IGF-2* & *p57^{KIP2}*.

Denys-Drash syndrome (AD)
- Intersex disorders, nephropathy, and Wilms' tumour.
- *WT1* mis-sense mutation – heterozygous.
- More severe phenotype with mutation than *WT1* deletion.

Four-monthly abdomen ultrasound (US) scan recommended for these syndromes until 8 years of age.

Hereditary DNA repair defects

Usually autosomal recessive (AR)

Xeroderma pigmentosum (XP) (AR)
- Defective nucleotide excision repair, including thymidine dimer repair following UV irradiation.
- Leads to skin cancers in sun-exposed areas.

Fanconi anaemia (AR)
- Defect in *BRCA2* predisposes to early onset solid malignancies in FANC-D1 complementation group.
- Other complementation groups associated with AML, often preceded by bone marrow failure.
- Congenital abnormalities common.

Ataxia telangiectasia (AR)

- Defective double strand break repair due to chain terminating mutations in *ATM*.
- Ataxia, choreoathetosis, and telangiectasia develop by 3–5 years of age.
- Immunodeficiency, leukaemia, and lymphoid malignancy common.
- Increased sensitivity to cytotoxic agents. Need care with treatment.
- Increased frequency of breast cancer in carriers (1–2% population).

BRCA1 and BRCA2 germline mutations

Predispose to familial breast and ovarian cancer.

HNPCC (AD)

- Increased risk of colon cancer without polyps, manifesting in 2nd decade of life.
- Extra-colonic malignancies may occur, including uterine, ovarian, upper GI.

Inherited immunodeficiency (ID) syndromes

- Severe combined immunodeficiency.
- Wiskott-Aldrich syndrome.
- X-linked lymphoproliferative syndrome.
- Selective IgA deficiency.

All associated with ↑ risk of lymphoid malignancy (non-Hodgkin) or leukaemia. Compare with ↑ risk in acquired ID patients with organ allografts (especially EBV driven), HIV, prior treatment with cytotoxics, and some chronic viral infections.

Targeted treatments for molecular defects in childhood cancers

Therapies are aimed at targeting the 4 main events in tumourigenesis and progression:
- Regulation of cell cycle progression.
- Apoptosis.
- Differentiation.
- Angiogenesis and metastasis.

Regulation of cell cycle progression
Growth factor receptor inhibitors
- **EGFR inhibitors:**
  - Trastuzamab (Herceptin);
  - anti-Erb-B2 antibody, used in breast cancer, glioma;
  - cetuximab – metastatic colorectal cancer.
- **IGFR inhibitors:** IGF2 over-expression occurs in Wilms' tumours and RMS. IGF2 inhibitors are under development.

Intracellular tyrosine kinase inhibitors
- **BCR/ABL tyrosine kinase inhibitors:** CML, c-kit+ GIST, Ph+ ALL:
  - Imatinib (Glivec);
  - Dasatinib.
- **TRK inhibitors:** CEP-701 – AML, NBL, MBL.
- **Aurora kinase inhibitors:**
  - ↑ expression in *MYCN* amplified NBL;
  - undergoing clinical trials in adult cancers.
- **Other tyrosine kinase inhibitors:**
  - Erlotinib (Tarceva) – metastatic non-small cell lung cancer, glioma;
  - Sunitinib (Sutent) – Metastatic renal cell cancer, GIST.

Other kinase inhibitors
- PI3 kinase inhibitors.
- mTOR (mammalian target of Rapamycin) kinase inhibitors: sirolimus (used in immunosuppression).
- Farnesly transferase inhibitors: inhibit RAS activity. Potentially useful for NF1-associated tumours.
- CDK inhibitors, e.g. flavopiridol.
- Multiple kinase inhibitor: sorafenib (advanced renal cell carcinoma).

HDAC inhibitors
- Inhibit histone deacetylation, leading to less chromatin condensation and enhanced transcription of growth inhibitory and apoptotic genes.
- Vorinostat (SAHA), romidepsin (depsipeptide, FK-228), belinostat (PXD101), and LAQ824/LBH589:
  - active in T cell lymphoma;
  - undergoing trials in NBL.

Demethylating agents
- Inhibit DNA methylation leading to tumour suppressor gene re-expression and inhibition of cell growth.
- Decitabine is undergoing clinical trials, e.g. in NBL.
- Enhanced effects when combined with HDAC inhibitors.

DNA repair inhibitors:
- PARP inhibitors.
- Potentiate cytotoxic therapy, e.g. temozolamide (TMZ) in melanoma.
- Preclinical studies of AG1699 combined with topotecan and TMZ in NBL and MBL.
- ATM and DNA-PK inhibitors under development.

Proteasome inhibitors:
- Bortezomib (Velcade).
- Inhibits NF kappa B signalling. Involved in growth control and p53 degradation. Also active in p53 mutant cells.
- Used in multiple myeloma, but active in NBL and other paediatric tumours.

Blocking antibody therapy
- Anti-CD20 (Rituximab) → apoptosis, used in NHL.
- Anti-GD_2:
  - disialoganglioside GD_2 over-expressed on NBL and osteosarcoma, also weakly on peripheral nerves;
  - anti-GD_2 kills cells by antibody dependent cytotoxicity;
  - possible additive effects when combined with other immunotherapies;
  - e.g. activation of the innate immune system with GM-CSF (neutrophils, macrophages) + IL-2 (NK cells) may have anti-tumour activity and activate cells expressing Fc receptors.

Drug-antibody conjugates
E.g. gemtuzumab ozogamicin (Mylotarg) = anti-CD33 antibody and cali-cheamicin, used in AML.

Apoptosis
Apoptosis inducers
- **Anti-sense** = oligonucleotides that bind to RNA via complementary base pairing and prevent translation.
- **Anti-sense X inhibitor of apoptosis protein** (XIAP): preclinical studies in paediatric oncology.
- **Anti-sense BCL2:** used in adult follicular NHL.
- **Aplidine:** a natural substance from the marine tunicate induces apoptosis, e.g. in small cell lung cancer.
- Some kinase inhibitors block anti-apoptotic effects of kinases, e.g. imatinib.
- **Fenretinide:** novel retinoid that ↑ apoptosis, active in NBL and ES.

Differentiation:

- Main role of differentiation agents is in chemoprotection/chemoprevention or in the treatment of minimal residual disease.
- Not active against actively growing tumours.
- Retinoids are derivatives of vitamin A (retinol).
- Following retinoid treatment NBL cells *in vitro* undergo morphological differentiation with extension of neurites (Fig. 2.1a).
- Retinoids (retinoic acid, RA) mediate their activity via nuclear receptors (RAR and RXR $\alpha\beta\gamma$), which bind to DNA sequences called retinoic acid response elements (RARE) and exert biological effects (Fig. 2.1b,c).
- In NBL cell lines, RA → ↓ *MYC*, *MYB* + cell cycle gene transcription + ↑ TGFβ.
- 13 *cis*-RA (isotretinoin) is used in minimal residual disease treatment of high risk NBL.
  - 13 *cis*-RA ↑ 3 year EFS to 46%, cf 29% in controls;
  - 13 *cis*-RA ↓ basal cell carcinoma in XP patients;
  - All *trans*-retinoic acid (ATRA) used in treatment of APML – 90% CR rate, ATRA relieves transcriptional repression of mutant *PML/RAR*α;
  - bexarotene – retinoid X receptor agonist, used in cutaneous T cell lymphoma.

Angiogenesis and metastasis

- Neovascularization involved in initial tumour growth and development of metastases.
- Angiogenesis begins when VEGF interacts with VEGFR → endothelial cell proliferation.
- Hypoxia induces VEGF expression and selects for mutant p53.
- Other factors, e.g. matrix metalloproteinases (MMPs) involved.
- Metastasis begins with loss of tumour cell–cell contact and migration by proteolytic degradation of the basement membrane to enter the circulation.
- This is followed by capillary trapping, extravasation, and proliferation.
- Key processes are:
  - *cell adhesion* – involves integrins, laminins, cadherins, focal adhesion kinase, and CD44;
  - *epithelial (E) cadherin function* disrupted by β-catenin alterations and APC (regulates β-catenin);
  - *proteolysis* – involves proteases (plasminogen activators), cathepsins (cysteine proteases), MMPs, and TIMPs (tissue inhibitors of MMPs);
  - *motility* – involves pseudopodia, dynamic polymerization, and depolymerization of cytoskeleton;
  - inhibition of endothelial cells by endostatin, is used in preclinical models of paediatric tumours;
  - *MMP inhibitors* – marimastat, neovastat;

- *VEGF inhibitors* – anti–VEGF antibodies, e.g. bevacizumab (Avastin) used in:
  - renal cell cancer, colon cancer;
  - paediatric solid tumour clinical trials;
  - inhibitors of VEGF, e.g. interferon;
  - blockage of VEGF-kinase activity using small molecule inhibitors.

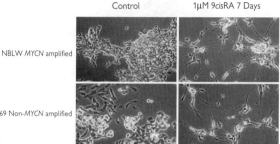

(a)

Fig. 2.1 (a) NBL cells *in vitro* undergo morphological differentiation with extension of neurites. Reprinted with permission from Chen *et al.* 2007, Cell Cycle: 6(21), 2685–96.

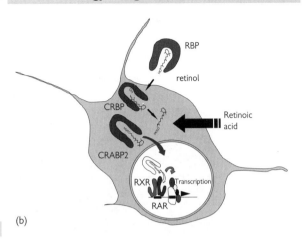

(b)

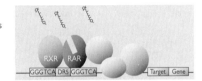

Retinoids bind to
retinoic acid receptors
(RARs)

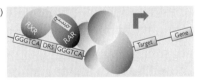

Activating (or repressing)
gene expression

(c)

Fig. 2.1 (cont.) (b) RBP = retinol binding protein; CRBP = cellular retinol binding
protein; CRABP2 = cellular retinoic acid binding protein. (c) Retinoid acid in the
nucleus. Fig. 2.1b Courtesy of C.P. Redfern, Northern Institute for Cancer Research,
Newcastle University. Fig. 2.1c Courtesy of B. Goranov, Northern Institute for
Cancer Research, Newcastle University.

Practical considerations

It is vital to make every effort to obtain a fresh sample of tumour tissue (solid tumours) or bone marrow (leukaemias) before treatment is commenced. In addition to allowing a histological/haematological diagnosis, this provides material for cytogenetic investigations that may:

- Play a major or even crucial role in establishing or clarifying the precise diagnosis, especially in cases where the histological diagnosis is very difficult or uncertain (e.g. some cases of Ewing's sarcoma or rhabdomyosarcoma).
- Provide important prognostic information, e.g. by identifying poor risk malignancies, such as Philadelphia-positive ALL or alveolar rhabdomyosarcoma.
- This prognostic stratification may also determine treatment, e.g. intensive chemotherapy ± haemopoietic stem cell transplantation in Philadelphia-positive ALL.

Very occasionally, tumour or bone marrow biopsy may not be appropriate, when:

- Biopsy is very hazardous, e.g. in the presence of a large mediastinal mass. In some of these children the diagnosis may be made and sufficient material obtained for biological studies by other means, e.g. peripheral blood blasts in T-cell ALL, pleural effusion in NHL.
- The diagnosis has been established with certainty from initial investigations (e.g. neuroimaging in tectal plate glioma) and in whom a biopsy may carry a high risk of further morbidity.

Genetic information may offer very important clues about the likely diagnosis and behaviour of a tumour, e.g. a visual pathway tumour in a patient with NF1 is nearly always a low grade glioma and more likely to behave in a relatively indolent manner. This permits an 'observation' policy in some patients whose vision is not under significant threat. Furthermore, radiotherapy should be avoided if at all possible in patients with NF1, due to the increased risk of second malignancies secondary to DNA damage.

Diagnosis of a familial cancer predisposition syndrome may provide important information to facilitate management of the whole family, e.g. by:

- Informing screening recommendations in asymptomatic individuals.
- Guiding treatment decisions in patients, e.g. avoiding radiotherapy wherever possible in patients with Li-Fraumeni syndrome or neurofibromatosis.

An ever-increasing array of cytogenetic and genetic techniques may be used to assist the investigation of paediatric malignancies. Those used most commonly include:

- Karyotype analysis
- Fluorescent *in situ* hybridization (FISH).
- Polymerase chain reaction (PCR).
- Comparative genomic hybridization (CGH).
- Genotyping.

Biological testing is becoming more important for guiding treatment. *Real time* biology is being used to guide treatment in neuroblastoma (*MYCN*) and, soon, a number of biological markers will be used to stratify treatment in medulloblastomas. It is anticipated that similar strategies will be introduced in more disease types in the future.

The future

- More targeted drugs to use in combination with conventional chemotherapy to prevent emergence of drug resistance.
- Harness the power of RNA interference to inhibit oncogenes, currently used *in vitro* only.
- Individualized therapy depending on the patient's tumour biology.

Paediatric oncology in the developing world

Paediatric oncology in resource-rich countries relies heavily on detailed investigation with high technology machinery and expensive tests. It also relies on intensive chemotherapy, radiotherapy, and delicate, but extensive, surgery to achieve the high cure rates that are now expected in the so called western world.

In resource-limited countries, the expectations are different and the level of infrastructure varies enormously. Paediatric oncology has to redefine its traditional goals and tailor treatment according to available resources and infrastructure. Many resource-limited countries achieve excellent results given the limited resources available to them. Examples of diseases that are treated well include Burkitt's lymphoma and Wilms' tumours. On the other hand, ALL is difficult to treat in the resource challenged world as the treatment is long in duration and requires multiple visits to hospital (despite excellent outcome in most western countries). Some observations on how this has been achieved are given below:

- Inspired and visionary leadership is essential. Ideally, this should arise from local individuals at a local level, although outside help may be necessary to start the process. However, longevity of the process is best achieved by nurturing local medical and nursing staff. A realistic, but sustainable, service should be provided as a basic, but essential, building block.
- The maximum possible benefit should be achieved by using the available resources wisely. Treatment should be provided initially for common and potentially treatable malignancies before trying to cure all patients.
- Protocols used in the resource-rich world should be adapted to ensure a tolerable level of side effects in accordance with the underlying infrastructure and facilities, e.g. it is unhelpful trying to perform bone marrow transplants if the patient does not have running water at home.
- It may be useful to twin with a centre from a resource-rich country to provide educational resources and moral support.
- Co-operative groups within countries or regions may be very useful to enable basic trials or at least a consistent approach, and may also help promote a higher standard of care.
- Records of patients and their progress should be kept to enable audit of outcomes to measure progress.
- Patient follow-up is essential to monitor long-term effects of the protocols or treatments. For example, some countries have used a clinical officer on a motorbike to go to the patients' homes. Another centre takes a photograph of children receiving treatment so that health workers going out to the villages may more accurately find the child, since the addresses given are often inaccurate.

It is the responsibility of the whole paediatric oncology community to help each other and, in so doing, benefit children with cancer all over the world. How that is achieved is open to interpretation, and may differ in different countries and areas around the world. The International Society of Paediatric Oncology (SIOP) and the Children's Oncology Group (COG), from the USA both have programmes to help less wealthy countries and a large number of charities also exist with specific aims in providing some support for paediatric oncology teams in resource-limited countries.

General approaches to suspected cancer

Chapter 4

Abdominal mass

Abdominal mass

The presence of a palpable mass in the abdomen of a child is a serious finding because of the possibility of malignant disease. Even benign conditions can be a cause of concern and warrant prompt evaluation. Careful initial assessment, including a full history, examination, and limited investigations can provide sufficient evidence to determine the diagnosis, and enable swift referral to the appropriate specialist.

The differential diagnosis for a child with an abdominal mass is extensive. The age and sex of the patient, site of origin of the mass, presence or absence of other related symptoms and signs, and specific examination findings will narrow the list of possible diagnoses.

Malignant neoplasms are more commonly encountered as the cause of abdominal masses in children than in infants. The most common abdominal malignancies diagnosed in the paediatric population include:
- Neuroblastoma.
- Wilms' tumour.
- Hepatoblastoma.
- Lymphoma.
- Germ cell tumours.

History

- Patient age is one of the most important factors in directing the diagnostic workup. Differential diagnoses of abdominal masses in neonates and in infants and children are shown in Table 4.1.
- Length of time since mass was first noticed (reflects speed of growth).
- Symptoms and signs of gastrointestinal (GI) or genitourinary obstruction.
- **Constitutional symptoms:** pallor, fever, night sweats, weight loss, anorexia (suggestive of malignancy, but not specific).
- **Antenatal and birth history:**
  - prenatal US scan revealing poly/oligohydramnios, suggestive of developmental abnormalities of the urinary tract;
  - increasing number of tumours are diagnosed prenatally, including germ cell tumours and neuroblastoma;
  - a foetus with one congenital abnormality is at greater risk of having another.
- **Infections/bruising/bleeding:** may be an indication of bone marrow involvement.
- **Systemic symptoms due to metabolic effects of tumours:** high levels of catecholamines, and occasionally vasoactive intestinal peptide (VIP), associated with neuroblastoma can cause bouts of sweating, pallor, watery diarrhoea, and hypertension.
- Known congenital syndromes, familial cancer syndromes and chromosomal abnormalities (see associations with malignancy in Table 4.2).
- **Older females:** remember possibility of pregnancy.
- Family history of cancer, particularly familial cancer syndromes.

Table 4.1 Differential diagnosis of abdominal masses in neonates, infants, and children

Neonates	Infants/children
Retroperitoneal	**Retroperitoneal**
Renal	*Renal*
Hydronephrosis (urinary tract obstruction, urethral valves, ectopic urethrocele)	Wilms' tumour
	Hydronephrosis
Multicystic dysplastic kidney	Cyst
Infantile polycystic kidney	Congenital malformation
Mesoblastic nephroma	*Non-renal*
Wilms' tumour	Neuroblastoma
Renal vein thrombosis (may → haematuria)	Teratoma
Horseshoe kidney	Rhabdomyosarcoma
Ectopic kidney (usually in pelvis)	Other neoplasm
Bilateral renal enlargement (hypoxia/ischaemia)	
Single, benign renal cyst	
Non-renal	
Adrenal haemorrhage	
Neuroblastoma (adrenal primary)	
Teratoma	
Gastrointestinal	**Gastrointestinal**
Duplication	Appendiceal abscess
Mesenteric or omental cyst	Other neoplasms (e.g. lymphoma)
Complicated meconium ileus	
Dilated bowel proximal to atresia	Congenital malformation
Hepato-spleno-biliary	**Hepatic**
Haemangioma	Haemangioma
Haemangioendothelioma	Haemangioendothelioma
Hepatoblastoma	Hepatoblastoma
Hepatic cyst	Hepatocellular carcinoma
Splenic haematoma	Other neoplasm
Splenic cyst	
Choledochal cyst	
Hydrops of gallbladder	
Genital	**Genital**
Ovarian cyst	Ovarian cyst or teratoma
Hydrocolpos	Hydrometrocolpos
Hydrometrocolpos	Other neoplasm

Examination

- Perform thorough examination of all systems (but especially GI).
- Assess for organomegaly:
  - liver and/or spleen may be enlarged as part of malignant process (e.g. lymphoma, leukaemia, neuroblastoma);
  - primary liver or renal tumour.
- Evaluate size and character of mass if possible:
  - solid masses or fluid filled cysts are dull to percussion;
  - air-filled bowel is tympanic.
- **Abdominal distension:** the mass may be obvious on inspection or palpation.
- Lower pole of normal kidneys may be palpable on examination in children.
- **Bowel sounds:** high-pitched ('tinkling') in intestinal obstruction.
- Assess for ascites.
- **Measure blood pressure:** hypertension common in Wilms' tumour, neuroblastoma, phaeochromocytoma.
- **Lymphadenopathy:** suggests haematological malignancy or neuroblastoma.
- **Skin nodules:** e.g. 'blueberry muffin' skin nodules in neuroblastoma.
- **Skin rash:** e.g. eczema-like skin rash over napkin area and/or back may be seen in children with hepatosplenomegaly due to multisystem Langerhans cell histiocytosis (LCH).
- Features suggestive of a syndrome (see Table 4.2).
- **Full neurological assessment:** to exclude signs of spinal cord compression secondary to invasion of vertebral canal, e.g. neuroblastoma.

Genetic cancer syndromes

The majority of tumours in children occur sporadically but rarely (<5% of childhood tumours) they are associated with recognized congenital syndromes, familial predisposition syndromes, or chromosomal abnormalities. The same tumour may also occur in more than one member of the family in which case it is assumed that there is a genetic predisposition. These families should be referred for genetic counselling (see Table 4.2).

WAGR is a congenital malformation syndrome characterized by aniridia (congenital absence of the irises), genitourinary malformation and mental retardation, and is associated with the development of Wilms' tumour in 30–50% of cases. This group of patients have a constitutional deletion of 11p13, which encompasses the gene loci for both Wilms' tumour (*WT1*) and aniridia (*PAX6*). The *WT1* gene deletion is also responsible for the development of genitourinary malformations.

A number of other syndromes are associated with an increased risk of developing Wilms' tumour, including:

- Overgrowth syndromes, e.g. Beckwith-Wiedemann syndrome (BWS), X-linked Simpson-Golabi-Behmel syndrome.
- Syndromes associated with nephrotic syndrome, e.g. Denys-Drash syndrome (DDS), Perlman syndrome.

Hemihypertrophy, either alone or as part of BWS, is also associated with hepatoblastoma and adrenocortical carcinoma (ACC), in addition to Wilms' tumour.
- A second Wilms' tumour gene (*WT*2) has also been identified, which carries an increased risk of neuroblastoma and hepatoblastoma.

Table 4.2 Congenital syndromes, familial cancer syndromes and chromosomal abnormalities

Congenital syndromes	
Neurofibromatosis	(N.B. CNS tumours commoner than abdominal) Soft tissue sarcoma (rhabdomyosarcoma)
Beckwith-Wiedemann	Wilms' tumour
Hemihypertrophy	Wilms' tumour
WAGR	Wilms' tumour
Sporadic aniridia	Wilms' tumour (loss of 11q)
Turcot	Colon cancer and CNS tumours
Denys-Drash	Pseudohermaphroditism and nephrosis
Gonadal dysgenesis with Y chromosome	Gonadoblastoma, dysgerminoma
Peutz-Jegher	Cancer of GI tract and many other sites
Genitourinary abnormalities	Wilms' tumour
Familial cancer syndromes	
Familial adenomatous polyposis	Hepatoblastoma, hepatocellular carcinoma
Chronic hereditary tyrosinaemia	Adrenocortical tumours (also brain tumours, soft tissue sarcomas and breast cancer)
Li-Fraumeni (p53)	
Chromosomal abnormalities	
11p13 chromosome deletion	Wilms' tumour
1p deletion	Neuroblastoma
Trisomy 21	Leukaemia

Investigations

- First step is a plain abdominal X-ray to exclude gastrointestinal tract (GIT) or genitourinary tract obstruction. Identification of obstruction should lead to early involvement of the paediatric surgical team and consideration of contrast studies (oral contrast study or barium enema for upper and lower GIT obstruction, respectively).
- Abdominal X-ray may also detect calcification of the mass.
- US scan is an invaluable adjunct in investigating an abdominal mass in children, since it is inexpensive, readily available, seldom requires sedation, and can provide information on site of origin, characteristics (solid or cystic), and vascularity of the mass.
- More specific anatomical and detailed tissue architectural information can be obtained from magnetic resonance imaging (MRI) or computed tomography (CT) scanning.
- Laboratory investigations will generally be carried out in parallel to radiological imaging. Baseline blood tests include full blood count/film, electrolytes, uric acid, and lactate dehydrogenase. Abnormalities in these will guide subsequent investigations:
  - *Anaemia, thrombocytopenia, neutropenia* – suggestive of marrow failure or infiltration. Bone marrow aspiration and trephine indicated.
  - *Elevated uric acid and lactate dehydrogenase levels* – indicators of rapid cell turnover associated with malignancy, particularly lymphomas. Elevated uric acid levels and abnormal electrolytes may be caused by tumour cell lysis and warrant prompt management to prevent renal impairment (Tumour lysis syndrome 📖 pp.94–95).
  - *Tumour markers may aid in the diagnosis of certain tumours* – teratomas (α-fetoprotein, AFP), liver tumours (AFP), some carcinomas (carcinoembryonic antigen, CEA).
  - *Urinary catecholamines* (homovanillic acid [HVA] *and vanillylmandelic acid* [VMA]) – elevated in >90% of cases of neuroblastoma and phaeochromocytoma.
- Viral serology should be performed in all new presentations of malignancy and bone marrow failure:
  - *Varicella-zoster virus (VZV), measles* – to guide post-exposure prophylaxis in susceptible patients) (Immunization 📖 pp.270–274).
  - *Herpes simplex virus (HSV)* – to assist differential diagnosis and management of mouth ulcers.
  - CMV ± EBV are performed routinely in some units.
  - In high risk areas, hepatitis B/C and HIV screening will usually be performed.
  - The blood sample should be taken *before* any blood product transfusion to avoid passive transfer of antibodies giving a false positive result.
- If malignancy is suspected after initial investigations have been performed, refer the children to the regional paediatric oncology unit for further management.
- The subsequent diagnostic work up involves detailed imaging to determine the local extension and infiltration of the primary mass, and the stage of the disease by identifying the presence of distant metastases.

Histological evaluation of the mass is essential to confirm the diagnosis. Fresh tissue material should also be sent for cytogenetic studies.

Table 4.3 Summary of investigations to be performed or considered in a child with an abdominal mass

Laboratory/tests	Findings	Disease
Haematology		
FBC/film	Cytopenia	Leukaemia, marrow infiltration by non-haemopoietic malignancy (e.g. neuroblastoma)
	Blasts on film	Leukaemia
Clotting screen	Acquired coagulation disorders	Haematological malignancies
	Acquired von Willebrand disease	Wilms' tumour
Bone marrow aspirate/biopsy	Infiltration by malignant cells	Marrow infiltration – leukaemia, non-haemopoietic malignancy (e.g. neuroblastoma, rhabdomyosarcoma, Ewing's)
Biochemistry		
Electrolytes (including K/Ca/PO$_4$/Mg/urate)	Hypercalcaemia	Solid tumours, leukaemia
	Hyperkalaemia, hyperphosphataemia	Tumour lysis syndrome
Lactate dehydrogenase	Rapid cell turnover	Any cancer, especially non-Hodgkin lymphoma
Tumour markers		
α-fetoprotein (AFP)	Used in diagnosis and monitoring response to treatment	Hepatoblastoma, germ cell tumours
β-human chorionic gonadotrophin (HCG)		Hepatoblastoma, germ cell tumours
Carcinoembryonic antigen (CEA)		Disseminated adenocarcinoma
Urine		
Catecholamines	Elevated HVA/VMA	Neuroblastoma Phaeochromocytoma
Urinalysis	Haematuria	Renal tumours

Table 4.3 (cont.) Summary of investigations to be performed or considered in a child with an abdominal mass

Laboratory/tests	Findings	Disease
Radiology		
Abdominal X-ray	Calcification	Neuroblastoma, hepatoblastoma, teratoma (N.B. may diagnose urinary or biliary tract lithiasis)
	Fluid levels/dilated bowel	Gastrointestinal obstruction
Ultrasound scan	Identify origin/vascularity of mass Organomegaly	
MR imaging	Characterize solid tumours, volume, extension, etc.	
CT scan	Assess tumour extent and staging	
PET CT scan	Used to evaluate metabolically active tumours	Hodgkin lymphoma
MIBG scan	Sensitive radio-isotope scan used to measure disease extent in neuroblastoma, and to monitor response to treatment. Also has therapeutic use in neuroblastoma	Neuroblastoma, phaeochromocytoma
Bone scan	Focal lesions ('hot spots')	Bone tumours, staging of solid tumours e.g. neuroblastoma, soft tissue sarcoma
Pathology		
Tissue biopsy (open/laparascopic/trucut)	Staging of disease/cytogenetics	Histological tissue diagnosis essential
Bone marrow trephine biopsy	Identification of leukaemia or infiltration by non-haemopoietic malignancy	Bone marrow involvement
Cytogenetics	Detection of specific cytogenetic abnormalities is of therapeutic and prognostic benefit	e.g. neuroblastoma (MYCN amplification, 1p loss, 17q gain)

Diagnosis

Abdominal masses in neonates

- Neonatal tumours are rare. <2% of all childhood cancers.
- Over half of abdominal masses found in neonates are genitourinary in origin with hydronephrosis and multicystic dysplastic kidney accounting for over 40% of masses overall. The majority of tumours are benign, with the exception of Wilms' and neuroblastoma, both of which have an excellent prognosis in this age group.
- Neonatal abdominal tumours constitute an interesting group that differ in incidence, history, and response to treatment when compared with those seen in older children. It is important to know the natural history as even large tumour masses or disseminated disease may regress completely.
- Mesoblastic nephroma (arising from nephrogenic mesenchyme) is the most common solid renal tumour and presents with an abdominal mass, or occasionally haematuria, and is managed surgically by nephrectomy. Other renal tumours, e.g. Wilms' and rhabdoid, are rare in the neonatal period.
- Ovarian cysts in the neonatal period are relatively common, often diagnosed prenatally and generally benign. The majority regress spontaneously. Malignant transformation of benign abdominal masses arising from the GI tract is extremely rare.

Abdominal masses in infants and children

The most common abdominal tumours seen in infants and children are neuroblastoma, Wilms' tumour and lymphomas in decreasing order of frequency. Rarer malignancies include germ cell tumours, liver tumours and soft tissue sarcomas. These tumours are described fully in the specific disease chapters (Lymphomas 📖 pp.443–450, Neuroblastoma 📖 pp.453–464, Renal tumour 📖 pp.469–476, Extracranial germ cell tumours 📖 pp.485–489, Soft tissue sarcomas 📖 pp.491–497, Liver tumours 📖 pp.499–506).

Summary

Prompt clinical evaluation is essential in a child presenting with an abdominal mass. History, particularly the child's age, careful examination and abdominal US scan may quickly narrow the possible diagnoses. Neuroblastoma, Wilms' tumour and lymphoma are the most common causes of abdominal tumours seen in children.

Once a cancer diagnosis is suspected the child should be referred to a paediatric oncology principal treatment centre for further investigation, including staging and histological diagnosis of their disease.

Chapter 5

Initial diagnosis of brain tumours

Brain tumour: initial management

- Children and young people with brain tumours present with a variety of symptoms, including raised intracranial pressure, focal seizures, neurological signs, and endocrinopathies.
- Children with brain tumours should be treated in an institution that is used to treating such children.
- If the child is to be transferred, dexamethasone should be given to reduce tumour swelling prior to transfer.
- A multidisciplinary team approach is essential for the complex management of such children.
- If a *biopsy* is performed, the results should be seen initially or reviewed by a neuropathologist with significant experience of paediatric brain tumours before further treatment is started (see Fig. 5.1).

(1) Raised intracranial pressure headaches

- Typically, but not exclusively present in the early morning.
- Vomiting may occur in isolation and a high index of suspicion should be maintained.
- The headaches typically get worse over time and last for longer each day.
- Papilloedema is a relatively late sign.
- In extremis, the child will show signs of coning (drowsiness and even loss of consciousness, hypertension, bradycardia, neck extension) and become obtunded.
- Children with raised intracranial pressure should be seen immediately by a medical professional.

(2) All *unexplained focal seizures* in children require CNS imaging as do unexplained neurological signs.

Further information
Stills, R.H. (Ed) (2003) *Practical algorithms in pediatric hematology and oncology.* S. Karger AG, Basel.

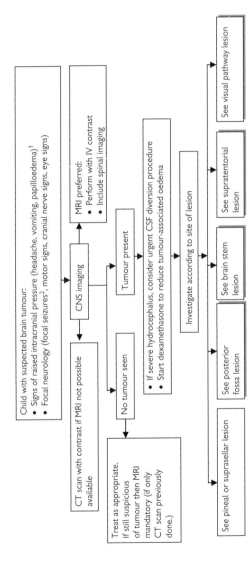

Child with suspected brain tumour:
- Signs of raised intracranial pressure (headache, vomiting, papilloedema)[1]
- Focal neurology (focal seizures[2], motor signs, cranial nerve signs, eye signs)

CT scan with contrast if MRI not possible

CNS imaging

MRI preferred:
- Perform with IV contrast
- Include spinal imaging

No tumour seen

Tumour present

Treat as appropriate. If still suspicious of tumour then MRI mandatory (if only CT scan previously done.)

- If severe hydrocephalus, consider urgent CSF diversion procedure
- Start dexamethasone to reduce tumour-associated oedema

Investigate according to site of lesion

See pineal or suprasellar lesion

See posterior fossa lesion

See brain stem lesion

See supratentorial lesion

See visual pathway lesion

Fig. 5.1 The initial approach to a child thought to have a newly diagnosed brain tumour. Adapted with permission from Stills, R. H. (Ed) Practical Algorithms in Pediatric Hematology and Oncology (2003) ©S. Karger AG, Basel.

Pineal, suprasellar, and atypical tumours

(1) Basic pre-operative endocrine workup is essential

- Both anterior and posterior pituitary function:
  - growth hormone, IGF1, LH/FSH, T_4/TSH;
  - diabetes insipidus must be considered; it is commonly the presenting feature in germinomas.
- It is advisable to involve a paediatric endocrinologist prior to surgery.

See Fig. 5.2.

(2) Germ cell tumours

- Typically found in the pineal or suprasellar region.
- A high index of suspicion of these tumours must be maintained, especially if the lesion is not typical for any other type of tumour.
- Secreting germ cell tumours will have raised serum markers (α-feto-protein [AFP] and/or human chorionic gonadotrophin [HCG]) in both the serum and/or the CSF. A diagnosis can be made on raised markers and biopsy is not needed. These tumours respond well to a combination of chemotherapy and radiotherapy. Germinomas may have marginally raised markers but do not reach 50µg/L for AFP and 50IU/L for HCG level. These tumours respond very well to radiotherapy.

(3) Craniopharyngiomas

These are usually cystic. Children may present with raised ICP, visual changes, disorders in pituitary function, and sometimes mental abnormalities. Most centres use post-operative radiotherapy.

Further information

Stills, R.H. (Ed) (2003) *Practical algorithms in pediatric hematology and oncology.* S. Karger AG, Basel.

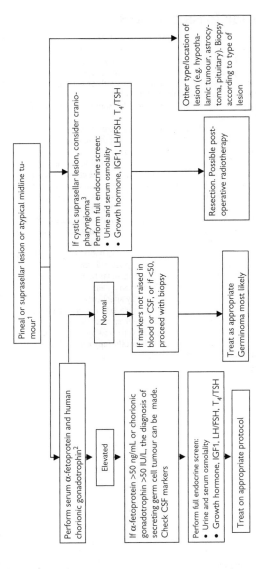

Fig. 5.2 Pineal, suprasellar or atypical midline tumour. Adapted with permission from Stills, R. H. (Ed) Practical Algorithms in Pediatric Hematology and Oncology (2003) ©S. Karger AG, Basel.

Pineal or suprasellar lesion or atypical midline tumour[1]

Perform serum α-fetoprotein and human chorionic gonadotrophin[2]

Elevated

If α-fetoprotein >50 ng/mL or chorionic gonadotrophin >50 IU/L, the diagnosis of secreting germ cell tumour can be made. Check CSF markers

Perform full endocrine screen:
• Urine and serum osmolality
• Growth hormone, IGF1, LH/FSH, T$_4$/TSH

Treat on appropriate protocol

Normal

If markers not raised in blood or CSF, or if <50, proceed with biopsy

Treat as appropriate Germinoma most likely

If cystic suprasellar lesion, consider craniopharyngioma[3]
Perform full endocrine screen:
• Urine and serum osmolality
• Growth hormone, IGF1, LH/FSH, T$_4$/TSH

Resection. Possible postoperative radiotherapy

Other type/location of lesion (e.g. hypothalamic tumour, astrocytoma, pituitary). Biopsy according to type of lesion

Posterior fossa tumours

(1) Very important to have spinal imaging with contrast in posterior fossa lesions, especially if medulloblastoma or ependymoma is suspected. Presence of metastases confers worse prognosis.

(2) If hydrocephalus is present, CSF diversion usually necessary:
   • removal of tumour alone may suffice (with or without temporary external ventricular drain [EVD]);
   • third ventriculostomy preferable to VP shunt if more permanent measure needed;
   • if an experienced paediatric neurosurgeon is not initially available, EVD, followed by resection a few days later may be best.

(3) Intraoperative frozen section mandatory where ependymoma suspected. Ependymomas require radical excision for cure. A more aggressive surgical approach is needed even if it causes increased morbidity. It is not as critical to remove all the tumour in a patient with medulloblastoma or low grade glioma, since the presence of a small amount of residual tumour does not alter prognosis.

(4) Low grade astrocytomas often have a typical MRI appearance with a small enhancing nodule and large cystic component. Treatment is by surgical resection alone.

(5) Medulloblastomas are treated with a combination of chemotherapy and craniospinal radiotherapy, with a posterior fossa boost. CSF staging alters the prognosis, but not necessarily the treatment. CSF should be examined for medulloblastoma cells 7–10 days post-surgery since their presence may affect prognosis.

(6) Other posterior fossa tumours are rare, but include high grade gliomas and their variants, which are treated similarly to high grade gliomas elsewhere. Chordomas are very slow growing skull base tumours, which are resistant to chemotherapy and radiotherapy, and are best cured by surgery alone.

See Fig. 5.3.

Further information
Stills, R.H. (Ed) (2003) *Practical algorithms in pediatric hematology and oncology.* S. Karger AG, Basel.

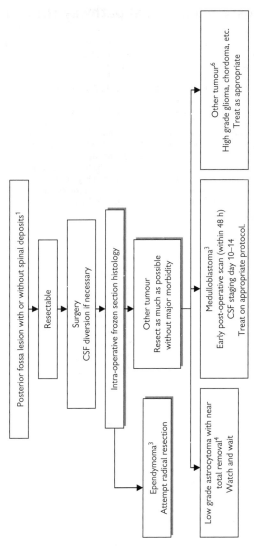

Fig. 5.3 Posterior fossa tumours. Adapted with permission from Stills, R. H. (Ed) Practical Algorithms in Pediatric Hematology and Oncology (2003) ©S. Karger AG, Basel.

Posterior fossa lesion with or without spinal deposits[1]

Resectable

Surgery
CSF diversion if necessary

Intra-operative frozen section histology

Ependymoma[3]
Attempt radical resection

Other tumour
Resect as much as possible without major morbidity

Low grade astrocytoma with near total removal[4]
Watch and wait

Medulloblastoma[3]
Early post-operative scan (within 48 h)
CSF staging day 10–14
Treat on appropriate protocol.

Other tumour[6]
High grade glioma, chordoma, etc.
Treat as appropriate

Brain stem and visual pathway tumours

(1) If brain stem lesions have typical appearance of an infiltrating high grade diffuse pontine glioma on MRI scan, most centres do not biopsy these lesions, but treat on their current protocol. Radiotherapy +/− chemo-therapy is the mainstay of treatment. These children have a very poor outlook with a survival rate <1%. Usually present with cranial nerve palsies and pyramidal signs. Radiologically atypical lesions need a tissue diagnosis.

(2) Visual pathway tumours are common in children with neurofibro-matosis type 1 (NF1), but also occur in non-NF children. Biopsy is not usually necessary unless a lesion is radiologically atypical. Visual pathway tumours, especially in NF1 patients, often remain static with no further treatment, although regular imaging, as well as opthalmo-logical assessment, is mandatory. In those children needing treatment, chemotherapy or radiotherapy is used depending on age and site of lesion (Central nervous system tumours, low grade glioma 📖 pp.512–515, Brainstem glioma 📖 pp.538–539).

See Fig. 5.4.

Further information
Stills, R.H. (Ed) (2003) *Practical algorithms in pediatric hematology and oncology*. S. Karger AG, Basel.

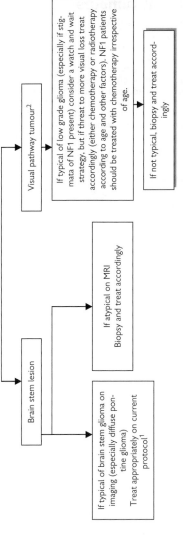

Fig. 5.4 Brain stem and visual pathway lesions. Adapted with permission from Stills, R. H. (Ed) Practical Algorithms in Pediatric Hematology and Oncology (2003) ©S. Karger AG, Basel.

Brain stem lesion

If typical of brain stem glioma on imaging (especially diffuse pontine glioma) Treat appropriately on current protocol[1]

If atypical on MRI Biopsy and treat accordingly

Visual pathway tumour[2]

If typical of low grade glioma (especially if stigmata of NF1 present) consider a watch and wait strategy, but if threat to more visual loss treat accordingly (either chemotherapy or radiotherapy according to age and other factors). NF1 patients should be treated with chemotherapy irrespective of age.

If not typical, biopsy and treat accordingly

Supratentorial tumours

(1) May present in a variety of ways:
  • Focal seizures, headaches and neurological deficits commonest.
  • If not typical of any tumour type on imaging, then germ cell markers need to be performed prior to biopsy/resection (since a positive result may negate the need for initial surgery).
(2) Low grade gliomas can be management by observation with serial MRI scanning, unless resection has not been possible. Chemotherapy or radiotherapy are good treatment options, dependant on site and age of child (Low grade glioma 📖 pp.512–515). High grade gliomas (anaplastic astrocytomas and glioblastoma multiforme) need adjuvant treatment with radiotherapy +/– chemotherapy. Survival rates for high grade gliomas are poor.
(3) Primitive neuroectodermal tumours (PNETs), germ cell tumours and meningeal tumours are treated according to the current treatment recommendations for those tumours.
(4) Choroid plexus tumours are usually recognizable on MRI scan. They are treated initially with surgery. If papillomatous and complete resection has been achieved, no further treatment is needed. Choroid plexus carcinomas need adjuvant treatment with chemotherapy and radiotherapy.

See Fig. 5.5.

Further information
Stills, R.H. (Ed) (2003) *Practical algorithms in pediatric hematology and oncology.* S. Karger AG, Basel.

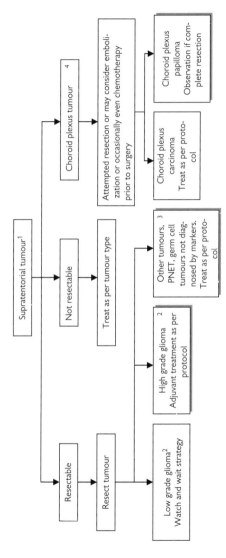

Fig. 5.5 Supratentorial tumours. Adapted with permission from Stills, R. H. (Ed) Practical Algorithms in Pediatric Hematology and Oncology (2003) ©S. Karger AG, Basel.

The bleeding or bruising child

Excessive bleeding or bruising in childhood is a relatively common presentation in paediatric medicine and general practice. Although no pathological cause is found in some otherwise healthy children, bleeding and/or bruising may be the harbinger of serious or life-threatening illness. A systematic approach to history-taking and clinical examination will narrow the differential diagnosis, and careful investigation should enable an accurate diagnosis to be reached.

History

This should include:
- **Type and site of bleeding:** pattern of bleeding may suggest a particular causative mechanism, although the associations listed below are not invariable:
  - *bruises* – how many, where, spontaneous, or explainable;
  - *Petechiae* – how many lesions and where (palpable petechial lesions predominantly on lower limbs are typical of Henoch-Schönlein purpura);
  - *mucosal* – oral, epistaxis, GI, urinary tract, menorrhagia suggestive of thrombocytopenia or von Willebrand disease);
  - *superficial* – following minor trauma;
  - *haematomas* – multiple/repeated deep haematomas may be suggestive of clotting factor deficiencies;
  - *internal* – e.g. haemarthroses (suggestive of clotting factor deficiencies), intracranial;
  - after dental procedure, surgery, or injury (suggestive of clotting factor deficiencies).
- **Length of history:**
  - *long* (months/years) – suggests hereditary (e.g. haemophilia) or chronic acquired (e.g. constitutional bone marrow failure) illness;
  - *short* (days/weeks) – suggests acute acquired illness (e.g. idiopathic thrombocytopenic purpura [ITP], acute leukaemia).
- **Enquire about other features of:**
  - *bone marrow failure* – e.g. lethargy (anaemia), leucopenia (infection);
  - *systemic illness* – e.g. the seriously ill infected child (suggesting the possibility of disseminated intravascular coagulation [DIC]), liver failure (leading to clotting factor deficiency);
  - *congenital abnormalities* – raises the possibility of an inherited bone marrow failure syndrome (e.g. Fanconi anaemia);
  - *other symptoms* – e.g. abdominal pain (Henoch-Schönlein purpura, organomegaly in acute leukaemia).
- **Take a careful family history:** if positive, suggests hereditary illness, e.g. von Willebrand disease, several rare clotting factor deficiencies; a history in males only suggests haemophilia A or B.
- **History of recent infection** (last few weeks or months): may be present in acute leukaemia (due to leucopenia), bone marrow failure (either due to leucopenia, or occasionally as a possible cause of acquired aplastic anaemia), or idiopathic thrombocytopenic purpura (preceded by a recent viral infection in about 80% of cases).

- **Drug history:** occasionally, relevant as a possible cause of acquired aplastic anaemia.
- **History of exposure to chemicals or other toxins:** theoretically relevant as a possible cause of acquired aplastic anaemia, but in practice very rare.

Examination

Pay particular attention to:
- Site, number, and severity of bruises/petechiae.
- Evidence of mucosal bleeding, site, and severity.
- Signs of major acute haemorrhage (▶▶ may need urgent investigation and emergency treatment).
- **Signs of systemic illness/infection:**
    - *acute* – e.g. sepsis, viral infection (VZV, CMV, EBV), malaria;
    - *chronic* – e.g. connective tissue disease, HIV.
- Signs of anaemia.
- Presence of lymphadenopathy.
- Presence of hepatosplenomegaly.
- Presence and nature of congenital abnormalities, e.g. limb defects, congenital cardiac disease.

Investigation and initial management

- Full blood count (FBC).
- **Coagulation profile:** initially prothrombin time (PT), activated partial thromboplastin time (APTT), thrombin time (TT); more extensive investigation may be required subsequently depending on clinical picture and initial results (Haemostasis and thrombosis 📖 pp.327–360).
- Biochemical profile (including liver function tests).

Other investigations/initial management steps are required in appropriate clinical circumstances:
- **Major haemorrhage:**
  - urgent cross-match, volume replacement to maintain circulatory status followed by red cell transfusion;
  - identify and correct remediable aggravating factors (thrombocytopenia, DIC);
  - identification and local treatment (if possible) of source of bleeding (Haemorrhage 📖 pp.108–109).
- **DIC:**
  - blood cultures/infection screen;
  - history, examination, and investigations for other underlying causes, e.g. malignancy (especially acute promyelocytic leukaemia), trauma, microangiopathic diseases (including haemolytic-uraemic syndrome);
  - treat underlying cause and any aggravating factors;
  - correct coagulopathy;
  - Haemostasis and thrombosis 📖 pp.327–360.
- **Sepsis:**
  - blood cultures/infection screen;
  - consider meningococcal (or less commonly other bacterial) septicaemia in the severely ill septic child with petechiae – these children may or may not have laboratory evidence of thrombocytopenia ± DIC;
  - a similar, but usually less severe picture may result from viral infection;
  - a petechial rash that become necrotic suggests purpura fulminans, which may be associated with protein C, protein S, or antithrombin (i.e. natural anticoagulant) deficiency.
- Hereditary coagulation disorders:
  - history, especially family history, very important;
  - further investigations (e.g. clotting factor assays, platelet aggregation studies) needed to establish precise diagnosis and inform subsequent management;
  - Haemostasis and thrombosis 📖 pp.327–360.
- **Thrombocytopenia:**
  - *numerous potential causes* –
    - *inherited* – e.g. Wiskott-Aldrich syndrome (male, eczema, small platelet size on blood film and ↓ mean platelet volume [MPV] on FBC), metabolic (storage) disease (e.g. Gaucher's disease – Gaucher cells seen in bone marrow);
    - *acquired* – e.g. ITP, hypersplenism with splenic sequestration/ destruction of platelets, acute leukaemia, aplastic anaemia
    - Bone marrow failure 📖 pp.361–378.
  - Haemostasis and thrombosis 📖 pp.327–360.

- **Acute leukaemia:**
  - *biochemical profile* – looking for evidence of tumour lysis (Tumour lysis syndrome ▢ pp.94–95);
  - *chest X-ray* – vital to exclude mediastinal mass before undertaking general anaesthetic (Superior vena cava syndrome ▢ pp.102–103);
  - *bone marrow aspirate and biopsy* – morphology, immunophenotype, immunocytochemistry, cytogenetics;
  - *lumbar puncture* – looking for leukaemic blasts in CSF (central nervous system leukaemia);
  - further management usually follows national treatment trials or protocols;
  - Acute lymphoblastic leukaemia ▢ pp.345–404, Acute myeloid leukaemia ▢ pp.405–418.
- **Bone marrow failure:**
  - history and examination findings that may suggest a cause of acquired aplastic anaemia (e.g. exposure to potentially myelotoxic drugs or chemicals) or presence of an inherited bone marrow failure syndrome (e.g. longer history, congenital abnormalities);
  - investigations for a potential cause of acquired aplastic anaemia (e.g. infection);
  - bone marrow aspirate and biopsy;
  - specific investigations to exclude rare causes of bone marrow failure, e.g. Fanconi anaemia (chromosomal fragility test), paroxysmal nocturnal haemoglobinuria (flow cytometry for red and white blood cell CD 55/59);
  - Bone marrow failure ▢ pp.361–378.
- Viral serology should be performed in all new presentations of malignancy and bone marrow failure:
  - *VZV, measles* – to guide post-exposure prophylaxis in susceptible patients) (Immunization ▢ pp.270–275);
  - *HSV* – to assist differential diagnosis and management of mouth ulcers;
  - CMV ± EBV are performed routinely in some units;
  - in high risk areas, hepatitis B/C and HIV screening will usually be performed;
  - the blood sample should be taken *before* any blood product transfusion to avoid passive transfer of antibodies giving a false positive result;
- Apparently normal and otherwise healthy child with significant or suspicious unexplained bruising:
  - *history* – trauma, social history;
  - *examine pattern of bruises* – number, site, size;
  - consider non-accidental injury and seek appropriate advice.

Lymphadenopathy

Introduction

Lymphadenopathy is a common finding in paediatric practice. The causes of lymphadenopathy are myriad and a systematic approach is necessary.

- Lymph nodes expand, becoming palpable and often visible, during the immune system's response to infections.
- As the acute response subsides, the nodes normally decrease in size slowly, but they may not disappear completely.
- The majority of well children have sub-centimetre nodes palpable in the neck and groin, which reflect past infections and should be regarded as normal.
- In general, lymph nodes greater than 1 cm in any direction can be considered as enlarged and described as lymphadenopathy.
- As there are literally hundreds of causes of lymph node enlargement, a pragmatic 'oncological approach' to diagnosis is described below.

In general lymphadenopathy is either:

- Localized or generalized.
- With or without systemic symptoms.

History

- It is common for lymphadenopathy to be reported as 'suddenly appearing', but this should not be taken to mean the same as rapidly growing.
- The parents' or patient's assumption that the nodes were not present until the moment they were discovered does not necessarily mean that they had not been steadily increasing in size unnoticed over a period of weeks.
- Nevertheless, eliciting the timing of the appearance and the rate of progression of lymphadenopathy can be very helpful in making the diagnosis.
- A localized, rapidly increasing nodal mass suggests acute local bacterial infection, EBV infection, or Burkitt's lymphoma (BL). In each case there may be pain owing to stretching of the nodal capsule.
- Slower, but sustained, progression in size over weeks is more suggestive of mycobacterial infection, lymphoblastic lymphoma (LL) or diffuse large cell lymphoma (DLCL).
- Progression over months, often interspersed with periods of apparent improvement, is suggestive of Hodgkin disease (HD).
- Associated systemic symptoms of pruritis (suspicious of HD), fever, night sweats, weight loss, and malaise suggest significant disease.

Examination

- The distribution of the lymphadenopathy can be helpful. Nodal groups involved, including Waldeyer's ring, and the presence or absence of splenomegaly should be carefully documented. In particular, any supraclavicular or epitrochlear nodes should set oncological alarm bells ringing.
- Redness of the overlying skin and tenderness suggest that acute infection is the most likely cause.
- Skin overlying the non-tender nodes found in non-tuberculous mycobacterial (NTM) infection often has a brawny texture.
- Apart from fluctuance pointing to bacterial infection, the characteristics of how the nodes feel is generally unhelpful in making a diagnosis.
- Localized malignant causes of lymph node enlargement include HD, neuroblastoma, nasopharyngeal carcinoma, and melanoma. Langerhans cell histiocytosis (LCH) may also present with localized nodes as single system or part of multisystem disease. Generalized lymphadenopathy is found in leukaemia and NHL (non-Hodgkin lymphoma).

Investigation

The direction and depth of investigation is dictated by the history and the examination findings. Initial blood tests should include:

- **FBC and film:**
  - *cytopenias* – bone marrow failure;
  - *peripheral blasts* – acute leukaemia;
  - *atypical lymphocytosis* – acute EBV infection;
  - left shifted – acute infection;
  - microcytic anaemia – HD;
  - normocytic anaemia – chronic disease.
- **ESR and CRP:** significant inflammatory response.
- **IM screening test:** acute EBV infection.
- **LFTs:** infection.
- **LDH:** increased cell turnover in ALL or NHL.

If the cause is not clearly malignant, but there are no other aetiological clues and the patient is relatively well, the following should be performed: serology +/– PCR, for:

- EBU
- CMU
- Toxoplasmosis
- Bartonella (cat scratch fever).
- HIV (if clinically indicated).
- **Chest X-ray:** effusions, mediastinal nodes, and airway patency.
- **Ultrasound:** appearance can be suggestive of malignancy.
- Additional viral serology should be performed in all new presentations of malignancy and bone marrow failure.
- **VZV, measles:** to guide post-exposure prophylaxis in susceptible patients) (Immunization 📖 pp.270–275).
- **HSV:** to assist differential diagnosis and management of mouth ulcers.
- In high risk areas, hepatitis B/C and HIV screening is usually performed.
- The blood sample should be taken *before* any blood product transfusion to avoid passive transfer of antibodies giving a false positive result.
- If the patient is not well enough to go home, or if the lymphadenopathy is of such a degree that malignancy is considered likely, a node should be biopsied.
- Although FNA (fine needle aspiration) and core biopsies may be diagnostic in some infections, carcinoma, and other solid tumours, they are not sufficiently representative of nodal architecture to diagnose lymphoma.
- The largest easily accessible node should be excised whole and sent fresh to histopathology.
- In addition, either at the same time as pre-biopsy airway assessment (suspicious chest X-ray or any respiratory compromise) or as part of staging, all nodal areas should be imaged by CT or MRI.
- Depending on the level of suspicion, bone marrow examination and diagnostic lumbar puncture can be performed at the same time as the initial biopsy, or subsequently, once a malignant diagnosis has been established, during the same anaesthetic used for central line insertion.

Chapter 8

Imaging of brain tumours

Brain tumours are a diverse group of lesions, the correct diagnosis of which depends on three factors:
- Age of the child.
- Location of the lesion.
- Imaging characteristics of the lesion.

Imaging modalities

- **CT:** usually the first imaging modality because of easy accessibility and rapid acquisition. CT characterisation depends on tissue density. It is very good for identifying calcification, acute haemorrhage, and characterizing the lesion in terms of general density.
- **MRI:** imaging time is much longer and requires thorough safety checks to exclude contraindicating factors like implanted electronic devices and metallic foreign bodies *in situ*. Represents the best imaging modality because of the better characterization of tissues, as well as multi-planar capabilities allowing accurate localization of lesions and determining the full extent of the lesion, which will help in surgical and radiotherapeutic planning. All tumours should ideally be imaged with cranial MRI prior to surgery. All lesions that potentially spread via CSF dissemination should have pre-surgical spinal MRI for staging.
- **Digital subtraction cerebral angiography:** this modality is very rarely required for lesion characterization. May be required for pre-operative embolization of very vascular tumours.

MRI imaging sequences

These may vary from centre to centre, but the general principles remain the same, requiring different sequences in different imaging planes. The following are generally accepted:

Cranial imaging
- **Axial T1W SE:** T1 sequence provides good anatomical detail. Gray matter appears gray and white matter appears white. T1 is good for identifying blood (methaemoglobin), fat, and proteinaceous fluids, all of these being bright on T1.
- **Axial T2W SE:** T2 sequence is generally good for pathology as most abnormalities tend to be brighter relative to normal brain on T2. CSF and other similar fluids are very bright on T2.
- **Coronal FLAIR:** very similar to T2W SE, being very good for identifying pathology, most lesions being bright. CSF signal is suppressed and appears dark; similarly, truly cystic lesions may appear dark.
- **Diffusion-weighted imaging (DWI):** used increasingly often. Good for differentiating an abscess from a centrally necrotic tumour and also to exclude an acute infarction mimicking a tumour.
- **Post-gadolinium T1W SE in two planes:** usually acquired in the axial and coronal planes for cerebral or cerebellar hemispheric tumours. For midline tumours involving the corpus callosum, suprasellar/hypothalamic regions, pineal region, and midline posterior fossa tumours, axial, and sagittal planes are appropriate.

Spinal imaging
Post-gadolinium sagittal T1W SE +/− axial T1W SE
To look for leptomeningeal disease in the spinal canal resulting from CSF dissemination. This is best performed pre-operatively to avoid misinterpretation.

MRI evaluation of the tumour will:
- Determine if it is arising from the brain parenchyma (intra-axial) or outside the brain (extra-axial), either from the meninges, choroid plexus, or the subarachnoid space.
- Reveal the full extent of the tumour in all three orthogonal planes.
- Show the tissue characteristics, i.e. solid tumour, cysts, fat, haemorrhage, or calcification.
- Identify the adjacent structures, which may be eloquent areas (i.e. vital for higher functions), invaded by the tumour, e.g. motor strip, optic pathways, etc.
- Reveal:
  - mass effect, e.g. midline shift, transtentorial herniation, cerebellar tonsillar herniation, and hydrocephalus;
  - other synchronous lesions, representing multifocal disease, e.g. bifocal germinoma or metastatic spread, e.g. leptomeningeal deposits;
  - other associated features in syndromic conditions, e.g. optic pathway glioma and myelin vacuolation in neurofibromatosis type I, bilateral vestibular schwannomas and meningiomas in neurofibromatosis type II, haemangioblastomas in von Hippel-Lindau disease.

Immediate post-operative imaging of the brain and spine

This is often performed to determine if there is a significant residuum requiring second-look surgery to achieve complete tumour removal. An MRI scan within 72h optimizes the chance to differentiate iatrogenic post-surgical enhancement from residual enhancing tumour. Post-surgical enhancement becomes maximal at around 6 weeks, and has usually resolved by 12 months. Beware of pachymeningeal (dural) enhancement that can occur following surgery, or even lumbar puncture and which is different from the leptomeningeal enhancement usually seen in CSF seeding.

Post-operative spinal imaging for staging should not be performed in the first two post-operative weeks as blood products and tumour cells dispersed from tumour surgery often result in leptomeningeal enhancement on the cord surface, which subsequently disappears.

Follow-up imaging post-surgery or chemotherapy

The need for and frequency of this is determined entirely by the clinical oncology team, depending on the histology of the lesion and the overall management strategy. MRI is often employed and the sequences used should be similar to those obtained pre-operatively for effective comparison.

Imaging of non-CNS tumours

Tumours outside the brain and spine include a wide range of lesions in all parts of the body, but some general principles regarding the radiological approach apply to all paediatric masses. Suspected abdominal and pelvic masses must be examined by ultrasound (US) first, and this may be all that is necessary to evaluate benign lesions. Superficial masses or palpable lumps should also be assessed by US initially. Further cross-sectional imaging will be guided by the US findings, tumour location, and local availability of MRI.

The *differential diagnosis* is largely governed by the age of the child, and the organ of origin or location of the lesion. Calcification (neuroblastoma) or fat plus calcium (teratoma) are useful in suggesting a diagnosis, but in general the imaging characteristics of the majority of tumours are relatively non-specific. Most tumours are, for example, hypovascular on contrast-enhanced CT with areas of low attenuation and heterogeneity. Homogeneous imaging appearances of a paediatric mass usually suggest a benign cause. Tumours are typically of low T1 and high T2 signal on MRI, again with variable contrast enhancement after gadolinium administration.

Imaging modalities

Plain radiography

Plain films play a very limited role in the diagnostic work-up of new paediatric mass lesions. The major exception to this is bone tumours (both benign processes and malignant lesions). In this setting, the plain X-ray probably often has a bigger role in suggesting the proper diagnosis than other techniques.

- Bone lysis with ill-defined margins is highly suggestive of an aggressive process, such as an osteomyelitis or tumour (which may be indistinguishable on imaging). A lytic lesion with well-defined margins is very likely a benign bone cyst or benign tumour.
- Although the chest X-ray (CXR) is performed routinely, it usually plays a minor role in staging for metastatic disease at diagnosis, as reliance is generally placed on chest CT to detect or exclude pulmonary metastases with a new presentation of a malignancy. The exception to this rule is neuroblastoma, which does not routinely merit chest CT at diagnosis as metastatic disease is easily detected with scintigraphy (see Glossary of terms ☐ p.88).
- An important role for the plain CXR, including the lateral film, is assessing for airway compression in the setting of a new mediastinal mass. Significant airway compression should be excluded prior to CT or anaesthesia, in particular with an anterior mediastinal tumour.
- Later follow-up and surveillance for metastatic relapse of most tumours is, of course, performed with serial CXRs.
- CXR is also useful in detecting superadded infection or other less common complications of treatment during follow-up, such as rib osteochondromas or rib hypoplasia secondary to irradiation.
- At presentation of a new chest mass, rib changes should be sought. Posterior rib changes with a chest mass are virtually pathognomic of a neurogenic tumour, such as neuroblastoma, whilst anterior rib erosion suggests Ewing's sarcoma or primitive neuroectodermal tumour (Fig. 9.1).

- As the osseous lesions of Langerhans cell histiocytosis (LCH) tend not to show much uptake on bone scans, skeletal surveys are preferred in the overall assessment of the skeleton in LCH.

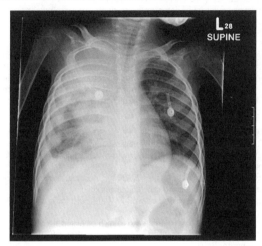

Fig. 9.1 CXR showing a right pleural effusion. A posterior mediastinal mass in the right apex is also confirmed by the separation of the posterior aspects of the right 2nd and 3rd ribs. This is typical of a neuroblastoma, which has also resulted in erosion of some of the medial aspect of the 2nd rib.

Ultrasound

- Entails no radiation burden and so can be performed repeatedly without harm.
- Soft tissue masses can be easily evaluated to assess their cystic or solid nature, and presence of calcification.
- US is a dynamic real-time examination. With large abdominal masses invasion into other organs can be difficult to interpret on CT or MRI, but may be easily evaluated with US. For example, movement of the liver separate from a renal mass is a reliable sign of non-invasion of the liver by the adjacent renal mass.
- With additional Doppler assessments, the degree of vascularity of a tumour can be identified. US is the best technique for detecting and excluding tumour thrombus extension into the IVC from a renal or adrenal tumour.
- Most radiological-guided biopsies can be performed simply with US guidance.
- US is, however, an operator-dependent technique. Selected hard copy images are entirely at the discretion of the person scanning. Consequently, later review of US images by a third party is of limited value. For this reason, in clinical trial settings US images are largely ignored in favour of CT or MRI images.

Computed tomography

- The size and extent of large masses are easily assessed with CT, but with the added considerable radiation burden of CT.
- However, newer multi-detector CT scanners are extremely fast at examining any body region avoiding the need for sedation or anaesthesia in many circumstances.
- CT is the optimal method for assessing the lung parenchyma.
- Calcification in a mass, often not apparent on MRI, is easily detected with CT.
- Bone detail is very well demonstrated on CT such that, for example with many head and neck tumours, an MRI to assess soft tissue extent and a CT to assess erosion of the skull base or facial bones may be necessary.

Magnetic resonance imaging

- MRI is the ideal imaging modality because of its excellent characterization of various tissues, multi-planar capabilities and lack of ionizing radiation.
- A typical MRI examination takes 20–30min, necessitating sedation or anaesthesia for the uncooperative younger child.
- Tumour extent is best assessed with MRI, although for large masses CT can be as accurate.
- As MRI is sensitive to oedema (seen as high or bright signal on T2 sequences), tumour margins from oedema are often difficult to differentiate.
- At the end of treatment or after surgery, MRI frequently cannot distinguish residual fibrosis or benign residual tissue from residual tumour.

Nuclear medicine scintigraphy

- Wilms' tumour and hepatoblastoma seldom metastasize to bone and so do not merit routine bone scanning with technetium ^{99m}MDP (Tc^{99m}MDP).
- Suspected neuroblastoma metastases are best assessed with iodine ^{123}MIBG (meta-iodobenzylguanidine) scans – if the primary neuroblastoma tumour is not avid for MIBG then a Tc^{99m}MDP bone scan is recommended to evaluate for skeletal metastases in this setting.
- Most sarcomas and other solid tumours usually require routine bone scans for staging at diagnosis.

Glossary of terms

Ultrasound General terms used include echogenicity or reflectivity. A lesion may thus be of low reflectivity or it may be described as *hypoe-choic* (dark). *Hyperechoic* foci are bright on US. Water, e.g. CSF or uncomplicated ascites are typically *anechoic* (no echoes). Acoustic shadowing occurs beyond dense calcification (the area beyond the calcification is dark, lacking echoes).

CT Density or *attenuation* are the terms used. Low attenuating lesions appear darker than high attenuating lesions, e.g. calcification has high attenuation and appears bright on CT. Contrast media contain iodine and it is the iodine that renders contrast media in blood vessels as high attenuation on CT (Fig. 9.2). Fluid-filled or cystic lesions have low attenuation.

MRI (Figs 9.3 and 9.4) *Hyperintense* lesions are bright, *hypointense* foci are dark because they lack signal. T1-weighted (T1W) sequences show fat as a hyperintense structure and water is hypointense (dark) on T1. Additional fat suppression (also called fat saturation) will suppress the signal from fat and will make fat appear dark on that sequence – fat suppression can be used with either T1W or T2W imaging sequences. Water, oedema, and tumours are all typically hyperintense (bright) on T2W sequences. Calcium usually has no signal on MR sequences and so appears dark on MR or is invisible.

Scintigraphy Lesions that take up a radioisotope are '*hot*' or show intense uptake on scintigraphic studies. A photopenic lesion does not absorb the isotope, and appears '*cold*' or shows reduced uptake of the radiopharmaceutical.

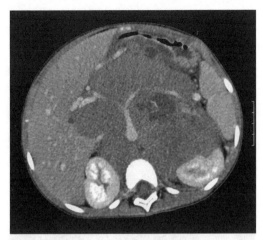

Fig. 9.2 Axial contrast-enhanced CT demonstrates a large midline mass lesion encasing the aorta. The aorta is of higher attenuation due to intravenous contrast-enhancement, with this typical neuroblastoma tumour clearly seen surrounding the coeliac artery and its major branches.

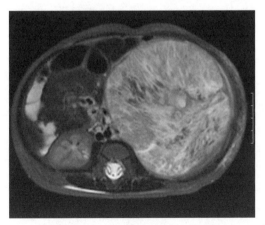

Fig. 9.3 Sagittal T1W MRI after gadolinium administration. A large enhancing pelvic neuroblastoma, of higher signal than vertebral marrow, is seen in the pre-sacral region posterior to the bladder. Note that on T1W images CSF is of low signal (dark).

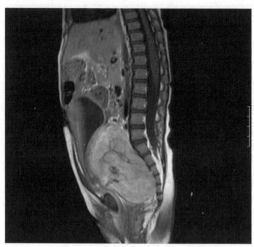

Fig. 9.4 Axial T2W MRI showing a large hyperintense left renal Wilms' tumour. Note on T2W images, CSF and most tumours are hyperintense.

Haematological and oncological emergencies

Chapter 10

Haematological and oncological emergencies

Tumour lysis syndrome

Tumour lysis syndrome (TLS) is a life-threatening emergency due to metabolic derangements secondary to tumour cell necrosis. Can occur prior to initiation of therapy or after hydration alone.

Possible end results if untreated include:
- Death.
- Acute renal failure.
- Hyperkalaemia, hyperphosphataemia and hyperuricaemia
- Hypocalcaemia (2° to hyperphosphataemia).

Mainly occurs in haematological malignancy, but may occur occasionally with solid tumours. Patients at *high risk* of TLS include those with:
- **Burkitt's lymphoma** and other non-Hodgkin lymphomas (especially if high LDH reflecting bulky disease).
- Acute lymphoblastic leukaemia (particularly *high white cell count [WCC] >50 x 10^9/L* and bulky disease such as hepatosplenomegaly or mediastinal mass).
- Acute myeloid leukaemia (particularly high WCC >100 x 10^9/L).
- High serum uric acid (>0.4mmol/L) at diagnosis.
- Pre-existing renal compromise.

Clinical and biochemical features

Onset of TLS may be rapid. Careful clinical observation and regular analysis of electrolytes is essential. Biochemical derangements occur 2° to high cell turnover and death, releasing intracellular contents into the circulation, with the following clinical consequences:
- Hyperuricaemia → renal colic and arthralgia. Acidosis decreases solubility of urate.
- Hyperphosphataemia → CaPO$_4$ deposition in tissues, which is increased by aggressive alkalinization.
- Hyperkalaemia → muscle weakness, arrythmias, paraesthesia.
- Acute renal failure due to intravascular volume depletion, hyperuricaemia, acute nephrocalcinosis, fluid overload, cardiac failure. May necessitate dialysis/ultrafiltration.
- Hypocalcaemia (usually 2° to hyperphosphataemia) → paraesthesia, tetany, carpopedal spasm, seizures, arrhythmias, altered mental state.

Management

- Identify patients at high risk of tumour lysis.
- Patients at very high risk (poor renal function at diagnosis + Burkitt's or high count ALL) should have a central venous catheter (capable of supporting haemofiltration/haemodialysis) inserted before commencing therapy. However, this may not always be possible if the child's clinical condition is poor.
- Stabilize electrolytes prior to commencement of therapy.
- Hydration fluid and xanthine oxidase inhibitors/urate oxidase should be given for at least 12h before starting chemotherapy. Occasionally, special circumstances warrant earlier chemotherapy, e.g.
  - mediastinal mass compromising airway patency;
  - leucostasis.

- **Fluid management:**
  - IV hydration fluid at $3L/m^2/24h$ (maximum 4L/24h);
  - fluid should contain NaCl and dextrose, but no potassium;
  - check fluid balance 6-hourly and weight twice daily;
  - maintain urine output at ≥2ml/kg/h and, if necessary, use diuretics (frusemide or mannitol);
  - monitor blood pressure closely.
- **Xanthine oxidase** inhibitors (allopurinol) ($100mg/m^2$/dose tds) block conversion of hypoxanthine to xanthine (only available in oral format in UK) and of xanthine to uric acid. *Urate oxidase* (rasburicase, IV formulation only; 100U/kg od) should be used for high risk patients if available. This converts uric acid to allantoin (more soluble) and is more effective than xanthine oxidase inhibitors.
- **Electrolyte management:**
  - Check serum electrolytes, creatinine, phosphate, calcium, and urate 4–6-hourly in high risk patients for first 24h. Monitor lower risk patients 12-hourly.
  - **If serum potassium** >6mmol/L, give kayexelate (calcium resonium) (1–2g/kg/day oral 6-hourly, or retention enema in 20% sorbitol). If ECG changes present, bicarbonate (0.5mmol/kg bolus), calcium gluconate (0.5ml/kg of 10% solution IV over 10min), and glucose and insulin (0.5g/kg 10% glucose IV with 0.3U of insulin per g glucose) should be given to stabilize cardiac membrane and reduce serum potassium. If this fails to reduce serum potassium, dialysis may be necessary.
  - **If serum phosphate** >3mmol/L, contact nephrologists. Aluminium hydroxide (50–150mg/kg/day) may reduce hyperphosphataemia. Calcium × phosphate product >4.6mmol/L implies higher risk of renal calcium phosphate deposition. *Hypocalcaemia* often occurs in association with hyperphosphataemia. Care should be given before giving calcium due to risk of calcium phosphate deposition. If necessary (symptomatic hypocalcaemia), give calcium gluconate (0.5ml/kg of 10% solution IV over 10 min).
  - **Hyperuricaemia** rarely occurs in isolation to a degree requiring treatment (especially if urate oxidase used). If levels continue to rise >0.5mmol/L, consider dialysis.
  - If dialysis is necessary, haemofiltration/haemodialysis more effective than peritoneal dialysis. Dialysis usually only needed for short period (days), unless established renal failure develops.

Spinal cord compression

Spinal cord compression may be defined as extrinsic compression of the spinal cord leading to disturbance of normal neurological functioning. It may occur as a direct consequence of malignant disease or, rarely, its treatment.

Epidemiology

Spinal cord compression is a potential complication of nearly all paediatric malignancies, including leukaemia.

- May occur at initial diagnosis, at relapse or during subsequent disease progression.
- Occurs at some stage in about 5% of all children with cancer or leukaemia.

Causes

Spinal cord compression is commoner in solid tumours than in haematological malignancies. It occurs at some stage in:

- 10–20% of patients with:
  - Ewing's sarcoma;
  - medulloblastoma.
- 5–10% of patients with:
  - neuroblastoma;
  - germ cell tumours (e.g. dysgerminoma);
  - soft tissue sarcomas;
  - osteosarcoma.
- <5% of patients with other solid tumours, e.g. Wilms' tumour.
- 1–2% of patients with haematological malignancies, e.g. lymphoma, leukaemia.

In about 65% of patients with spinal cord compression, it is the main clinical feature at the initial presentation of their malignancy. Most other cases occur at relapse or during disease progression, but a small proportion of cases are due to a complication of treatment, e.g. vertebral body collapse due to prolonged steroid treatment.

Spinal cord compression may result from different pathological processes:

- Invasion from paravertebral disease via intervertebral foramina, e.g neuroblastoma – ~40% cases extradural.
- Vertebral body compression – ~30%.
- CSF seeding – ~20% intradural, extraspinal.
- Direct invasion – ~10% intraspinal.

Clinical presentation

The symptoms of spinal cord compression vary with the level of the lesion, but may include:

- Motor dysfunction (weakness) – occurs in >90% of cases.
- Radicular or back pain – occurs in 55–95%.
- Sensory changes – 10–55%.
- Sphincter dysfunction – 10–35%.

A very small proportion of patients (2–3%) remain asymptomatic despite clinical signs of spinal cord compression.

Other potential causes of these symptoms should be considered, particularly vascular events or transverse myelitis.

A complete neurological examination should be undertaken to both confirm signs which suggest cord compression and to provide a baseline for evaluating response to therapy.

The imaging modality of choice is spinal MRI.

Management

Start dexamethasone urgently to reduce peri-tumour oedema and hopefully expedite neurological recovery.

Definitive treatment with chemotherapy is appropriate when rapid response is expected (e.g. neuroblastoma, lymphoma/leukaemia), and causes fewer long-term side effects than surgery and/or radiotherapy. However, these latter treatment modalities remain essential in less chemosensitive tumours.

Outcome

The most important feature determining neurological outcome of spinal cord compression is the severity of impairment, rather than the duration between symptoms and diagnosis. Full neurological recovery may occur in over 90% of patients with milder neurological impairment, but is seen only in up to 65% of initially paraplegic patients.

Raised intracranial pressure

Introduction

Raised intracranial pressure (ICP) is a common presenting feature of brain tumours in children. Most commonly caused by posterior fossa tumours, compressing 4th ventricular outflow, resulting in raised ICP from obstructive hydrocephalus. Rarely caused by tumours secreting CSF (e.g. choroid plexus papillomas) or poor reabsorption (communicating hydrocephalus). Masses in non-midline supratentorial regions can cause raised ICP due to mass effect .

Normal ventricular system (Fig. 10.1)

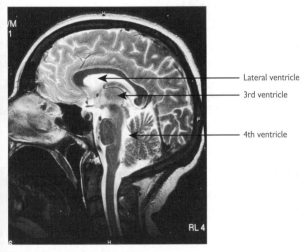

Lateral ventricle

3rd ventricle

4th ventricle

Fig. 10.1 Normal ventricular system.

Presenting signs and symptoms

Early

- Early morning headache, improving over course of morning. Worse on lying down. Pain usually frontal or occipital.
- Early morning nausea and vomiting (may be the only symptom) especially significant if no other gastrointestinal (GI) disturbance.
- Rapidly increasing head circumference in infants.
- Tense fontanelle in babies, shrill cry.
- Non-specific symptoms, e.g.
  - declining academic performance;
  - fatigue;
  - personality changes;
  - failure to thrive.
- By 6 months from onset of headache, nearly all children have developed additional focal neurological symptoms/signs.

Late
- Headaches may be constant and unrelieved by analgesics.
- **Papilloedema:** not always easy to detect, especially in younger children.
- Diplopia due to VI nerve palsy is the most common eye sign. Other eye signs include:
  - strabismus;
  - nystagmus;
  - *Parinaud syndrome* – loss of upward gaze, impaired accommodation, abnormal papillary reflexes;
  - IV nerve palsy;
  - sunset eyes in babies (rare; sclera seen above the pupil due to extreme lack of upward gaze).
- Neck stiffness (glass neck) and altered neck posture. Head tilt may occur due to herniation of cerebellar tonsils.
- Status epilepticus.
- Reduced conscious level.
- Bradycardia/hypertension suggests incipient herniation of tentorium cerebri.

Imaging
- CNS imaging mandatory if suspected raised ICP.
- CT scan is a good screening procedure.
- MRI best for more accurate diagnosis.

Symptoms needing urgent management
- Severe headaches.
- Neck pain and stiffness especially with extension of head and neck.
- Decreased level of consciousness.
- Decerebrate posture.
- Respiratory changes, e.g. Cheyne-Stokes respiration.
- Hypertension and/or bradycardia.
- Worsening vision.

Hydrocephalus due to tumour (Fig. 10.2)

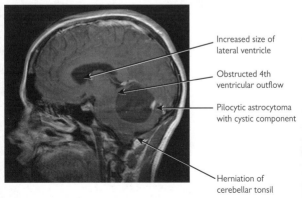

Increased size of lateral ventricle

Obstructed 4th ventricular outflow

Pilocytic astrocytoma with cystic component

Herniation of cerebellar tonsil

Fig. 10.2 Hydrocephalus due to tumour.

Treatment
- If hydrocephalus is due to the tumour, dexamethasone should be given immediately to reduce oedema and, hence, increase opportunity for CSF flow (250µg/kg as single dose best given as IV dose; thereafter 125µg/kg/dose bd).
- If there are any danger signs (see Symptoms needing urgent management, p.99), urgent CSF diversion is necessary.
- CSF diversion usually performed by one of three methods depending on site of obstruction. Surgery of primary lesion alone is often sufficient to re-establish CSF flow.
  - *ventriculostomy* – hole made in membrane at base of 3rd ventricle with endoscope (preferred method where possible);
  - external ventricular drain as a temporary procedure;
  - ventriculo-peritoneal (VP) shunt.

Superior vena cava syndrome

Definitions
- Superior vena cava (SVC) syndrome (SVCS) – clinical picture caused by compression or complete obstruction of SVC by a mediastinal mass.
- Superior mediastinal syndrome (SMS) – association of SVCS with tracheal compression.

Epidemiology
SVCS is rare, occurring in <1% of newly diagnosed paediatric malignancies.

Causes
Several paediatric malignancies may present, relapse, or progress with mediastinal masses leading to SVCS. The commonest causes are:
- **Anterior superior mediastinal mass:**
  - *non-Hodgkin lymphoma* (NHL) – approximately 30% of all mediastinal masses in children;
  - *acute lymphoblastic leukaemia* (ALL) (especially T cell) – 25%;
  - *thymoma* – rare.
- **Posterior mediastinal mass:**
  - *Hodgkin disease* (HD) – 10–20%;
  - *germ cell tumour* (teratoma) – <10%;
  - *neuroblastoma* – <10%.
  - *middle mediastinal mass* – sarcoma (heart, great vessels) – <10%.

Most cases of SVCS presenting at initial diagnosis are due to haematological malignancies. Children with solid tumours are more likely to develop SVCS at disease relapse.

Non-malignant causes of SVCS include:
- CVAD-associated thrombosis.
- Disseminated infection (e.g. candidiasis) – rare.

Diagnosis
SVCS has a characteristic clinical presentation, often with rapid onset and progression (especially in NHL or T-ALL):
- Facial, neck, and upper thoracic plethora, oedema, cyanosis.
- Distended jugular and collateral chest wall veins.
- Ill patient.
- Anxious, impaired conscious level (cerebral oedema).
- Less frequent symptoms/signs of SVCS include:
  - dysphagia;
  - hoarse voice (vocal cord paralysis);
  - Horner's syndrome.
- Symptoms/signs of tracheal/main bronchus compression (SMS):
  - dyspnoea, tachypnoea, cough, wheezing, stridor;
  - *orthopnoea* – avoid placing patients in supine position (may precipitate complete tracheal obstruction);
  - effects of SMS in younger children are exacerbated by their relatively smaller tracheal diameter.

Radiology
- *Chest X-ray* – mediastinal mass, sometimes with associated pulmonary collapse/consolidation, pleural, or pericardial effusion.
- *CT scan* – shows extent of tracheal compression more accurately.
- *Echocardiography or Doppler US* – indicated for suspected CVAD-associated thrombosis.

Management
- Ideally, urgent biopsy should be performed to give a tissue diagnosis, but not at the cost of catastrophic respiratory collapse precipitated by general anaesthetic (GA) in patients with incipient large airways obstruction.
- Such patients should be managed in an upright position.
- Important diagnostic information may be obtained by other means without GA, e.g.
  - FBC;
  - bone marrow aspirate/biopsy or lymph node biopsy under local anaesthetic;
  - pleural aspirate.
- ▶▶ Definitive treatment is required urgently.
- Chemotherapy, guided by the underlying histological diagnosis, is usually rapidly effective
- Occasionally, presumptive treatment (e.g. with steroids) may need to be commenced to reduce a mediastinal mass in the absence of a definite histological diagnosis. If so, definitive investigations, based on the likely differential diagnosis (e.g. including lumbar puncture for suspected ALL), should be performed as soon as deemed safe, although histology may have been rendered uninterpretable.
- Radiotherapy is effective, but may cause initial increased respiratory distress due to tumour swelling and is now seldom employed.
- Rarely, surgery may be required in less chemo- or radiosensitive malignancies.
- CVAD-associated thrombosis should be treated by thrombolytic therapy (which may be delivered via the CVAD). Usually followed by systemic anticoagulation (often with low molecular weight heparin).

Patients with mediastinal masses due to T-cell ALL or NHL are at high risk of tumour lysis syndrome (TLS), and should be managed accordingly (Tumour lysis syndrome 📖 pp.94–95). Although central venous access should ideally be placed before commencing treatment, this is not always feasible. Since these malignancies are usually very chemosensitive, most contemporary treatment protocols incorporate a 'gentler' cytoreductive prephase of prednisolone +/– low dose cyclophosphamide for a few days to reduce the size of the mediastinal mass, whilst avoiding significant TLS. This is then followed by full dose combination 'induction' chemotherapy.

Outcome
SVCS/SMS is potentially life-threatening, but most of the underlying malignancies have a good prognosis.

Hypertension

Hypertension is defined as raised systolic blood pressure (rSBP) recorded as being above the 95th centile for age, gender, and height (see Table 10.1) on three or more occasions (National High Blood Pressure Education Program Working Group, 2004). If left untreated, rSBP may result in cerebrovascular and cardiovascular disease. It is a common cause of morbidity and mortality in children with renal diseases.

Table 10.1 95th centile for systolic blood pressure (mmHg)

Sex	Age	Height percentile		
		5th	50th	95th
Male	1 year	98	103	106
Female		100	104	107
Male	5 years	108	112	116
Female		107	110	113
Male	10 years	115	119	123
Female		116	119	122
Male	15 years	126	131	135
Female		124	127	131

Causes

When assessing rSBP in a child with malignancy or undergoing cytotoxic treatment, it is important to exclude:
• Pain.
• Fear/stress.
• Urinary tract obstruction (e.g. tumour).
• Intrarenal tumour extension.
• Drug-induced (e.g. steroids).
• Fluid overload.

rSBP could be also due to one of the following underlying diagnoses:
• *Renal* – scarred kidneys 2° to vesico-ureteral reflux, renal failure (acute or chronic), glomerulonephritis, renal artery stenosis, polycystic kidney.
• *Endocrine* – phaeochromocytoma, hyperthyroidism, hypothyroidism, Cushing syndrome, congenital adrenal hyperplasia.
• *Drugs* – calcineurin inhibitors (e.g. ciclosporin), non-steroidal anti-inflammatory drugs, oral contraceptive pills.
• *Others* – coarctation of aorta.

▶ Always ensure that rSBP is not 2° to ↑ intracranial pressure (Raised intracranial pressure 📖 pp.98–100).

Presentation

Most cases of mild to moderate hypertension are picked up during routine measurements in apparently asymptomatic children. Symptoms/signs include headaches, nose bleeds, fatigue, vomiting, confusion, blurred vision, facial palsy, or failure to thrive.

▶▶ If rSBP is associated with decreased conscious level, seek immediate senior help.

History

- Decreased urine output.
- Haematuria.
- Puffiness.
- Previous urinary tract infection.
- Current medications.
- Family history of polycystic disease, hypertension, renal disease.

Examination

The most important examination is recording an *accurate* blood pressure (BP). Ensure the bladder of the cuff is the largest that can be applied to the proximal part of the upper limb and that it extends round 80–100% of the arm circumference. Use a reliable, properly calibrated sphygmomanometer with either a stethoscope over the brachial artery or detection of vascular Doppler flow of brachial or radial artery (which is reliable and easy to perform in smaller children and babies). Many automatic machines are unvalidated and unreliable in children, especially when SBP is outside the normal change. Repeated measurement is essential to determine if the SBP is truly elevated. This will also exclude reactive rises in SBP ('white coat hypertension').

<u>Always</u> look for signs of end organ damage irrespective of the severity of hypertension (although it is more common with severe rSBP):

- **Eye:** papilloedema.
- **Cardiovascular:** left ventricular hypertrophy.
- **Kidney:** proteinuria.
- **Central nervous system:** seizures, encephalopathy, stroke.

Investigations

1st line

- **Blood:** U&Es, creatinine, bicarbonate, Ca^{2+}, urate, parathyroid hormone (PTH), renin, aldosterone, (complement C3, C4, auto-antibody screen if glomerulonephritis suspected).
- **Urine:** dipstick (protein and blood), microscopy.
- **Imaging:** Doppler renal US, DMSA scan, ECG, echocardiogram, chest X-ray.
- Ophthalmology review.

2nd line investigations guided by initial results

- ACTH, thyroid function tests.
- Urine VMA, catecholamines, steroid profile, free cortisol.
- Renal angiography, renal vein renin sampling, MIBG.

Treatment
- **Remove underlying cause**: drugs, pain, etc.
- **Lifestyle advice if appropriate**: salt restriction, healthy diet, physical exercise, weight reduction, smoking advice.

Management
The treatment goal is to maintain SBP below 95th centile for age, gender, and height, or below 90th centile if concurrent conditions or risk factors (National High Blood Pressure Education Program Working Group, 2004). Specific treatment depends on the cause, duration and severity of hypertension. High BP of unknown duration must be *lowered slowly*.

Accelerated/malignant hypertension

▶▶ Seek expert help; manage in specialist centre.

Emergency intravenous treatment (e.g. labetolol, nitroprusside, hydralazine) Although this is potentially life-saving, it may also be dangerous since a rapid decrease in BP can result in occipital blindness.

Monitor BP very frequently, e.g. every 15min or continuously during treatment, and titrate dose according to response. Aim to decrease SBP only by a third every 24h.

Investigations should be commenced once BP is stable.

Oral antihypertensives should be started once the acute rise in BP has been treated.

Table 10.2 Medications for acute and chronic management of hypertension

Drug	Dose/route	Dose interval	Comments
Acute management			
Nifedipine	0.1–0.2 mg/kg/dose Route: sublingual	As needed (PRN)	Short-acting calcium channel blocker
Hydralazine	0.1–0.5mg/kg/dose (up to 3mg/kg/day) Route – slow IV	4-hourly PRN	Potent vasodilator and could cause sudden fall in SBP
Frusemide	0.5–4.0mg/kg/dose Route: oral or IV	1–4-hourly	Used if patient is fluid overloaded
Chronic management			
Amlodipine	0.1–0.2mg/kg/dose (up to 10mg/day) Route: oral	1	Long-acting calcium channel blocker
Atenolol	1–2mg/kg/day Route: oral	1	Cardioselective beta-blocker Use with caution in asthma
Enalapril	0.2–0.5mg/kg/day Route: oral	1	Can cause reversible hyperkalaemia and raised creatinine Contraindicated in renal artery stenosis

Further information

National High Blood Pressure Education Program Working Group on High Blood Pressure in Children and Adolescents (2004) *Pediatrics* **114:** 555–76.

Haemorrhage

Before the introduction of effective platelet transfusion support in the early 1960s, acute thrombocytopenic haemorrhage accounted for up to 60% of deaths in leukaemic patients. Now that transfusion support is readily available, life-threatening bleeding is rare in children with malignancy.

Causes

Clinical scenarios associated with a high risk of haemorrhage include:
- **Leukaemia:** at initial presentation, relapse, or during progression:
  - especially acute promyelocytic leukaemia (APL, M3 AML), and (to a lesser extent) M5 AML;
  - associated risk factors include:
    - hyperleucocytosis;
    - thrombocytopenia;
    - infection.
- Severe thrombocytopenia following intensive chemotherapy or haemopoietic stem cell transplantation (HSCT). Often in context of mucosal damage, e.g. mucositis, haemorrhagic cystitis.
- Rarer causes of bone marrow failure, e.g. aplastic anaemia.
- **Invasive solid malignancies:** may complicate progressive disease.
- Disseminated intravascular coagulation (DIC), usually complicating newly diagnosed acute leukaemia (especially APL) or severe infection.
- Rarely, severe invasive infection, especially moulds (e.g. aspergillosis).

Severe thrombocytopenia is the commonest underlying factor, but clotting factor deficiency may complicate APL or DIC. Although major vascular invasion by tumour or infection is rare, it is often life-threatening. Many episodes of severe haemorrhage are multifactorial.

Diagnosis

The diagnosis of major haemorrhage is usually clinically obvious:
- Site of overt blood loss, especially GI, haemorrhagic cystitis, respiratory.
- Hypovolaemic shock.

It is important to maintain a high index of suspicion of more subtle presentations of incipient major bleeding, especially in the appropriate clinical context, e.g. otherwise unexplained tachycardia and/or hypotension and/or falling haemoglobin.

Management

Prevention is preferable to treatment, e.g. by H_2-receptor or proton-pump inhibition for upper GI protection, or prophylactic platelet transfusions in severe thrombocytopenia (Blood transfusion, platelets 📖 p.241).

The management of major haemorrhage includes:

- Urgent volume replacement (crystalloid and/or colloid) followed by red cell transfusion. No consistent evidence for superiority of colloids over crystalloids in hypovolaemic shock.
- Optimizing haemostasis:
  - *thrombocytopenia* – platelet transfusion(s);
  - *coagulopathy* – clotting factor support, especially in DIC and APL.
- In appropriate clinical circumstances, identification, and management of a specific bleeding source may occasionally involve:
  - *endoscopy, cystoscopy* (with bladder irrigation) – may allow local measures to control bleeding;
  - *interventional radiology* – may permit embolization;
  - *surgery* – arterial ligation or resection of bleeding tissue;
  - use of local or systemic haemostatic agents.
- In addition, any underlying cause(s) should be treated (e.g. the malignancy, infection or mucosal damage).

Outcome

In most cases, the outcome depends on the underlying cause(s), and how easily this can be corrected. Despite modern supportive care, haemorrhage can cause considerable morbidity and may even lead to occasional deaths.

Seizures

Introduction

Seizures are serious episodes of impaired cerebral function. Presenting features may include repetitive involuntary movements, impairment of consciousness, and disturbance of the sensorium. Patients in the oncology setting without underlying epilepsy are likely to present with acute symptomatic seizures, which have a number of possible causes:

• Structural CNS abnormailities, e.g. brain tumours, brain haemorrhage.
• Hypoglycaemia.
• Electrolyte disturbance, e.g. low serum sodium.
• Acute hypoxia: respiratory or cardiac including cardiac arrhythmias.
• CNS infection.
• Toxic effects of drugs, e.g. intrathecal methotrexate.

Convulsive seizures lasting more than 5min are likely to continue and require treatment (see Assessment 🕮 p.110). Convulsive status epilepticus is currently regarded as continuous convulsive seizure lasting 30min or more, or recurrent convulsive seizures without recovery of consciousness lasting 30min or more. Convulsive status epilepticus may be generalized or focal.

Assessment

Whatever the cause of the seizure, the assessment is always the same.

• **A (Airway):** establish airway and give high flow oxygen, attach oxygen saturation monitor.
• **B (Breathing):** ensure adequate ventilation and oxygenation. Use 'bag and mask' ventilation if spontaneous ventilation inadequate.
• **C (Circulation):** check pulse and blood pressure. Establish IV access, check blood glucose by BM stick and treat hypoglycaemia with 5ml/kg of 10% dextrose. Give fluid bolus if shocked.
• **D (Disability):** assess conscious level and pupillary responses. Observe posture: decorticate or decerebrate posturing, acute dytonic reactions and psychogenic attacks can be confused with seizures and require different treatment.

Management

Treatment follows the algorithm taught and published by the APLS course (see Fig. 10.3).

Investigations

The cause of the seizure must be sought and investigations can be considered as follows:

• **Mandatory:** glucose, calcium, phosphate, magnesium, full blood count, arterial blood gas.
• **Consider:** cranial CT scan, septic screen (lumbar puncture only after discussion with senior medical staff and in the absence of contraindications, e.g. raised intracranial pressure, focal neurological signs), LFTs, ammonia, lactate, toxicology, other metabolic tests, chest X-ray.

Continuing care

Once seizure has ceased, continue to monitor ABCD, maintain normoglycaemia, treat pyrexia, and give antibiotics if appropriate.

Continuing treatment of seizures should be guided by a neurologist (there are many different drugs and combinations), as well as attempting to remove or treat the cause of the seizures if possible.

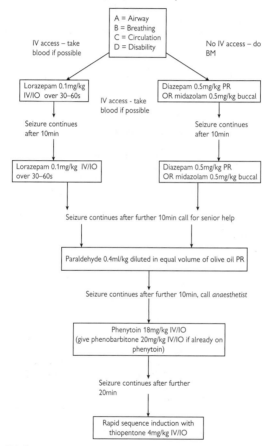

Fig. 10.3 Treatment algorithm for status epilepticus.

Severe sepsis

Background

A significant proportion of morbidity seen in children with cancer is due to infectious complications, which usually require hospital admission. Sepsis is a common and often serious complication of treatment for cancer, especially in neutropenic patients. The absence of neutrophils may diminish the symptoms and signs of infection, and it may be impossible to identify a focus. Frequently, non-specific symptoms, such as fever and lethargy may be the only presenting features of impending severe sepsis. Awareness among medical and nursing staff about the potential seriousness of infection is imperative for a successful outcome:

- Severe sepsis can be a complication in any patients with malignancy. Although more likely to occur in neutropenic patients (absolute neutrophil count [ANC] $<1 \times 10^9$/L), it may also occur in the absence of neutropenia.
- Neutropenia is most common in patients receiving chemotherapy, but may also occur in patients during radiotherapy if large areas of bone marrow are irradiated.
- Neutropenia may be a presenting feature in haematological malignancies and bone marrow failure syndromes, whilst marrow infiltration by malignant cells may cause neutropenia/pancytopaenia in some advanced solid tumours.
- Presence of in-dwelling catheters (e.g. central venous access devices [CVADs]) or prosthetic implants may increase risk of severe sepsis.
- During cyclical chemotherapy, the neutropenia nadir occurs typically 10–14 days after the start of each cycle, at which time patients are at greatest risk of developing severe sepsis.

If sepsis is untreated or there is significant delay in instituting appropriate antibiotic therapy, more serious complications may develop including:

- Septicaemic shock.
- Multi-organ dysfunction.
- Death.

High risk patients

Patients at high risk of severe sepsis include:

- Patients on high intensity multi-agent cyclical chemotherapy (e.g. treatment of acute myeloid leukaemia, bone, and other solid tumours).
- Patients with ANC $<0.5 \times 10^9$/L and absolute monocyte count $<0.1 \times 10^9$/L at the time of the febrile episode.
- Prolonged neutropenia lasting >7 days.
- Patients with mucosal inflammation (e.g. mucositis, diarrhoea after chemotherapy).
- Patients undergoing high dose chemotherapy regimens with autologous stem cell rescue.
- Patients undergoing allogeneic haemopoietic stem cell transplantation.
- Fever greater than 39°C.

Causes of sepsis

Multiple Gram −ve and +ve organisms can cause infections in oncology patients. Although it is common for no organisms to be isolated despite careful investigation, those organisms that are commonly implicated in causing severe sepsis in children with malignancy include:

- *Pseudomonas aeruginosa*.
- Other non-fermenting Gram −ve bacteria previously grouped together in the Pseudomonas family, e.g. *Stenotrophomonas maltophilia*
- Enterobacteriaciae:
  - *Escherichia coli*;
  - *Klebsiella oxytoca*;
  - *Enterobacter*;
  - *Serratia*.
- *Streptococcus pneumoniae*.
- Other α-haemolytic streptococci.
- Enterococci.
- *Staphylococcus aureus*.
- Coagulase −ve staphylococci (rarely cause severe sepsis).
- Fungi:
  - *Candida* spp.;
  - *Aspergillus* spp.

Up to date knowledge of the common organisms isolated in the hospital is useful to plan empirical antimicrobial therapy.

Clinical presentation

Severe sepsis in immunocompromised patients has a wide spectrum of clinical presentations. At one end of the spectrum are patients in whom there may be a paucity of clinical signs and symptoms, especially in the neutropenic setting. In these patients generalized or non-specific symptoms may be the only indicator of an underlying serious infection. Medical and nursing staff need a high index of suspicion in these scenarios.

In this situation, a child may present with features such as:

- Fever *or* low temperature (<35°C).
- Aches and pains, myalgia, headaches.
- Irritability.
- Lethargy, drowsiness.
- Poor appetite.
- Vomiting, bowel disturbances.

At the other end of the spectrum are patients who may present in septicaemic shock or overt organ dysfunction. These patients may present with:

- Drowsiness or loss of consciousness.
- **Cardiovascular compromise:** tachycardia, low blood pressure, poor peripheral perfusion (prolonged capillary refill time).
- **Respiratory signs:** tachypnoea, hypoxia.
- Oliguria/anuria.
- Metabolic acidosis.

In addition patients may also have symptoms or signs specific to a particular organ system, which may guide further investigation.

In any patient with suspected severe sepsis, an emergency assessment should be performed and therapy instituted without any delay and without waiting for the results of investigations. Rapid clinical deterioration is not uncommon, and patients need to be monitored carefully and meticulously.

Whenever possible, a thorough history and detailed physical examination should be performed on all patients. Special attention should be paid to areas such as oropharynx, ears, respiratory tract, peri-anal area, CVAD sites, and any sites of recent surgery.

Essential investigations
- FBC, coagulation profile.
- Serum biochemical profile, including renal and liver function tests.
- Inflammatory markers (e.g. C-reactive protein).
- Blood cultures (ideally from both peripheral blood and CVAD if present, although most UK units seldom take peripheral blood cultures).
- Blood sample for cross-match.
- Urine microscopy and culture.
- Throat swab.
- Chest X-ray (if clinical symptoms or signs of lower respiratory tract infection, or if severe sepsis present).

Other investigations which may be necessary as dictated by the patient's clinical status include:
- Lumbar puncture.
- Stools for virology/bacteriology/parasitology/*Clostridium difficile* toxin.
- Ultrasound/CT imaging of abdomen/chest or head.
- Swabs from sites of infection or inflammation (e.g. CVAD exit site, recent surgical wounds).
- Bronchoalveolar lavage/endotracheal aspirates for microbiology/virology.
- Blood for viral PCRs, fungal antigens/PCRs.

Management
Emergency assessment
Assess patient's airway, breathing, and circulation, and institute appropriate emergency management as required (refer to local resuscitation guidelines). Consider contacting paediatric intensive care or anaesthetic team.

The immediate management of any patient with severe sepsis should include the following:
- Establish airway and provide 100% oxygen. Consider ventilatory support if necessary.
- Establish intravenous access (or access existing CVAD) and start fluid resuscitation if patient shows any evidence of shock (remember to take blood cultures and other essential investigations at this stage).
- Fluid boluses (crystalloids/colloids) should be given in aliquots of 20ml/kg. If no response to two fluid boluses of 20ml/kg, consider inotropic support (contact paediatric intensive care team if not already present).
- Antimicrobial therapy (Antimicrobial therapy, p.115).

Carefully monitor the patient's vital parameters for any deterioration and respond to changes rapidly.

Obtain a detailed history and perform a full examination when the patient's clinical condition has stabilized.

Antimicrobial therapy

Broad spectrum antibiotic therapy should be instituted as soon as venous access is established.

Most centres have local guidelines for the management of neutropenic sepsis. The choice of antibiotics should be guided by the predominant organisms and the antibiotic sensitivity patterns at the centre in which the patient is being treated. Various combinations of antibiotics have been reported in the literature, essentially the combination should provide broad cover against both Gram +ve and −ve organisms.

Possible combinations include:

- A carbapenem, in combination with either an aminoglycoside or a glycopeptide.
- An antipseudomonal penicillin with an aminoglycoside.
- A 3rd/4th generation cephalosporin with an aminoglycoside.
- A 3rd/4th generation cephalosporin with a glycopeptide (teicoplanin or vancomycin) with or without an aminoglycoside.

Appropriate changes to antibiotics may be made subsequently, based on sensitivity patterns if an organism is isolated by microbiological cultures.

The duration of therapy should be guided by the clinical response and local policies.

Other measures

- **Intensive care support:** patients may need transfer to a high dependency unit or the paediatric intensive care unit. Therapeutic interventions that may be needed include oxygen therapy, mechanical ventilation, inotropic support, dialysis, blood product support, etc.
- Careful attention should be paid to fluid and electrolyte balance, with regular monitoring of urine output and serum electrolytes.
- Nutritional support is important particularly in patients with severe infection.
- The patient may need packed red cell and/or platelet transfusion support. If any signs of disseminated intravascular coagulation (DIC) are present, consider giving fresh frozen plasma (liaise with transfusion haematologist).
- In the setting of prolonged neutropenia with severe sepsis, consider growth factors such as granulocyte colony stimulating factor (G-CSF).
- Request a surgical opinion if an abscess is suspected, although abscess formation is unusual whilst a patient remains neutropenic. Surgical intervention may also be required in dealing with bowel complications (e.g. perforation, obstruction, etc.), and in the management of any tissue necrosis or gangrene.
- If CVAD infection is suspected, the device may need to be removed urgently.
- Consider antifungal therapy in the setting of prolonged neutropenia or if fungal infection is suspected.
- Consider antiviral therapy if any 'viral' rash is observed or if virology tests suggest infection.

Acute biochemical abnormalities

Causes

Several acute biochemical derangements may complicate childhood malignancy or its treatment. Collectively, they are common, although the prevalence of the individual disorders is variable and, in some cases, poorly documented. Those most frequently observed in children with malignancy include:

- Derangements of phosphate and potassium due to tumour lysis syndrome (Tumour lysis syndrome 📖 pp.94–95).
- Hyper- or hyponatraemia.
- Hypercalcaemia.
- Consequences of acute nephrotoxicity.

Many other biochemical abnormalities may occur less frequently, with numerous possible causes.

Hypernatraemia

Uncontrolled central diabetes insipidus (CDI) causes polyuria, polydipsia, and a risk of severe hypernatraemic dehydration. Several tumours may cause CDI in children:

- **Suprasellar/chiasmatic tumours** (or complicating their surgical treatment): collectively account for up to 50% of cases of CDI:
  - craniopharyngioma;
  - pineal tumours;
  - intracranial germinoma;
  - optic tract (visual pathway) glioma – a rarer cause of CDI.
- **Langerhans cell histiocytosis** (LCH): responsible for 10–15% of CDI (even though only occurs in ~1% of patients with LCH).

Hyponatraemia

Potential causes include:

- Syndrome of inappropiate antidiuretic hormone secretion (SIADH) – ADH secretion and, hence, urine osmolality and sodium are inappropriately high (urine sodium >50mmol/L) in relation to the low/normal serum osmolality and sodium concentrations, leading to increased water reabsorption with dilutional hyponataemia. SIADH may complicate:
  - *chemotherapy* – vincristine, vinblastine, cyclophosphamide, ifosfamide, cisplatin, melphalan;
  - *other drugs* – e.g. morphine, carbamazepine, thiazide diuretics;
  - CNS tumours;
  - rarely HD, NHL;
  - pulmonary infection.
- Iatrogenic (over-hydration with hypotonic fluids).
- Renal tubular sodium leakage:
  - *chemotherapy* – especially platinum drugs (cisplatin, carboplatin);
  - *cerebral salt wasting* – especially post-neurosurgery;
  - failure to give stress doses of corticosteroids.

Hypercalcaemia

Hypercalcaemia associated with malignancy is much less common in children (<1%) than in adults (5–20%).

It may occur at diagnosis, relapse, or during disease progression, due to:
- Reduced renal calcium loss or
- Increased bone resorption, often caused by humoral factors (especially PTH-related peptide).

Many childhood malignancies may cause hypercalcaemia:
- **Acute leukaemia:**
  - 40–50% of cases of malignancy-associated hypercalcaemia in children;
  - predominantly ALL;
  - usually at initial presentation;
  - respond well to anti-leukaemic chemotherapy and specific treatment for hypercalcaemia.
- **Solid tumours:**
  - 50–60% of cases;
  - variety of diagnoses:
    - rhabdomyosarcoma commonest;
    - association with infantile renal tumours reported.
  - often occurs later in disease course;
  - less responsive to treatment.

Nephrotoxicity

Several cytotoxic and anti-infective drugs may cause acute renal toxicity. The acute presentation is usually due to:
- Acute renal (glomerular) impairment:
  - *may be subclinical* – revealed only by an elevated serum creatinine concentration; or
  - *may lead to clinical manifestations* including:
    - hypertension;
    - fluid retention;
    - consequences of hyperkalaemia.
- Reduced renal tubular electrolyte reabsorption, with a number of patterns typical of individual drugs:
  - platinum drugs (cisplatin, and to much lesser extent, carboplatin) → hypomagnesaemia (very common), hypocalcaemia;
  - ifosfamide → hypophosphataemia (common), renal tubular acidosis, other electrolyte deficiencies, very rarely nephrogenic diabetes insipidus;
  - amphotericin B → hypokalaemia (very common, but may be reduced by use of amiloride), hypomagnesaemia (common); less common and severe with liposomal preparations;
  - aminoglycosides → electrolyte deficiencies, especially hypomagnesaemia (usually occurs only after prolonged treatment);
  - ciclosporin A, tacrolimus → hypomagnesaemia (common).

Diagnosis

Most biochemical abnormalities are detected initially by routine biochemical monitoring. However, they may sometimes present with characteristic clinical manifestations, e.g.:

- **Hypernatraemia:** anorexia, nausea, weakness, altered mental status, irritability, progressing to stupor, fits, and coma. Signs of dehydration and volume depletion may be present if treatment is delayed or inadequate.
- **Hyponatraemia:** nausea, lethargy, progressing to confusion, fits, coma.
- **Hypokalaemia:** muscle weakness, cardiac arrhythmias.
- **Hyperkalaemia:** cardiac arrhythmias.
- **Hypocalcaemia or hypomagnesaemia:** tetany, convulsions, cardiac arrhythmias.
- **Hypercalcaemia:** nausea, constipation, abdominal pain, anorexia, irritability, muscle weakness, polyuria leading to dehydration, renal damage (risk of nephrocalcinosis).
- **Hypophosphataemia:** muscle weakness, rickets.
- **Renal tubular acidosis:** acidotic breathing.

Management

- Try to treat or remove the underlying cause. Seldom justifiable to stop potentially curative chemotherapy, but the regimen may be modified (e.g. dose reduction, or changing nephrotoxic drug, e.g. ifosfamide for a less toxic alternative such as cylophosphamide).
- Specific treatment strategies include:
  - Avoid excessively rapid correction of hyper- and hyponatraemia, since it may cause irreversible neurological damage.
  - Hypernatraemia in CDI should be corrected carefully and slowly (≤12mmol/l per 24h), usually with IV 0.45% NaCl:
    - may need initial resuscitation with IV isotonic fluid if hypovolaemic at presentation;
    - DDAVP (desmopressin) may be needed acutely, especially in immediate post-neurosurgical CDI;
    - endocrine input is essential, and intensive care may be required.
  - *SIADH* – fluid restriction, with nephrology input (± intensive care if neurological symptoms present). Serum sodium concentration should be raised slowly (<2mmol/l/h).
  - *Hypercalcaemia* – vigorous hydration with intravenous saline +/– frusemide (given with care to avoid hypovolaemia) to improve renal calcium clearance. Additional specific strategies may include:
    - *bisphosphonates* (e.g. pamidronate) – reduce bone resorption and osteoclast activity;
    - *calcitonin* – inhibits bone resorption and renal tubular calcium reabsorption.
  - *Renal tubular electrolyte leakage* – regular oral electrolyte supplementation (dose titrated as necessary) usually sufficient for prevention of complications, but intravenous treatment often necessary in acutely ill children.

Outcome

Most acute biochemical derangements can be readily treated, although hypercalcaemia may be refractory in the presence of progressive solid tumours. Chemotherapy-induced nephrotoxicity may persist long after treatment withdrawal.

Hyperleucocytosis

Definition

Conventionally defined as peripheral white cell count (WCC) >100 × 10⁹/L.
Occurs at presentation or during relapse/progression of leukaemia.

▶▶Oncological emergency – may → death rapidly.

Threshold for development of clinical symptoms varies between patients
and with underlying disease:
- Lower in acute myeloid leukaemia (AML) due to larger size of
  myeloblasts – typically WCC >200 × 10⁹/L
- Higher in acute lymphoblastic leukaemia (ALL) and chronic myeloid
  leukaemia (CML) – typically WCC >300 × 10⁹/L.

Although patients with higher WCCs may be asymptomatic, they should
still be observed very carefully, and specific treatment instituted rapidly if
symptoms arise or WCC continues to increase.

Frequency

In childhood, hyperleucocytosis:
- Occurs in most patients with chronic phase CML.
- Is more common in:
  - AML (up to ~20% of new presentations) compared with ALL (~10%);
  - infantile AML and ALL;
  - blast phase CML;
  - T cell ALL (+/– mediastinal mass);
  - Philadelphia positive ALL.

Pathogenesis

- Increased blood viscosity.
- Aggregations of blast cells with thrombi.
- Endothelial damage → leucostasis.

Clinical features

- **Central nervous system (CNS)**
  - **Numerous symptoms:** may include altered mental status, headache, visual disturbances (diplopia, blurring), impaired hearing, vertigo, tinnitus, seizures, somnolence/impaired consciousness (may → coma), limb weakness/paralysis/paraesthesia, ataxia.
  - **Signs:** of cerebrovascular accident (CVA), visual field defects, cranial nerve palsies, fundoscopy → papilloedema, retinal vessel engorgement, haemorrhages.
- **Pulmonary:** tachypnoea, dyspnoea, hypoxia, 2° pulmonary haemorrhage; → respiratory failure, CXR shows widespread pulmonary infiltrates.
- **Cardiovascular:** congestive cardiac failure, arrhythmias.
- **Haematological:** coagulopathy, bleeding (CNS, pulmonary, mouth, epistaxis, uterine).
- **Renal:** acute renal failure.
- **Others:** priapism, clitoral enlargement, dactylitis.
- **Metabolic:** tumour lysis syndrome (Tumour lysis syndrome 📖 pp.94–95).

Commonest causes of death

- CNS haemorrhage or thrombosis – AML > ALL.
- Pulmonary leucostasis – AML > ALL.
- Metabolic consequences of tumour lysis (rare, but ALL > AML).

Management

▶▶ Commence anti-leukaemic treatment ASAP.
- Prevention preferable to treatment
- Prevention of tumour lysis (Tumour lysis syndrome 📖 pp.94–95).
- If platelets <20 × 10⁹/L, give platelet transfusion to decrease risk CNS haemorrhage (platelets do not ↑ blood viscosity significantly).

▶ Avoid blood transfusion (risk of ↑ viscosity) if at all possible. Consider leucopheresis or exchange transfusion in patients with very high WCC (>200 × 10⁹/L), especially if symptoms/signs of hyperleucocytosis, but benefit is only temporary.

Central venous access device-associated venous thrombosis

Definitions
- **Thrombosis:** pathological presence of intravascular coagulation.
- **Embolism:** vascular obstruction due to dislodgement of a thrombus.

Venous thromboembolism (VTE) in children with malignancy occurs in two main clinical scenarios:
- **Central venous access device** (CVAD)-associated (develops in ~1.5% of CVADs) – arising at the CVAD tip or within its lumen.
- **Tumour-related** (rare): due to large vein obstruction, e.g. by mediastinal, pelvic or extremity tumours.

Arterial thromboembolism is rare in childhood malignancy, but may occasionally complicate asparaginase treatment.

Epidemiology and pathogenesis
CVAD-associated VTE is commonest in children with ALL, especially during induction therapy, occurring in 3–5% of patients (but with wide variability in frequency between different treatment protocols), due to:
- Increased thrombin generation due to ALL itself.
- Suppression of endogenous anticoagulants (especially anti-thrombin) by asparaginase.
- Promotion of factor VIII/von Willebrand factor complexes and increased plasminogen activator inhibitor levels due to steroids.
- Use of CVADs.

Although individual studies of the relevance of inherited prothrombotic disorders in the pathogenesis of VTE in ALL have given conflicting findings, it is likely that there is a relationship between the presence of at least one prothrombotic factor and the development of VTE. This risk is probably modulated by the treatment regimen used (particularly the dose, exact type, and timing of steroid and asparaginase treatments).

Diagnosis
- CVAD-associated thrombosis may be asymptomatic or may lead to characteristic clinical symptoms and signs, e.g.:
  - oedema;
  - warmth;
  - collateral circulation;
  - impaired venous return.
- Several imaging modalities may reveal venous thrombosis at the site of, or adjacent to, a CVAD, e.g.:
  - linogram;
  - venogram;
  - Doppler US, echocardiogram;
  - magnetic resonance venography (MRV).

The investigation strategy varies considerably between centres and the optimal approach is not clear. Major CVAD-related thromboembolic events include:
• CNS venous thrombosis.
• SVC thrombosis.
• Right atrial thrombosis.
• Pulmonary embolism.

Management

Prevention is preferable to treatment.
• Most CVADs in children with malignancy are placed in the upper venous system; in this context, the risk of thrombosis may be lower when the device is placed on the right side and in the jugular (rather than subclavian) vein.
• In ALL, the importance of the timing of CVAD insertion is uncertain, and may be modulated by the type, dose and scheduling of asparaginase and steroid treatment. Many UK centres delay insertion until after induction therapy in an effort to reduce the risk of thrombosis.

The treatment of established CVAD-associated VTE varies greatly between centres:
• Most centres remove the CVAD unless this is impractical (e.g. if alternative venous access is very difficult), but there is much uncertainty about the need for and nature of additional strategies, which include:
  • systemic anticoagulation (low molecular weight heparin and warfarin have both been used);
  • thrombolysis (used less often, but may be delivered via the CVAD itself).
• Particular uncertainty about the optimum management of asymptomatic CVAD-associated thrombosis, which may be present in up to 40% of children undergoing elective removal of vascular ports.

Outcome

The consequences of CVAD-associated thrombosis include:
• Distress to patient/family: due to CVAD malfunction.
• Inconvenience to staff: due to CVAD malfunction.
• Requirement to remove (+/– replace) CVAD.
• Delay or impairment in ability to deliver planned and optimum chemotherapy.
• Risk of:
  • deep venous thrombosis (may be recurrent);
  • SVC syndrome;
  • pulmonary embolism;
  • post-thrombotic syndrome (pain, swelling, ulceration of affected limb);
  • death (the average reported case fatality of symptomatic VTE in ALL is 15%).

Pleural and pericardial effusions

Definition

Pleural or pericardial effusions are pathological collections of fluid in the pleural or pericardial sacs. In the context of malignancy, they may be caused by:

- Local malignant disease.
- Systemic malignant disease.
- Complications of treatment.

Effusions due to malignancy itself usually occur at diagnosis or relapse, and may become persistent in the context of progressive disease.

Epidemiology

Pleural effusions are relatively common presentations of malignancy or complications of its treatment in children, but pericardial effusions are rarer. There are no published data concerning their overall frequency.

Causes

The commoner causes of effusions in children with malignancy include:

- **The malignancy itself:**
  - *Leukaemia* – may present or relapse with pleural and/or (less commonly) pericardial effusions; commoner in acute lymphoblastic leukaemia (ALL) (especially T-cell), but may occur rarely in acute myeloid leukaemia (AML) (especially M5).
  - *Lymphoma* – may cause pleural effusions, commoner in NHL (especially T-cell) than Hodgkin lymphoma (HL).
  - *Solid tumours* – pleural and/or pericardial effusions may occur in a wide variety of malignancies, including sarcomas (rhabdomyosarcoma, soft tissue, Ewing's, osteosarcoma, neuroblastoma, medulloblastoma).
- **Treatment:**
  - Pericardial and/or (less commonly) pleural effusions may be caused by radiotherapy or colony stimulating factors (CSFs).
  - Rare reports of pleural effusions associated with chemotherapy (e.g. cyclophosphamide, methotrexate) or tyrosine kinase inhibitors (e.g. dasatinib).
- **Infection:** tuberculosis, pneumococcal, or aspergillus may all → pleural and/or pericardial effusions.
- **Graft-versus-host disease** (GvHD) may rarely → pleural and/or pericardial effusions.

Diagnosis

Both pleural and pericardial effusions may present with:
- Dyspnoea.
- Orthopnoea.
- Chest pain.
- Irritable cough.

Clinical signs, although usually obvious in larger effusions, may be difficult to detect in younger children. Small effusions may only be detected radiologically (including echocardiography). Large pericardial effusions may lead to cardiac tamponade.

Investigations depend on the clinical context (the cause may be obvious in progressive disease) and include aspiration of effusion fluid, with evaluation of:
- Protein.
- Cell count.
- Microscopy.
- Culture.
- Cytology.
- Immunophenotyping.

Effusions due to malignancy or infection are usually exudates (fluid protein >25g/L, or >50% of serum protein concentration).

A chylous pleural effusion implies obstructed lymphatic drainage.

Management

This includes:
- Treatment of the underlying cause with, e.g. cytotoxic or anti-infective treatment, but this may not be feasible for advanced malignancy.
- Relief of the consequences of the effusion(s). This may not be necessary if rapid and effective treatment of the cause is possible.

Although 'emergency' fluid aspiration may be necessary to relieve severe symptoms or complications (e.g. cardiac tamponade), timely institution of effective chemotherapy leads to rapid improvement in most pleural and pericardial effusions occurring at initial presentation of malignancy, without the need for or risks of invasive procedures.

Effusions may be persistent or recurrent in progressive disease, leading to severe symptoms, and necessitating repeated aspiration procedures or continuous catheter drainage.

Most information about chemical pleurodesis or intrapleural chemotherapy is derived from adult literature, but doxycycline or cisplatin have been shown to be effective in many malignant effusions in children. Rarely, surgical pleurectomy or pericardiectomy may be required.

Outcome

Most effusions are amenable to medical or surgical treatment, except in progressive malignant disease.

Long-term prognosis depends on the underlying cause.

Section 4

General principles

Multimodality treatment

Multimodality treatment is therapy that combines more than one modality of treatment. This is true for most malignant tumours seen in childhood and adolescence. The most established modes of treatment are:
• Chemotherapy.
• Surgery.
• Radiotherapy.

Often a combination of two or more of these modalities is used to treat children with cancer.

Individual chapters on chemotherapy, radiotherapy, and surgery follow this chapter (Chemotherapy 📖 pp.131–147, Paediatric radiotherapy 📖 pp.149–158, Surgery 📖 pp.160–162). Other modalities of treatment sometimes used in children with cancer include:
• Biological therapy (e.g. immunotherapy in the form of antibodies or vaccines).
• Molecularly-targeted therapy.
• Anti-angiogenic therapy.
• Other more specific therapies.

Multimodality treatment has potential advantages:
• Different treatment modalities have different mechanisms of action, which may potentially increase the chance of cure.
• One modality may enhance the chance of success of the other, e.g. initial chemotherapy may allow easier surgery and a higher chance of complete removal, whilst surgery may allow radiotherapy or chemotherapy to work more effectively on a smaller tumour residuum.

Multimodality treatment, whilst often effective, may result in more side effects since a combination of two modalities can often increase the severity of toxicities to a greater degree than the sum of the individual side effects. An example is cranial radiotherapy without cochlear sparing combined with platinum agents, which increases the chance of hearing loss.

One treatment modality may also potentiate the effect of another and increase the side effect profile. One example of this is the combination of actinomycin D and radiotherapy, where the actinomycin potentiates the effects of radiation ('radiation recall') with potentially severe consequences. It is important to consider any potential interactions beforehand when planning multimodality treatment.

The timing of the different modalities, and when to use each one, must also be considered carefully. It is important to decide whether initial surgery is better than delayed surgery (children with brain tumours usually have surgery first, whereas those with sarcomas have it later) and to consider when each modality is maximally effective.

There is often a difference of opinion and emphasis between different protocols or countries, e.g. children with Wilms' tumour in US have surgery prior to other treatment, whereas in Europe chemotherapy is given for 6 weeks prior to surgery.

Multimodality therapy must be used with thought and caution, but it has considerably enhanced the efficacy of treatment of children with cancer. Other modalities will become more prevalent in the future with individualized targeted therapy the ultimate goal.

Chemotherapy

General principles

Combination chemotherapy

Most chemotherapy protocols for childhood malignancies employ combinations of two or more cytotoxic drugs. Combination chemotherapy aims to take advantage of:

- Different mechanisms of action, which may be complementary.
- Non-overlapping side-effects to limit the toxicity profile, thereby offering the potential of improved cytotoxic action with less toxicity and a theoretically reduced risk of acquired resistance.

Differential cytotoxicity

Most cytotoxic drugs act by interfering with at least one aspect of nucleic acid (DNA or RNA) synthesis, metabolism, or function. Certain aspects of the malignant cell phenotype may render it more vulnerable to cytotoxicity than normal cells, thereby allowing differential cell kill. For example, mitosis of normal cells may be arrested in the G_1 phase (Phases of cell cycle 🕮 p.135) in response to cytotoxic-induced DNA damage, thereby allowing time for DNA repair, whilst this normal protective response may be lost in malignant cells, which are therefore killed.

Drug resistance

Drug resistance may be mediated by several mechanisms, including:

- **Reduced drug entry into malignant cells:** e.g. ↓ activity of folic acid transporter → ↓ methotrexate entry.
- **Increased drug elimination:** e.g. by P-glycoprotein transporter in 'multidrug resistance' (MDR) phenotype, which confers resistance to several cytotoxic drugs including anthracyclines, vinca alkaloids, taxanes.
- **Drug detoxification:** e.g. of alkylating agents or anthracyclines by glutathione-S-transferase (GST).
- **Increased DNA repair:** e.g. mediated by alkylguanine-DNA alkyltransferase, reducing sensitivity to temozolamide, dacarbazine, nitrosoureas.

Side effects

Cytotoxic drugs have numerous potential side-effects, most of which are predictable in nature, although often variable in severity. They can be broadly grouped as follows:

Acute toxicity

Usually (but not always) reversible.

- Damage to rapidly dividing cells:
  - bone marrow → anaemia, leucopenia, thrombocytopenia;
  - gastrointestinal tract/mucous membranes → mucositis;
  - skin/hair (→ alopecia).
- Nausea/vomiting.
- Organ toxicity, e.g.:
  - *neuropathy* – cisplatin, vincristine;
  - *hepatotoxicity* – actinomycin D, asparaginase;
  - *haemorrhagic cystitis* – cyclophosphamide, ifosfamide.
- Hypersensitivity.

Chronic toxicity

Often irreversible.

- Organ toxicity, e.g.:
  - *cardiotoxicity* – anthracyclines;
  - *nephrotoxicity* – cisplatin, ifosfamide;
  - *pulmonary* – bleomycin;
  - *gonadal* – alkylating agents.
- Secondary malignancies: alkylating agents, epipodophyllotoxins
  (Long-term follow-up, Secondary malignancy 📖 p.300).

Pharmacological principles

By the very nature of their mechanisms of action, the therapeutic index (the ratio between the clinically effective dose and the toxic dose) of cyto-toxic drugs is usually much smaller than that of most other drugs, and, indeed, may be close to one. Therefore, it is very important to have a good understanding of the underlying pharmacological principles and characteristics that guide optimal clinical use of chemotherapy agents.

Pharmacodynamics

In its widest sense, 'pharmacodynamics' is the interaction between the drug and the malignant cells (the 'target'), i.e. the effect that the drug has on the target (and, by extension, on the body as a whole).
- This may include an explanation of the drug's mechanism of action.
- In a stricter sense, the term describes the relationship between the drug's concentration in blood and its clinical effect.

Pharmacokinetics

This term describes the converse to pharmacodynamics, i.e. pharmacoki-netics documents the effect that the body has on the drug. This includes:
- **Absorption:** from the gastrointestinal tract, or after subcutaneous (SC) or intramuscular (IM) administration:
  - *bioavailability* – the rate and extent of absorption, usually quantified relative to availability of the drug when delivered intravenously (IV);
  - **NB.** Oral drugs are also exposed to *first pass metabolism*.
- **Excretion:** renal (glomerular ± tubular) and/or biliary.
- **Biotransformation:** enzymatic metabolism of the drug; although the liver is the major site of drug metabolism, other tissues (e.g. renal) may contribute.
- **Clearance:** the rate at which drug is eliminated from the body

  Total clearance = renal + non-renal (metabolic + biliary [faecal] + spontaneous breakdown

- **Half-life:** the time required to reduce plasma drug concentration by 50%.
- **Area under the curve** (AUC): a measure of total drug exposure over time, derived from the area under the plasma concentration–time curve (calculated as the integral of drug concentration with time).

Phases of cell cycle

Different chemotherapy drugs target different stages of the cell cycle (Fig. 12.1):

- **G$_1$**: pre-replicative phase (synthesis of cellular content, including RNA and protein, but not chromosomal material), targeted by, e.g. asparaginase.
- **G$_0$**: resting phase (cell cycle arrest, therefore very resistant to chemotherapy).
- **S**: DNA synthesis phase (with duplication of chromosomes), targeted by anti-metabolites, e.g. cytosine arabinoside, methotrexate, 6-mercaptopurine.
- **G$_2$**: premitotic interval (RNA and protein synthesis. The cell checks the duplicated chromosomes for errors and makes any necessary repairs), targeted, by e.g. bleomycin
- **M:** mitotic phase (cell division), targeted by, e.g. vincristine.

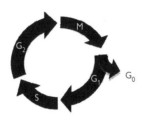

M = mitotic phase
G$_0$ = resting phase (cell cycle arrest)
G$_1$ = pre-replicative phase
S = DNA synthesis phase
G$_2$ = pre-mitotic interval

Fig. 12.1 Schematic representation of the cell cycle.

Classes of cytotoxic drugs

- **Alkylating agents:** cross-link DNA by forming covalent bonds with bases.
- **Anti-metabolites:** interfere with enzymes needed for production of purines, pyrimidines, DNA, or RNA by acting as fraudulent substrates.
- **Antitumour antibiotics:** impair DNA replication or transcription; in addition, anthracyclines act primarily by inhibiting topoisomerase II, causing DNA strand breaks.
- **Camptothecans:** inhibit topoisomerase I, leading to DNA strand breaks.
- **Epipodophyllotoxins:** inhibit topoisomerase II, resulting in DNA strand breakage.
- **Retinoids:** differentiation agents acting via nuclear retinoid receptors.
- **Taxanes:** inhibit mitosis by blocking microtubule depolymerization.
- **Vinca alkaloids:** block spindle formation during mitosis.
- **Miscellaneous:**
  - *amsacrine* – topoisomerase II inhibitor;
  - *asparaginase* – asparagine depletion;
  - *corticosteroids* – increase apoptosis of malignant lymphoblasts;
  - *dacarbazine* – atypical alkylating agent;
  - *imatinib* – tyrosine kinase inhibitor;
  - *procarbazine* – atypical alkylating agent.

Characteristics of cytotoxic drugs

The most important characteristics of individual cytotoxic drugs are summarized below. The lists of conditions in which they are used reflect recent or current Phase III clinical trials or other well established treatment protocols used in the UK, and may differ slightly from those in other countries. Some of the drugs currently used in Phase I and II clinical trials are mentioned, but not described in detail. Administration routes that are used rarely are not included, e.g. oral cyclophosphamide. Doses and detailed treatment schedules are not included since these depend greatly on specific treatment protocols for particular malignancies, and continue to evolve over time. Since most cytotoxic drugs cause at least some degree of myelosuppression, mucositis, nausea/vomiting, and alopecia, these side effects are not listed for each drug, unless exceptionally mild or severe. Predictable late toxicity, including gonadal toxicity and secondary malignancies, is not included, since it is covered in detail elsewhere (Long-term follow-up 📖 pp.293–314).

Drugs with steep dose-response curves, predominantly haemopoietic toxicity, but relatively tolerable non-haemopoietic toxicity, may allow high-dose treatment with haematological rescue by either autologous stem cell rescue procedure or allogeneic transplantation (Haemopoeitic stem cell transplantation 📖 pp.163–200).

Alkylating agents

Busulfan

- **Use:** haemopoietic stem cell transplant (HSCT) conditioning.
- **Route of administration:** oral or IV.
- **Toxicity:**
  - hepatotoxicity (veno-occlusive disease);
  - convulsions;
  - pulmonary fibrosis.
- **Elimination:** metabolism and chemical degradation. Very variable – therapeutic drug level monitoring often used.

Carboplatin

Cisplatin analogue, acts similarly by DNA binding.

- **Use:** brain tumours, germ cell tumours, hepatoblastoma, neuroblastoma, retinoblastoma, HSCT conditioning.
- **Dose:** may be calculated based on body surface area, weight, or by dose formula based on renal function.
- **Route of administration:** IV, no hydration fluid required.
- **Toxicity:** overall substantially less toxic than cisplatin (see 'Cisplatin', next page):
  - myelosuppression is predominant toxicity, especially thrombocytopenia;
  - nephrotoxicity mild compared to cisplatin;
  - significant ototoxicity uncommon.
- **Elimination:** renal excretion, predominantly of unchanged drug.
- Consider dose reduction or use of GFR dosing formula in renal impairment.

Carmustine (BCNU)

- **Use:** Hodgkin disease (HD), non-Hodgkin lymphoma (NHL), HSCT conditioning.
- **Route of administration:** IV.
- **Toxicity:**
  - Neurotoxicity;
  - pulmonary toxicity occasionally.
- **Elimination:** rapid spontaneous degradation.
- **N.B.** Carmustine is being withdrawn from production.

Chlorambucil

- **Use:** HD.
- **Route of administration:** oral.
  - **Toxicity:** nausea/vomiting and alopecia mild.
- **Elimination:** metabolism, with renal excretion of metabolites.

Cisplatin

Not a classical alkylating agent, but acts by binding to DNA.

- **Use:** brain tumours, germ cell tumours, hepatoblastoma, hepatocellular carcinoma, neuroblastoma, osteosarcoma.
- **Route of administration:** IV, usually as prolonged continuous infusion with pre-, intra- and post-hydration to reduce risk of nephrotoxicity.
- **Toxicity:**
  - severe nausea and vomiting;
  - mild hair loss;
  - mild/moderate myelosuppression (mostly with high dose);
  - *nephrotoxicity* – see Acute biochemical abnormalities, Nephrotoxicity 📖 p.117);
  - peripheral neuropathy (less severe than in adults);
  - *ototoxicity* – high frequency sensorineural hearing loss;
  - encephalopathy (usually with high dose).
- **Elimination:** rapid protein and tissue binding; renal excretion (slow terminal phase).
- Review further treatment very carefully if GFR <60mL/min/1.73m^2.

Cyclophosphamide

- **Use:** acute lymphoblastic leukaemia (ALL), brain tumours, HD, neuroblastoma, NHL, rhabdomyosarcoma, soft tissue sarcomas, HSCT conditioning.
- **Toxicity:** haemorrhagic cystitis caused by acrolein (toxic metabolite). Low dose cyclophosphamide (<300mg/m^2) seldom causes significant haemorrhagic cystitis, but urotoxicity is increasingly common after higher doses (especially ≥1000mg/m^2). May be prevented in most patients receiving <300mg/m^2 cyclophosphamide by maintaining adequate fluid input and frequent micturition (to reduce bladder mucosal exposure to acrolein). If cyclophosphamide dose 300–1000mg/m^2, IV hydration is usually given for 4–6h afterwards, and when dose >1000mg/m^2, IV hydration, and mesna (which inactivates acrolein) are given until at least 12h after last cyclophosphamide dose.

- **Elimination:** cyclophosphamide is an inactive pro-drug. Undergoes hepatic metabolism to active metabolites which are excreted renally. Considerable inter-patient variability in metabolism.
- Consider dose reduction when GFR <60mL/min/1.73m^2.

Ifosfamide
- Structural isomer of cyclophosphamide.
- **Use:** Ewing's sarcoma, HD, osteosarcoma, retinoblastoma, rhabdomyosarcoma, soft tissue sarcoma, HSCT conditioning.
- **Route of administration:** IV. Always used with mesna and IV hydration to reduce or prevent haemorrhagic cystitis.
- **Toxicity:**
  - haemorrhagic cystitis more severe than with cyclophosphamide – hence necessity for mesna;
  - encephalopathy;
  - *nephrotoxicity* – see Acute biochemical abnormalities, Nephrotoxicity 🕮 p.117).
- **Elimination:** like cyclophosphamide, ifosfamide is an inactive pro-drug, undergoing hepatic metabolism to active metabolites, which are excreted renally. Considerable inter-patient variability in metabolism. Metabolism is qualitatively similar, but quantitatively different to that of cyclophosphamide, which may explain different pattern of toxicities of the two drugs.
- Review further treatment very carefully if GFR <60mL/min/1.73m^2.

Lomustine (CCNU)
- **Use:** brain tumours (good blood–brain barrier penetration).
- **Route of administration:** oral (although absorption erratic).
- **Toxicity:**
  - usually no nausea and vomiting;
  - mild alopecia only;
  - *myelosuppression* – especially prolonged thrombocytopenia, with nadir at 3 weeks;
  - pulmonary toxicity occasionally.
- **Elimination:**– rapid hepatic metabolism.

Melphalan
- **Use:** HSCT conditioning.
- **Route of administration:** rapid IV injection (degrades in sunlight).
- **Toxicity:**
  - erythematous skin reaction;
  - occasionally, acute renal failure or convulsions.
- **Elimination:** rapid metabolism. Minor degree of renal excretion (about 20%).
- Consider dose reduction if GFR <60mL/min/1.73m^2.

Temozolomide
- **Use:** brain tumours, some investigational (Phase II) studies in paediatric solid tumours.
- **Route of administration:** oral.
- **Toxicity:** myelosuppression, especially prolonged thrombocytopenia, with nadir at 3 weeks.
- **Elimination:** metabolized to inactive metabolite.

Thiotepa
- **Use:** brain tumours, HSCT conditioning.
- **Route of administration:** IV.
- **Toxicity:**
  - *myelosuppression* – especially prolonged thrombocytopenia, with nadir at 3 weeks;
  - *hepatotoxicity* (veno-occlusive disease).
- **Elimination:** metabolized to active metabolite (TEPA).

Anti-metabolites

Cytosine arabinoside (Cytarabine)
- **Use:** ALL, acute myeloid leukaemia (AML), HSCT conditioning, NHL.
- **Route of administration:** usually IV. Can be given SC or IM. Low doses given intrathecally in AML, and sometimes in ALL and NHL (avoid intrathecal use at same time as high-dose intravenous use, due to increased risk of encephalopathy). Very wide range of doses and administration schedules.
- **Toxicity:**
  - cerebellar ataxia/encephalopathy;
  - fever, headache, arthralgia, myalgia, malaise may occur during treatment.
- **Elimination:** cytarabine is a pro-drug, which is activated to triphosphate form (araCTP) intracellularly. Hepatic metabolism, renal excretion of inactive metabolites.

Fludarabine
- **Use:** AML, HSCT conditioning.
- **Route of administration:** IV.
- **Toxicity:**
  - prolonged immunosuppression;
  - neurotoxicity (with high doses).
- **Elimination:** rapid metabolism, renal excretion.
- Consider dose reduction if GFR <60mL/min/1.73m^2.

6-Mercaptopurine (6MP)
- **Use:** ALL, Langerhans cell histiocytosis (LCH).
- **Route of administration:** oral.
- **Toxicity:** hepatotoxicity.
- **Elimination:** extensive metabolism to active thioguanine nucleotides (TGNs), inactivated by thiopurine methyltransferase (TPMT). Considerable inter-patient variability in metabolism, hence need to adjust dose in individual patient.

Methotrexate
Yellow colour.
- **Uses/route of administration:**
  - low oral dose (e.g. 20 mg/m^2 weekly) in ALL maintenance;
  - intermediate/high dose IV (e.g. 500–8000mg/m^2) in ALL, brain tumours, NHL, osteosarcoma;
  - low intrathecal dose in ALL, AML, NHL (age-related doses as specified in specific protocols).

- **Pharmacology:**
  - Intermediate/high doses usually given over 3–36h.
  - Intermediate/high doses always given with systemic folinic acid to rescue normal cells from methotrexate-induced inhibition of folinic acid production –
    - IV folinic acid is commenced 24–48h (depending on the protocol) after the start of methotrexate to prevent systemic toxicity, and continued at least until plasma methotrexate levels are <0.20–0.25µmol/L (according to the protocol);
    - normal cells, but not malignant ones, actively transport folinic acid to counter high intracellular methotrexate concentrations.
  - To prevent renal damage, IV hydration/alkalinization is given before methotrexate is commenced and continued until plasma methotrexate levels are <~1µmol/l – alkalinization prevents precipitation of methotrexate in renal tubules.
  - Beware of distribution of methotrexate into and slow release from 'third spaces' (e.g. pleural or ascitic fluid), which can delay the terminal phase of drug excretion.
  - Intermediate and high-dose methotrexate treatment can cause extremely severe, life-threatening toxicity if not administered correctly.
  - ⚠ It is vital to follow the administration protocol precisely.
  - Drugs that interfere with protein-binding and/or renal clearance of methotrexate (e.g. cotrimoxazole, non-steroidal anti-inflammatory drugs) may lead to delayed excretion and increased risk of toxicity, and should be avoided before and during high-dose methotrexate courses.
- **Toxicity:**
  - *low oral dose* – mouth ulcers, skin rashes;
  - *intermediate/high IV dose* –
    - no/mild nausea and vomiting;
    - no hair loss;
    - myelosuppression usually mild;
    - skin rashes;
    - rarely, acute renal failure, hepatotoxicity, or neurotoxicity;
    - systemic over-exposure to methotrexate (e.g. due to impaired clearance) results in a follicular skin rash, severe enteritis and myelosuppression;
  - *low intrathecal dose* – neurotoxicity.
- **Elimination:** hepatic metabolism, renal excretion (glomerular filtration and tubular excretion). In renal impairment, higher serum methotrexate concentrations will occur, which will need higher doses of folinic acid rescue.
- Consider dose reduction or avoid use if GFR <60mL/min/1.73m^2.
- Even low doses or intrathecal use of methotrexate can be lethal if given in the context of renal failure.
- Carboxypertidase G_2 may be used to inactivate methotrexate in accidental over dosage or severe delay in excretion with prolonged high levels.

6-Tioguanine
- **Use:** infantile ALL.
- **Route of administration:** oral.
- **Toxicity:** hepatotoxicity (veno-occlusive disease).
- **Elimination:** intracellular metabolism.

Antitumour antibiotics

Actinomycin D
Yellow colour.
- **Use:** Ewing's sarcoma, rhabdomyosarcoma, soft tissue sarcoma, Wilms' tumour.
- **Route of administration:** IV bolus.
- **Toxicity:**
  - skin rashes;
  - extravasation causes severe tissue necrosis;
  - radiation recall with severe reactions, so avoid use with or shortly after radiotherapy;
  - hepatotoxicity (veno-occlusive disease), rarely severe hepatic failure.
- **Elimination:** little metabolism. Rapid tissue binding with slow release. Biliary and renal excretion.

Bleomycin
- **Use:** germ cell tumours, HD, osteosarcoma.
- **Route of administration:** IV.
- **Toxicity:**
  - no nausea/vomiting, hair loss, or myelosuppression usually;
  - fever, chills, hypersensitivity a few hours after administration;
  - skin rashes, hyperpigmentation;
  - interstitial pneumonitis (especially if full dose given in patients with renal impairment).
- **Elimination:** renal excretion.
- Dose reduction when GFR <60mL/min/1.73m^2) is very important.

⚠ Beware of using high oxygen concentrations and/or repeated general anaesthetics in patients treated with bleomycin, both of which increase risk of potentially fatal interstitial pneumonitis.

Daunorubicin
Red colour.
- **Use:** ALL, AML.
- **Route of administration:** IV.
- **Toxicity:**– similar to doxorubicin.
- **Elimination:** hepatic metabolism with biliary excretion.
- Consider dose reduction if serum bilirubin >20μmol/l.

Doxorubicin
Red colour.
- **Use:** ALL, Ewing's sarcoma, HD, hepatoblastoma, hepatocellular carcinoma, NHL, osteosarcoma, retinoblastoma, rhabdomyosarcoma, soft tissue sarcoma, Wilms' tumour.

- **Route of administration:** IV.
- **Toxicity:**
  - Moderately severe mucositis and enteritis;
  - Extravasation causes severe tissue necrosis;
  - Red discolouration of urine;
  - *Cardiotoxicity* – need to monitor with echocardiogram. Total dose should not exceed 450mg/m^2, due to increased risk of cardiotoxicity above this dose (although it may also occur at lower doses, albeit less commonly);
  - May enhance radiation-induced damage. Therefore, avoid administration concomitantly or in post-irradiation period (risk of radiation recall).
- **Elimination:** hepatic metabolism with biliary and (minor) renal excretion.
- Consider dose reduction if serum bilirubin >20µmol/l.

Epirubicin

Red colour.
- **Use:** ALL.
- **Route of administration:** IV.
- **Toxicity:** similar to doxorubicin.
- **Elimination:** hepatic metabolism with biliary and renal excretion.
- Consider dose reduction if serum bilirubin >20µmol/l.

Idarubicin

Red colour.
- **Use:** ALL.
- **Route of administration:** IV or oral.
- **Toxicity:** similar to doxorubicin.
- **Elimination:** hepatic metabolism.

Mitoxantrone

Blue colour. Synthetic anthracenedione, closely related to anthracyclines.
- **Use:** AML, ALL.
- **Route of administration:** IV.
- **Toxicity:** similar to doxorubicin (blue/green discoloration of urine).
- **Elimination:** hepatic metabolism, biliary and (minor) renal excretion.
- Consider dose reduction if serum bilirubin >20µmol/l.

Camptothecans

Irinotecan

Topotecan

Use of these agents remains investigational (Phase I and II studies) in paediatric malignancies. Both cause myelosuppression and irinotecan may cause severe diarrhoea.

Epipodophyllotoxins

Etoposide (VP-16)
- **Use:** ALL, AML, brain tumours, Ewing's sarcoma, germ cell tumours, HD, haemophagocytic lymphophistiocytosis (HLH), HSCT conditioning, neuroblastoma, retinoblastoma.

- **Route of administration:** IV. Low doses sometimes used orally in palliative treatment.
- **Toxicity:**
  - extravasation can cause severe necrosis;
  - allergic reactions with generalized erythema and hypotension, rarely anaphylaxis.
- **Elimination:** extensive metabolism, but considerable inter-patient variability. Renal excretion (40%).
- Consider dose reduction if GFR <60mL/min/1.73m^2.

Retinoids

13-cis retinoic acid
- **Use:** neuroblastoma.
- **Route of administration:** oral.
- **Toxicity:**
  - usually no myelosuppression, nausea/vomiting, or alopecia;
  - dry skin and mouth, cheilitis.
- **Elimination:** hepatic metabolism, highly protein bound, excreted in faeces.

All-trans retinoic acid (ATRA)
- **Use:** AML (M3 – acute promyelocytic leukaemia).
- **Route of administration:** oral.
- **Toxicity:**
  - *retinoic acid syndrome* – fever, fluid retention, respiratory distress ± hyperleucocytosis;
  - headaches, pseudotumour cerebri ('benign intracranial hypertension');
  - hepatotoxicity.
- **Elimination:** rapid metabolism by cytochrome P450-dependent enzymes.

Taxanes

Docetaxel
Paclitaxel
Use of these agents remains investigational (Phase I and II studies) in paediatric malignancies. Both are myelosuppressive and can cause hypersensitivity; in addition, docetaxal may cause fluid retention and paclitaxel peripheral neuropathy.

Vinca alkaloids

Vinblastine
- **Use:** HD, LCH.
- **Route of administration:** slow IV bolus.
- **Toxicity:**
  - more myelosuppressive than vincristine;
  - severe tissue necrosis if extravasated;
  - less neurotoxic than vincristine.
- **Elimination:** hepatic metabolism, slow biliary excretion.
- Consider dose reduction if serum bilirubin >20µmol/L.

Vincristine
- **Use:** ALL, brain tumours, HD, neuroblastoma, NHL, rhabdomyosarcoma, retinoblastoma, soft tissue sarcoma, Wilms' tumour.
- **Route of administration:** slow IV bolus.
- **Toxicity:**
  - usually no nausea/vomiting or myelosuppression;
  - minimal hair loss;
  - extravasation causes severe tissue necrosis and inflammation;
  - *neurotoxicity* – may be dose-limiting:
    - peripheral neuropathy → painful, loss of tendon reflexes, weakness;
    - autonomic neuropathy → constipation;
    - rarely, convulsions;
  - inappropriate ADH secretion.
- **Elimination:** hepatic metabolism, rapid biliary excretion.
- Consider dose reduction if serum bilirubin >20μmol/L.

⚠ Vincristine is invariably fatal if inadvertently given intrathecally. Therefore, vincristine syringes should never be placed in any room or theatre where intrathecal chemotherapy is being administered.

Vinorelbine
- **Use:** rhabdomyosarcoma.
- **Route of administration:** IV over 10min.
- **Toxicity:**
  - more myelosuppressive than vincristine;
  - severe tissue necrosis if extravasated;
  - neurotoxicity.
- **Elimination:** hepatic metabolism, slow biliary excretion.
- Consider dose reduction if serum bilirubin >20μmol/L.

Miscellaneous

Amsacrine (m-AMSA)
- **Use:** AML.
- **Route of administration:** IV infusion (in 5% glucose precipitates on contact with saline).
- **Toxicity:** similar to anthracyclines
- **Elimination:** hepatic metabolism, biliary excretion.

Asparaginase
Depletes circulating pool of asparagine leading to apoptosis of cells that have an obligate requirement for exogenous asparagine, e.g. leukaemic lymphoblasts.
- **Use:** ALL.
- **Administration:** IM, SC, or IV (as specified in treatment protocol).
- **Toxicity:**
  - usually no myelosuppression;
  - allergic reactions, potentially severe anaphylaxis;
  - coagulation disturbances;
  - pancreatic damage (pancreatitis or diabetes mellitus);
  - hepatotoxicity;
  - encephalopathy (rare).
- **Elimination:** clearance appears to occur primarily via reticulo-endothelial system.

Corticosteroids (prednisolone, dexamethasone)
- **Use:** ALL (now predominantly dexamethasone), HD (prednisolone), HLH (dexamethasone), LCH (prednisolone).
- **Route of administration:** oral.
- **Toxicity:**
  - fluid retention;
  - weight gain;
  - hypertension;
  - hyperglycaemia;
  - hirsutism;
  - mood changes;
  - avascular necrosis (rare).
- **Elimination:** hepatic metabolism.

Dacarbazine
- **Use:** HD.
- **Route of administration:** IV infusion.
- **Toxicity:** extremely irritant to veins.
- **Elimination:** hepatic metabolism, renal excretion.

Imatinib
A tyrosine kinase (TK) inhibitor, specifically targeting the abnormal TK made by the *BCR/ABL* fusion gene. It is the prototype for a new class of molecularly-targeted drugs, and has already given rise to 2nd generation agents (e.g dasatinib).
- **Use:** chronic myeloid leukaemia.
- **Route of administration:** oral.
- **Toxicity:**
  - Myelosuppression;
  - *gastrointestinal symptoms* – nausea, vomiting, diarrhoea;
  - fluid retention;
  - bone pain.
- **Elimination:** metabolized by cytochrome P450-dependent enzymes, faecal excretion.

Procarbazine
- **Use:** brain tumours, HD.
- **Administration:** oral.
- **Toxicity:**
  - *neurotoxicity* – ataxia, headaches, paraesthesia;
  - alcohol intolerance;
  - monoamine oxidase inhibitor, therefore avoid tyramine-containing foods.
- **Elimination:** hepatic metabolism, renal excretion.

Paediatric radiotherapy

Radiotherapy is an effective modality of treatment that has a role in the management of many primary tumour sites. Radiotherapy is the therapeutic application of radiation. Usually the radiation source is a linear accelerator (Fig. 13.1), but radiation treatment can also be achieved by the administration of radioisotopes, e.g. MIBG in the treatment of neuroblastoma.

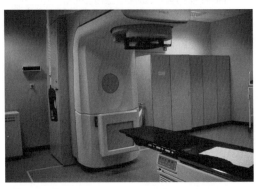

Fig. 13.1 Linear accelerator.

General principles of radiotherapy treatment

Radiotherapy works by causing cellular DNA damage from high energy X-rays. Tumour cells are either directly damaged or are rendered incapable of division, and therefore apoptose at the time the tumour cell attempts to divide.

- Allow margin around the tumour volume to take account of possible sub-clinical spread, e.g. as in the treatment of cerebral gliomas.
- Use conformal radiotherapy and, where there is a possibility of reducing normal tissue exposure to radiotherapy. Conformal radiotherapy usually employs 3D CT planning assisted techniques.
- In treatments aiming for cure, employ low daily doses of radiotherapy treatment over a 5–6-week period. This exploits the maximum therapeutic effect at minimum cost of long-term normal tissue damage, e.g. treatment of medulloblastoma.
- In palliative treatments, e.g. to help control pain from bone metastases single higher doses or lower number of treatments are effective. In this situation long-term affects are not a major consideration.
- Immobilization is necessary to ensure consistency of treatment position, e.g. the employment of custom-made plastic head shells for

the patients to lie in for head treatments (Fig. 13.2). Polystyrene mouldings can be used for other parts of the body and 'stocks' fixed to treatment table are helpful in the treatment of limbs. In some centres, vacuum devices to the trunk are used. Immobilization is particularly important for radical treatments. Radiotherapy units have a 'mould room' to assist with the issue of immobilization in preparation for radiotherapy.

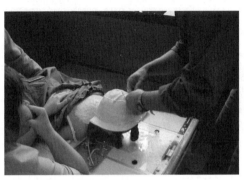

Fig. 13.2 Child having mould prepared for head immobilization shell.

- Radiotherapy treatments are planned with knowledge of the 'normal tissue tolerance' to radiotherapy of vital structures. If normal tissue tolerance is exceeded with radiotherapy dose damage to the function of these structures is threatened. For example if the dose to retina in radical treatments exceeds 45Gy visual function impairment is risked in the long term.
- In some circumstances it is acceptable to exceed normal tissue tolerance and, thus, anticipate toxicity if the consequences of avoiding the situation are thought to outweigh the loss of function risked, e.g. lens opacity risked if dose to lens exceeds 10Gy. This is deemed acceptable in the context of the treatment of medulloblastoma as priority is given to the adequate coverage of the meninges in the craniospinal component of the radiotherapy treatment. Cataracts can be subsequently managed surgically.
- There is a need to always take account of prior forms of treatment when planning radiotherapy as there may be enhanced toxicity risk from previous chemotherapy. For example, radiation after busulphan chemotherapy increases risk of lung toxicity occurring if lung is within subsequent radiotherapy field. If the patient has had prior radiotherapy to the same area careful consideration needs to be given to the tissue tolerance of the structures involved.

Special considerations in paediatric radiotherapy

- In children organs are developing and, therefore, more vulnerable than adults to the adverse normal tissue effects, e.g. premature epiphyseal end-plate fusion after bone irradiation resulting in shortened limb, cognitive loss/learning difficulties after cerebral irradiation.
- Normal tissue effects are greater in the younger child compared with the older child. There is a general reluctance to irradiate the brain in a child under the age of 3 years as significant neurocognitive disability is likely to result. In other parts of the body, there is concern about the effects of asymmetrical growth after radiotherapy in very young children, e.g. facial asymmetry after radiotherapy treatment for orbital rhabdomyosarcoma.
- In pre-pubertal boys it may not be possible to compensate for fertility loss as one would be able to do for adult males, since sperm banking is not feasible.
- Children require increased multidisciplinary team involvement (e.g. with play therapist) in preparation for radiotherapy treatments.
- If child is under 4 years of age it is likely that they will require daily anaesthetics for treatments, which ensure the child is still for treatment. This is necessary for assuring the accuracy of treatment delivery.
- Specialized staff and resources within the radiotherapy department are required to cater for the child's special needs compared with adults, this includes provision of play areas, specialized nursing staff, mould room staff, radiographers, anaesthetists, and doctor.
- Often the radiotherapy centre is a considerable distance from the child's home and, therefore, may need to provide family hostel accommodation.

Preparing child for radiotherapy treatment

- There must be discussion between members of the Paediatric Oncology/Clinical Oncology teams and child/parents. Informed consent should specifically include early (effects at the time of treatment) and late side effects predicted.
- Involvement with play therapist will help child in anticipating how treatment will feel (Fig. 13.3). Visits to the radiotherapy department and videos of other children having radiotherapy assist preparation.
- In planning steps parents are permitted to be in the room with the child, although this is not the case for treatment sessions. Having extra support and reassurance from a parent is extremely helpful in the early stages of planning.
- The child should be encouraged to bring in a favourite music/nursery rhyme or story CD to listen to whilst lying on the treatment couch.

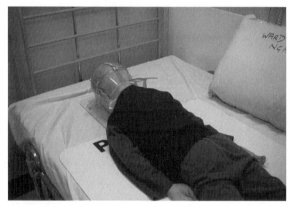

Fig. 13.3 Child practising lying still on ward in immobilization shell.

- Incentives, e.g. providing a personal radiotherapy diary that the child is encouraged to fill in and place stickers in after every treatment, are enthusiastically received by the younger child. At some centres patients requiring a shell for brain treatments are made a second shell (for play only) to keep and decorate as they wish (Fig. 13.4).

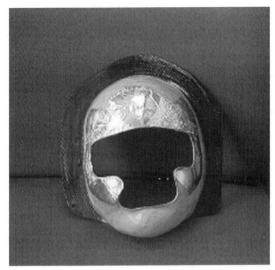

Fig. 13.4 Customized second shell with 'Power Rangers' for child to keep.

Acute side effects

It is important to discuss the expected side effects and prevent their occurrence if possible. In radical treatments (i.e. intention to cure), it is common to experience:

- **Tiredness:** usually improves within 1–2 weeks of finishing radiotherapy.
- **Nausea:** site of treatment influences the degree of anorexia or nausea experienced. Abdominal treatment increases risk. Prophylactic 5HT-3 inhibitors are effective.
- **Skin inflammation:** usually mild, tends to respond to simple aqueous cream, or if required hydrocortisone cream. Don't use creams containing metal ions.

Additional acute side effects are site dependent, e.g. in craniospinal radiotherapy:

- **Mild headache:** usually responds to paracetomol.
- **Diminished concentration:** results from the brain inflammation from the whole brain component of treatment. Tends to improve after 2 weeks of finishing treatment.
- **Hair loss:** occurs in first 2 weeks of treatment, grows back within 3–4 months of finishing radiotherapy unless chemotherapy delays regrowth.
- **Intermittent abdominal discomfort:** usually mild due to exit dose to intestines of spinal component of radiotherapy field.
- **Bone marrow suppression:** due to vertebral irradiation from spinal component of treatment. FBC should be monitored weekly as a precaution. Recovers within 1–2 months of radiotherapy. Rarely requires breaks in treatment or specific treatment such as platelet transfusion.

If the site of irradiation is the mediastinum, e.g. in the treatment of HD, acute side effects may occur such as:

- **Heartburn:** oesophagitis improved by antacids and proton pump inhibitors. Tends to recover after 2 weeks of completing radiotherapy.
- **Pneumonitis:** usually a dry cough, rarely a significant problem unless it is necessary to irradiate relatively large volume of lung. If it is thought appropriate to treat the pneumonitis, corticosteroids can be effective.

If the site of irradiation is the pelvis, e.g. in the treatment of prostatic rhabdomyosarcoma;

- **Urinary frequency/haematuria:** radiation cystitis, tends to improve after 2–3 weeks of finishing radiotherapy. Encourage good fluid intake and check that there is no evidence of UTI.
- **Bowel frequency/tenesmus:** proctitis secondary to radiotherapy. Resolves in 2–3 weeks after radiotherapy. If severe steroid enemas are helpful for proctitis symptoms.

Late effects of radiotherapy

- It is an important component of consent procedure to discuss with the child and parents any anticipated long-term effects of radiotherapy.
- In general, the younger a child is at the time of radiotherapy, the likelihood of significant late sequelae increases.

General categorization of late effects of paediatric radiotherapy

- Loss of normal **musculoskeletal growth**, e.g. vertebral radiotherapy in craniospinal radiotherapy will result in long-term truncal shortening. This is due to the effect of the radiotherapy on the vertebral epiphysis. In a child under 7 years this may make a difference of several centimetres in adult height. Use of growth charts and endocrinological assessments are important in follow-up.

- Loss of normal **endocrine function**, e.g. hypopituitarism after brain radiotherapy for medulloblastoma. This may well not manifest for 1–3 years until finishing radiotherapy and may lead to impaired growth hormone secretion (first and commonest), gonadotrophin deficiency, cortisol deficiency, secondary hypothyroidism.

- Loss of **cognitive potential**, for example, secondary to brain radiotherapy. The severity of anticipated cognitive impairment is inversely proportional to the age at treatment. The degree of cognitive effect is also proportional to the volume being treated and the dose applied. The effect of whole brain radiotherapy is greater than focal radiotherapy and the risk of cognitive impairment greater in a child under 7 years of age, rather than in an older child. Although children do not lose skills they have already acquired, it is in future education that the effects of their treatment can be seen. Children may require extra time and one-to-one assistance at school after formal statementing. The effects of the tumour prior to treatment, as well as the effects of neurosurgery and chemotherapy, can contribute to cognitive problems. It is helpful to undertake formal neuropsychological testing prior to and after radiotherapy treatment to characterize any deficits. The most common post radiation disability is in the area of complex new learning.

- **Cardiac disease**, for example, secondary to the combined affect of anthracycline therapy and radiotherapy in lymphoma treatment can occur. It is important in vulnerable patients to give lifestyle advice re diet and abstaining from smoking. Long term follow up in vulnerable patients can include regular ECG to monitor rhythm and ischaemic changes and echocardiograms if appropriate.

- **Secondary malignancy**, for example, in HD patients after radiotherapy, including breast tissue in adolescent females is a recognized risk. Breast cancer rates in such children are as high as 1 in 3, and thus formal follow-up programmes are in place starting several years after treatment for this purpose. Also meningiomas and secondary gliomas are recognized as a late tumour risk after cerebral irradiation, latent period is usually at least 10 years. Lung irradiation in childhood increases risk of later lung cancer in particular in individuals who later choose to smoke.

- In view of the recognized late effects of cancer treatments, children treated for cancer require follow-up in dedicated clinics. Within this structure, children/adults can have screening tailored to their individual needs aimed at maximizing their quality of life (Long-term follow-up 📖 pp.293–314).

Frequently asked questions

- **Will radiotherapy hurt?** No, it involves lying still on a firm bed for between 4 and 20min at a time. Children can't see or feel the treatment. Some children can smell a 'funny' smell that is actually caused by oxidation of the air.
- **Will my Mum be able to sit with me during radiotherapy?** It is not appropriate or acceptable to allow unnecessary irradiation of relatives. However, parents can provide encouragement and talk to their child over the intercom.
- **Will I get burns?** No, radiotherapy can cause mild skin inflammation, which normally settles well with aqueous creams. It is very unusual for skin complications to cause significant problems.

Chapter 14

Surgery

Surgical requirements and approach are usually best considered in a multidisciplinary meeting or tumour board.

This chapter refers to the usual practice in the UK, which is normally very similar to that in mainland Europe, but may differ from that advocated in North America.

Biopsy

Usually performed after full clinical and radiological work-up and staging:

- Tissue diagnosis is mandatory prior to treatment except in special/unusual circumstances, e.g. developing paraparesis in neuroblastoma. Tissue diagnosis is usually obtained by a biopsy of the primary site, but occasionally bone marrow aspiration/lumbar puncture/thoracocentesis/paracentesis may provide the diagnosis.
- Specimens should be fresh – **not in preservative** – and sent promptly to Pathology for appropriate histopathological processing, immunocytochemistry, cytogenetics, e.g. fluorescent *in situ* hybridization (FISH), assessment of ploidy, polymerase chain reaction (PCR).
- Procedures should be in place or arranged by a named pathologist, who facilitates processing, distribution to other laboratories and storage of the specimen.
- Adequate quantities of tumour material are required for a diagnosis and biological markers. The latter may influence treatment strategy.

Biopsy technique

- **Percutaneous:**
  - may need several 'passes' to obtain enough material;
  - allows embolization of track.
- **Radiological guidance:**
  - Ultrasound (US) (some necrotic tumours);
  - CT (e.g. lung, some bone).
- Laparoscopic/laparoscopic guidance.
- **Open:** may be a primary option or necessary when other methods have failed or are not available. Open biopsy usually provides a larger quantity of material, but often at the expense of increased morbidity. Sampling errors can be reduced by combining open biopsy with multiple needle biopsies.
- **Intact:** some biopsies, e.g. lymph nodes, should aim to provide an intact specimen, since often the final diagnosis will be influenced by the macroscopic or very low power magnification appearances of the architecture of the specimen.
- **Fine needle aspiration** (FNA): contrary to adult practice, FNA is rarely helpful in making the diagnosis or avoiding a formal biopsy. Complication rate of FNA is very low (<0.3%), but rises with the use of wider needles (up to 10% with Menghini needle). Complications include bleeding, viscus perforation, infection, and seeding of tumour along the track.

Vascular access

- Unpredictable, often urgent, timing dictated by chemotherapy protocols.
- Previously mainly open surgical procedure and part of the repertoire of most paediatric surgeons. Risk of injury to surrounding structures (vascular, neural, pleural, and lymphatic).
- Percutaneous US-guided insertion increasingly used. Radiologist involvement with the use of floppy wires may enable the use of much smaller veins, but time-consuming.
- Consider timely radiological assessment of patency of veins preoperatively in difficult situations, e.g. Doppler US, conventional, or MRI angiography.

Imaging

- Essential to inform potential resectability, either pre- or (usually) post-chemotherapy, e.g. MRI and angiography in liver tumours.
- Occasionally intra-operative imaging useful, e.g. US in liver resections.
- Multidisciplinary team (MDT) evaluation essential (oncologist, radiotherapist, surgeon, and radiologist).

Surgical aspects of specific sites/tumours

- Submandibular and cervical swellings: risk to the mandibular branch of the facial nerve, lingual and hypoglossal nerves. The accessory nerve is at risk in posterior cervical lymph node biopsies.
- 'Up front' surgery is rarely appropriate except when surgery alone is curative.
- Consider surgical management of secondaries, e.g. lung metastases in oesteosarcoma are often resectable.
- Involve other specialist disciplines as appropriate, e.g. hepatobiliary, ENT, orthopaedic, and gynaecological surgeons.
- Don't forget medical investigations, such as Mantoux, FBC with differential, platelet count, serology, CXR, and urinary catecholamines. In addition to sending the specimen for pathology, it is often important to send part for microbiological assessment (aerobic, anaerobic, mycobacterial, and fungal).

Preservation of gonadal function

Knowledge about and the techniques available for fertility preservation are advancing quickly. Although gonadal tissue preservation is still considered a research procedure, clinical practice, and guidelines are likely to evolve rapidly. Therefore, formal discussion, and consideration of gonadal tissue harvesting and cryopreservation may be required at the time of initial diagnosis of malignancy.

Treatment of complications of the tumour or its treatment

- Persistent abdominal ascites and pleural effusions. Simple drainage, consideration of valved shunt, e.g. Denver shunts.
- Treatment of GI, pelviureteric, ureteric, or urethral obstruction.

- Surgical management of haemorrhagic cystitis is controversial, but may include:
  - insertion of wide-bore suprapubic bladder catheter to enable high-flow bladder irrigation;
  - cystotomy and evacuation of clot.

Thoracic/thoracic wall tumours
- Rib resection usually leads to scoliosis.
- Thoracic and mediastinal tumours: mediastinoscopy rarely useful. Therefore, these tumours are usually approached by thoracotomy ± thoracoscopy, and occasionally sternal split.

Extra-gonadal germ cell tumours
Sacrococcygeal teratomas very rarely contain malignant tissue at birth, but frequency of malignancy rises rapidly to over 66% by 6 months. Therefore early, complete excision recommended with coccygectomy.

Rhabdomyosarcoma
Position the biopsy so that the track can be excised when definitive surgery is undertaken. It is important to remove these tumours with clear margins, which can be difficult, to avoid 'mutilating' surgery. For example, partial cystectomy may leave a low volume bladder reservoir.

Central nervous system tumours
- Where complete excision is technically impossible, surgery to debulk the tumour may influence prognosis.
- CSF diversion is often required after posterior fossa surgery (20–40% of cases; see General approaches to suspected cancer, initial diagnosis of brain tumours, Brain tumour: initial management 📖 pp.58–59).

Haemopoietic stem cell transplantation

Aims of haemopoietic stem cell transplantation

Haemopoietic stem cell transplantation (HSCT) was first used successfully in 1968 to treat a child with severe combined immunodeficiency, and developed further as a means of delivering high dose chemoradiotherapy to patients with advanced or resistant leukaemia. As the number of transplants performed annually has risen greatly (estimated at 50,000–60,000 in 2006, including nearly 20,000 allogeneic) and their safety has increased, the potential aims of HSCTs have diversified and may include:

- Rescue from high dose chemoradiotherapy given for cytotoxic effect in malignant disease, with additional benefit from graft-versus-leukaemia (GvL) or other graft-versus-malignancy effect.
- Provision of normal stem cells to replace or supplement diseased cells in serious disorders of:
  - haemopoietic system (correction of non-malignant haematological illness);
  - immune system (correction of immunodeficiency);
  - metabolic/enzymatic capacity (partial or complete correction of inborn errors of metabolism).
- Re-education of autologous stem/T cells (treatment of autoimmune disease).

Definitions

Types of haemopoietic stem cell transplantation

- **Autologous:** the patient's own haemopoeitic stem cells (HSCs) are harvested prior to delivery of intensive myeloablative 'conditioning' treatment, which is then followed by HSC reinfusion; nearly all conditioning protocols are scheduled over several days, necessitating cryopreservation of HSCs in liquid nitrogen, with subsequent thawing prior to reinfusion
- **Allogeneic:** HSCs from another individual (donor) are harvested and infused into the recipient on completion of conditioning therapy

Allogeneic transplants classification

Donor type

Related donors (RDs)

- **Syngeneic (identical twin):** HLA-identical by definition, but rarely available; much lower risk of graft-versus-host disease (GvHD), but this may be disadvantageous in certain high risk leukaemias where GvL effect is important
- **HLA-identical sibling:** genotypically HLA-matched; however, only ~25–30% of patients in UK have an HLA-identical sibling donor.
- **Phenotypically HLA-matched relative** (e.g. parent, aunt, or uncle, cousin): commoner in communities with higher frequency of consanguineous marriage, rare (but not unknown) in other populations.
- **Haploidentical (haplo) parent** (or less frequently sibling): increasing acceptability of this donor choice in high-risk patients (i.e. where other treatment options are unavailable or unsatisfactory) has widened donor availability (i.e. fewer patients unable to undergo HSCT due to lack of donor).
- **Other mismatched relative:** e.g. mismatched at 1 or 2 HLA antigens.

Unrelated donors (URDs)

- HLA-matched (matched unrelated donors, MUDs).
- HLA-mismatched (mismatched unrelated donors, MMUDs).
- Currently >12 million potential URDs registered on Bone Marrow Donor Panels (e.g. Anthony Nolan Bone Marrow Trust [ANBMT]).

Donors other than HLA-identical (or syngeneic) siblings are collectively regarded as *alternative donors*.

Stem cell source

- Bone marrow (BM).
- Peripheral blood stem cells (PBSC).
- Umbilical cord blood (UCB).

NB. BM or PBSC may be harvested for either autologous or allogeneic HSCT, whilst UCB is used only for allogeneic transplant (except for exceedingly rare case reports).

Conditioning regimen

- **Myeloablative:** utilizes steep dose–response relationship of chemo-therapy +/− radiotherapy to achieve high cytotoxicity against malignant cells, but at cost of considerable haemopoietic and systemic toxicity. It is also used in many non-malignant conditions, especially those with high rejection risk.
- **Non-myeloablative:** uses less intensive conditioning with aims of:
  - limiting regimen-related toxicity (RRT) by reducing direct toxicity and limiting inflammatory cytokine release; hence
  - diminishing likely severity of acute GvHD; but
  - retaining sufficient immunosuppressive action to prevent graft rejection and allow stable engraftment; thereby
  - allowing opportunity for graft-versus-malignancy effect.

Sometimes categorized (relatively arbitrarily) as:
- Reduced intensity conditioning (RIC); or
- Minimal intensity conditioning (MIC).

Indications for haemopoietic stem cell transplantation

The lists of indications below reflect current UK practice (2008), but are likely to evolve further over the next few years due to changes in survival rates after non-HSCT strategies and after HSCT.

Autologous haemopoietic stem cell transplantation

- **Non-Hodgkin lymphoma (NHL):**
  - relapsed Burkitt NHL;
  - relapsed diffuse large cell NHL;
  - **Hodgkin disease (HD):** relapsed or refractory HD (adolescents).
- **High risk solid tumours:**
  - Stage 4 (or other high risk) neuroblastoma;
  - high risk Ewing's sarcoma;
  - high risk or relapsed medulloblastoma;
  - selected patients with relapsed or refractory –
    - *Wilms' tumour* – usually performed in the context of a clinical trial;
    - *germ cell tumour* – usually performed in the context of a clinical trial.
- Selected autoimmune diseases [e.g. juvenile idiopathic arthritis (JIA)].

Allogeneic haemopoietic stem cell transplantation

Haematological malignancy

- **Acute leukaemia:**
  - acute lymphoblastic leukaemia (ALL):
    - high risk ALL in 1st complete remission (CR);
    - high- and intermediate-risk relapsed ALL in 2nd CR;
    - ALL in ≥3rd CR;
  - acute myeloid leukaemia (AML):
    - refractory AML (>2 courses to achieve remission) in 1st CR;
    - AML in 2nd CR (autologous HSCT may be appropriate in some patients with relapse >1 year from initial diagnosis).
- Chronic myeloid leukaemia (CML).
- Juvenile myelomonocytic leukaemia (JMML).
- Myelodysplasia (MDS) (selected patients).
- NHL:
  - relapsed anaplastic large-cell lymphoma (ALCL);
  - relapsed T-cell lymphoblastic NHL.
- Multiply relapsed HD (selected patients).

Non-malignant conditions

- Bone marrow failure (including inherited monocytopenias; see Bone marrow failure 📖 pp.361–378):
  - severe aplastic anaemia (SAA);
  - Fanconi anaemia (FA);
  - other constitutional bone marrow failure syndromes:
    - dyskeratosis congenita (DKC);
    - congenital amegakaryocytic thrombocytopenia (CAMT);
    - Schwachman-Diamond syndrome (SDS);
    - Diamond-Blackfan anaemia (DBA);
  - Kostmann syndrome.
- Haemoglobinopathy:
  - *thalassaemia* – selected patients;
  - *sickle cell disease* – selected patients.
- Primary immunodeficiency:
  - severe combined immunodeficiency (SCID);
  - Wiskott-Aldrich syndrome (WAS);
  - X-linked lymphoproliferative disease (XLP).
- Haemophagocytic syndromes.
- Osteopetrosis.
- Selected metabolic/storage diseases:
  - Hurler's disease (type 1H mucopolysaccharidosis) if <2 years age;
  - adrenoleucodystrophy (ALD) if performed before neurological impairment evident;
  - selected other rare, inborn errors of metabolism in presymptomatic children, depending on patient's age, condition, and availability (or not) of other therapy (especially enzyme replacement treatment).

Preparation for haemopoietic stem cell transplantation

Decision to perform haemopoietic stem cell transplantation
Sometimes straightforward, especially if patient has clear indication for HSCT (see Indications for haemopoietic stem cell transplantation 📖 p.168), is otherwise medically fit and has suitably matched donor, but:
- Often much more complex, particularly when other treatment options available [e.g. further chemotherapy for acute leukaemia, imatinib for CML, granulocyte colony stimulating factor (G-CSF) for Kostmann syndrome], presence of significant prior morbidity (e.g. cardiac or renal toxicity from previous treatment), or difficulty in identifying well matched donor.
- Timing of HSCT may be an important issue, e.g. in FA with slowly progressive bone marrow failure.
- Discussion and decision is facilitated by careful evaluation by multidisciplinary team (including experienced nurse and social worker) with appropriate consideration of what the aim of HSCT is in each individual patient.
- Active involvement of family and patient is vital.
- Ultimately depends on the views of the clinical team and family regarding the balance of:
  - *Potential benefits of HSCT* –
    - cure or control of disease that is otherwise unlikely/less likely to be cured by alternative treatment;
    - usually without need for protracted further treatment;
  - *risks of HSCT* – greater risk of early or late treatment-related morbidity or even mortality.

Selection of donor and stem cell source
Selection of donor
Indication for HSCT
Some diseases/disease stages (e.g. previously untreated SAA, thalassaemia) represent an indication for HSCT, but only if a HLA-identical sibling donor is available, whereas others (e.g. relapsed ALL) are considered suitable for HSCT with any appropriately matched (or even mismatched) donor (i.e. including alternative donors). This distinction may become much less clear as the results of alternative donor HSCT improve.

If more than one donor available, final donor choice influenced by donor characteristics:
- **HLA-type:**
  - Historically performed by serological detection of expressed antigens (denoted as, e.g. HLA-A), but now usually by DNA-based typing of HLA gene sequences (denoted as, e.g. HLA-A*) – at allele level where required.
  - Request both:
    - *Class I typing* – usually performed at 'allele group' level (corresponding to serologically detected antigens), e.g. HLA*02.

Some donor registries now require allele level typing of patients (e.g. HLA-A*0201), but this may reduce the number of matched donors available.
- *Class II typing* – DNA-based, usually, at allele level, i.e. DRB1*, DQB1* +/– DPB1*.
- Aim for 10/10 match (based on HLA-A,* B*, Cw* 'allele groups' and allele level typing for DRB1*, DQB1*) in most scenarios, but full 12/12 allele level match (based on HLA-A*, B*, Cw*, DRB1*, DQB1*, plus DPB1*) desirable for some indications (e.g. SAA, immunodeficiency).
- DRB1* mismatches are avoided if at all possible.
- Increasing use of 9/10 matched URD HSCTs with improving results.
- URD UCB donor units usually selected on basis of HLA-A, B, and HLA-DRB1* – no convincing evidence, yet that more detailed typing improves outcome in UCB HSCT.
- Consider the combination of HLA type, donor type and stem cell source (in descending order of preference):
  - HLA-identical sibling, or phenotypically HLA-matched RD (i.e. one haplotype is genotypically identical, but other is not), or HLA-identical RD UCB with adequate nucleated cell dose.
  - 10/10 HLA-matched URD, or 6/6 HLA-matched URD UCB with adequate nucleated cell dose.
  - 9/10 HLA-matched URD, or 5/6 HLA-matched RD, or ≥4/6 URD UCB with adequate nucleated cell dose.
  - 8/10 HLA-matched URD or haploidentical RD.

N.B. Options 3 and 4 are only used in poor risk patients with no feasible alternative treatment options:
- **Age:** in general, young adults preferred, ideally ≤40 years; in paediatric HLA-identical sibling HSCT, most siblings likely to be <18 years, in which case the oldest donor usually preferable.
- **Sex:** male usually preferred.
- **CMV status:** aim to match donor CMV serostatus to patient (i.e. CMV seropositive donor for CMV seropositive recipient, seronegative donor for seronegative patient).
- **ABO blood group:** aim for a match in heavily pre-transfused recipient to reduce risk of immune-mediated haemolysis.
- **Medical fitness:** ideally should be assessed by experienced clinician independent of HSCT team.

Choice of stem cell source
- **HLA-identical sibling:** BM preferred to PBSC in paediatric donors (to avoid exposing a healthy child to G-CSF).*
- **HLA-matched URD:** no preference between BM and PBSC.*
- **HLA-mismatched URD/RD:** PBSC preferred to BM (allows higher CD34 +ve cell dose).

*NB.** Adult RDs and URDs should be allowed a free choice between BM and PBSC donation after independent counselling.

Patient evaluation

History
- Diagnosis: stage, e.g. ALL in CR2.
- Previous treatment: especially radiotherapy to critical organs/tissues (e.g. brain, lungs), cumulative dose of anthracyclines and alkylating agents.
- Known organ/tissue damage from disease/treatment.
- Previous infections: especially in organs at risk of conditioning toxicity and/or GvHD (e.g. lungs, bowel).
- Transfusion history.
- Family history.
- Psychosocial status.
- School progress.
- Child (age appropriate) and family understanding of HSCT. Why is it being performed, what will it involve, what may happen?

Examination
- Evidence of active disease or its sequelae.
- Evidence of complications of disease or treatment.
- Evidence of infection or its sequelae.
- Careful systematic clinical examination, including neurological.
- Blood pressure.
- Dental examination (leave enough time before HSCT to permit dental procedures if required, e.g. extractions of carious teeth to reduce risk of infection during transplant).
- Height, weight.

Investigation
- Disease staging (e.g. BM aspirate/biopsy for leukaemia, CT scan/other imaging for lymphoma/other solid tumours).
- **Baseline bloods:**
  - FBC, coagulation profile;
  - biochemical profile, including liver function tests (LFTs), magnesium;
  - blood group;
  - sample for subsequent chimerism analysis.
- **Other baseline tests:**
  - *microbiological screening* – surface swabs for methicillin-resistant *Staphylococcus aureus* (MRSA), faeces for vancomycin-resistant enterococcus (VRE);
  - *chest X-ray;*
  - ?*thyroid function tests* – depending on previous therapy and planned conditioning treatment;
  - ?*echocardiogram* – depending on previous therapy and planned conditioning treatment;
  - ?*Pulmonary function tests* – depending on previous therapy and planned conditioning treatment;
  - ?*Glomerular filtration rate* – depending on previous therapy and planned conditioning treatment;
  - Urinalysis.

- **Evidence of infection (may be subclinical):**
  - *viral (and other) serology* – CMV, HSV, EBV, VZV, HIV, hepatitis B and C, toxoplasmosis;
  - microbiology/virology cultures/sensitive detection assays (e.g. PCR) as clinically indicated;
  - imaging as clinically indicated (e.g. high resolution CT chest if previous fungal pneumonia).

Potential donor evaluation

Related donors

- **Age-appropriate clinical assessment required:** ideally performed by a clinician independent of the transplant team (especially important for child donors).
- Should include:
  - assessment of donor's age-appropriate understanding of:
    - reason for HSCT;
    - what the harvest procedure involves;
    - potential HSCT outcomes for the recipient.
  - evaluation of medical and psychological fitness to donate.
- In UK, children who are not Gillick competent and adults who the lack capacity to consent for harvest procedure also require assessment by an Accredited Assessor [appointed by the Human Tissue Authority (HTA)] to ensure that donation is considered to be in their 'best interests'.
- Full medical/paediatric history to ensure no contra-indications to procedure (and to general anaesthetic in marrow donors). Should also include details of factors that may complicate the transplant:
  - previous blood product transfusions;
  - recent travel (infection risk);
  - pregnancy history in female donors.
- Full clinical examination.
- Investigation:
  - FBC, coagulation profile.
  - Biochemical profile.
  - Blood group.
  - Thyroid function tests (adult donors).
  - *Viral (and other) serology* – CMV, HSV, EBV, VZV, HIV, hepatitis B and C, toxoplasmosis (potentially blood-borne infections); positive hepatitis or HIV serology will usually contraindicate use of this donor in UK (may be necessary to use hepatitis seropositive donors in countries where hepatitis B and/or C are common, since it may be difficult to find a negative donor, but only after careful assessment of infectivity risk and of alternative donors or approaches).
  - Blood sample for subsequent chimerism analysis.
  - Chest X-ray (adult donors).
  - ECG (as clinically indicated in adult donors).
- Consent for harvest procedure: should be obtained by clinician independent of transplant team (ideally the same clinician who has evaluated the donor).

Unrelated donors
- Blood and marrow donor registries (e.g. ANBMT) arrange for detailed information provision and counselling to all potential URDs, followed by full clinical evaluation following above general principles.
- URDs are given non-directive information that they have a free choice to donate either BM or PBSC, and advised of the possibility of a request for a second donation for the same patient.
- Strict anonymity is maintained.
- After 2 years post-HSCT, a minority of BM donor registries still permit identified contact between URD and recipient, providing both parties agree, but most registries have now stopped this practice.

All donors

It is mandatory for the transplant team to be informed that donor has been given medical and virological 'clearance' to donate *before* the recipient starts conditioning treatment.

Stem cell harvest

Bone marrow harvest

Marrow is harvested under general anaesthesia by performing multiple aspirates from several bone puncture sites on each posterior iliac crest (usually accessed by one skin puncture site per side). Other bones (e.g. sternum) are used less commonly. A *maximum* of 30% blood volume is collected and less if this is sufficient to achieve the required cell dose.

Peripheral blood stem cell harvest

PBSC are harvested using leukopheresis techniques, usually after stem cell mobilization with chemotherapy (autologous harvest) or G-CSF (allogeneic harvest). Peripheral blood CD34 +ve cell count measured to guide optimum timing of PBSC harvest (rarely worth starting harvest until circulating CD34 count >20/µl). The use of G-CSF to stimulate the appearance of haemopoietic stem cells in allogeneic PB harvests allows collection of large stem cell (CD34 +ve) doses, which maximizes the likelihood of engraftment.

Umbilical cord blood harvest

UCB is harvested from the placenta at the time of birth and then cryopreserved for future use.

All harvests

After the harvest, cell dose is measured as NCC and CD34 +ve cell count, and quantified per kg of recipient weight. CD3 +ve and CD19 +ve counts are also often measured. NCC of first marrow bag is sometimes measured during adult BM harvest (especially when a large cell dose is desired) to guide the final volume harvested. Likewise, CD34 +ve cell count collected on 1st day of PBSC harvest guides decision about whether a 2nd day of collection is needed.

Target doses are:

Allogeneic
- **BMT (RD or URD):** NCC $\geq 2 \times 10^8$/kg (ideally ~4×10^8/kg), CD34 +ve cells $\geq 2 \times 10^6$/kg (ideally ~4×10^6/kg).
- **PBSCT:** CD34 +ve cells $\geq 2 \times 10^6$/kg (ideally ~5×10^6/kg).

- **Haplo PBSCT:** CD34+ cells $\geq 10 \times 10^6$/kg.
- **UCBT:** NCC $\geq 1.7 \times 10^7$/kg, CD34 +ve cells $\geq 1.5 \times 10^6$/kg.

Lower doses are accepted in some situations, whilst higher doses are preferred in mismatched allogeneic HSCTs, UCBTs (especially mismatched) and when there is particular concern about a higher risk of graft rejection or failure.

Autologous
- **BMT:** NCC $\geq 2 \times 10^8$/kg.
- **PBSCT:** CD34 +ve $\geq 2 \times 10^6$/kg.

As in allogeneic HSCT, lower doses may be accepted in some situations.

Conditioning treatment

- **Myeloablative conditioning:** classical (and still the most commonly used) regimens are CyTBI and BuCy, incorporating cyclophosphamide (Cy) given with either total body irradiation (TBI) or busulfan (Bu), respectively. Increasingly, other high-dose cytotoxic drugs, most commonly alkylating agents, especially melphalan (Mel), are used for alternative or additional myeloablative effect (e.g. BuMel, BuCyMel).
- **Non-myeloablative:** these regimens were developed to harness the GvL effect following observation of the efficacy of donor lymphocyte infusions (DLI), which may control leukaemia (especially CML) even in the absence of conventional cytotoxic therapy. The detailed mechanisms remain unclear, but GvL following DLI is mediated, at least in part, by allogeneic T cells, although GvL may occur even in the absence of overt GvHD. Most non-myeloablative regimens typically incorporate fludarabine in combination with low dose TBI or chemotherapy (e.g. melphalan or cyclophosphamide).
- **Immunosuppression:** intense immunosuppression is a vital component of conditioning for many alternative donor HSCTs to reduce the otherwise unacceptably high risk of graft rejection (e.g. MMUD or haplo RD HSCT). It is often provided by fludarabine and/or pre-transplant serotherapy (see Preparation for haemopoietic stem cell transplantation, Graft versus host disease prophylaxis 📖 p.176).

The type and intensity of conditioning regimen chosen for any given patient depends on several factors including:
- **Underlying disease:**
  - non-radiotherapy regimens usually employed for non-malignant diseases to reduce late adverse effects (especially secondary malignancy);
  - some diagnoses are conditioned with disease-specific regimens, e.g. low dose conditioning protocol in FA to prevent severe RRT.
- **Patient age:** radiotherapy avoided in infants (<2 years age), so chemotherapy-only conditioning used.
- **Nature and timing of prior treatment** (especially a previous HSCT):
  - chemotherapy-only conditioning used if TBI given during 1st HSCT;
  - non-myeloablative conditioning often used for 2nd HSCTs, especially if performed <12 months after 1st transplant.

- **Pre-transplant medical status:** non-myeloablative conditioning may be used in children in a poor medical condition, especially if a graft versus malignancy effect is anticipated to play a realistic role in achieving cure.
- **Indication for and type of HSCT:** more intensive conditioning, especially with immunosuppression, indicated for conditions or HSCTs with higher risk of graft failure.
- **Degree of HLA matching:** increased immunosuppression indicated in mismatched HSCTs.

Graft versus host disease prophylaxis

GvHD is a major cause of morbidity and mortality in allogeneic HSCT. The best way of reducing the risk or severity of GvHD is to use a well-matched donor, ideally an HLA-identical sibling donor. However, the use of alternative donors, especially mismatched RDs, and matched or mismatched URDs, has greatly increased the pool of available donors. Although donors can be found for most children in urgent need of a transplant, the increasing use of such alternative donors requires effective GvHD prophylaxis to reduce the risk of severe acute or disabling chronic GvHD. In addition, it is becoming very important to seek the optimal balance of GvHD and GvL in the context of HSCT for malignancy, where some degree of a GvL or other graft-versus-malignancy effect is important.

The three main methods used to achieve GvHD prophylaxis are:

Pre- and peri-HSCT serotherapy

Acute GvHD is caused by donor T lymphocytes reacting against antigenically different host tissues. Serotherapy involves the use of antibodies directed against these lymphocytes to achieve T-cell depletion. The antibodies used most commonly are:

- **Anti-thymocyte globulin** (ATG): polyclonal antibody made by injecting rabbits with human T lymphocytes.
- **CAMPATH:** a family of monoclonal antibodies directed against the CDw52 antigen (expressed on a wide range of B and T lymphocytes and monocytes).

In vivo ATG or CAMPATH serotherapy is usually given as daily intravenous infusions for 3–5 consecutive doses before (occasionally before and after – 'across the graft') HSCT. Both antibodies have long half-lives of up to 2–3 weeks and act on both host (thereby reducing risk of graft rejection) and donor (reducing GvHD) lymphocytes. Both ATG and CAMPATH may cause significant early reactions (fever, rash, cardiovascular, respiratory or gastrointestinal symptoms/signs), especially after the first dose, and/or later side effects (prolonged lymphopenia → risk of serious viral infections).

In vitro T-cell depletion

BM and PBSC harvests may be depleted of T cells *in vitro* by several physical or immunological techniques. Historically, physical methods have included sheep red blood cell rosetting, counterflow centrifugal elutriation, and fractionation on a density gradient.

Immunological techniques have included:

- Antibody-mediated purging, e.g. using CAMPATH 1M.
- Immunomagnetic positive selection, e.g. of CD34 +ve cells to give a stem cell population.
- Immunomagnetic negative selection, e.g. of CD3 +ve and CD19 +ve cells to remove T and B cells, whilst sparing haematopoietic precursor cells to a greater degree, thereby improving the speed and quality of early engraftment.

Post-HSCT immunosuppression

Many immunosuppressive drugs may be used, including ciclosporin A, methotrexate, tacrolimus, steroids, and mycophenolate mofetil (MMF).

The commonest immunosuppressive drug used post-HSCT has been ciclosporin, sometimes with the addition of short course methotrexate (3–4 IV boluses, low dose – typically 10–15mg/m^2/dose, given during first 6–18 days post-HSCT). IV ciclosporin is converted to oral administration (usually at approximately twice the IV dose) once mucositis has resolved. Dose adjustments are guided by trough blood levels. The duration of ciclosporin varies from 1–12 months (occasionally longer), depending on:

- Type of HSCT and, hence, the risk of GvHD (continued for longer when risk is higher).
- Indication for HSCT (withdrawn earlier in high-risk malignancies).
- Occurrence (or not) of acute or chronic GvHD (continued for longer).

Tacrolimus is increasingly used as an alternative to ciclosporin. In addition to the risks of immunosuppression, both ciclosporin and tacrolimus have many other potentially serious side effects, including nephrotoxicity (glomerular impairment, hypomagnesaemia), hypertension, neurotoxicity (including tremor, visual disturbance, seizures, and encephalopathy – commoner after ciclosporin) and impaired glucose homeostasis. Both, but especially ciclosporin, also commonly cause gum hypertrophy and hypertrichosis.

Corticosteroids, especially methylprednisolone, are used in many protocols (especially for UCB transplants), whilst MMF is increasingly used (often with ciclosporin).

Anti-infective prophylaxis

Potentially fatal bacterial, viral and fungal infections are frequent and significant complications of HSCT. The risk is proportional to the duration and severity of immunosuppression (both neutropenia and lymphopenia) post-transplant. Allogeneic HSCTs are associated with greater risk than autologous procedures. As well as physical isolation for recipients of allogeneic HSCTs, who are usually nursed in a HEPA (high efficiency particulate air) filtered cubicle with a restricted number of visitors and careful hand washing by healthcare workers and visitors, prophylactic anti-infective agents are used to decrease the risk of infection. Prophylactic regimens vary between units, but usually include:

Pneumocystis jiroveci pneumonia

Cotrimoxazole prophylaxis against *Pneumocystis jiroveci* (previously called *Pneumocystis carinii*) pneumonia is either started on admission for HSCT or (in some units) introduced at the time of engraftment (to avoid possibility of cotrimoxazole-induced delay in engraftment), and then continued until all immunosuppression is stopped and/or there is evidence of adequate immune reconstitution.

Fungal infections

Antifungal prophylaxis may be initiated with:

- **Azoles:**
  - Early trials found that fluconazole reduced invasive *Candida* infections post-HSCT, but few paediatric HSCT units use it for prophylaxis now in view of its poor activity against the increasing proportion of non-albicans *Candida* (especially *C. glabrata* and *C. krusei*), and lack of protection against *Aspergillus* and other filamentous mould infections.
  - Itraconazole offers protection against *Candida* and other yeasts, and against *Aspergillus* and some other filamentous fungi, but many children are intolerant of the oral preparation, whilst its use is complicated by a long half-life, drug interactions (e.g. leading to an increase in ciclosporin levels), and toxicity (especially abnormal liver function tests).
  - Voriconazole has a broad spectrum of activity against most fungi (except *Mucor*) and is increasingly used for prophylaxis, although it shares the drug interactions and toxicity of itraconazole (and may also cause visual disturbances), it is usually better tolerated.
- **Amphotericin** (used less commonly than azoles for prophylaxis):
  - Active against nearly all fungi, including *Mucor*.
  - Conventional amphotericin B is seldom used for prophylaxis due to its considerable toxicity (infusion-related reactions, glomerular and tubular nephrotoxicity).
  - Liposomal amphotericin preparations (e.g. AmBisome) have reduced toxicity compared to the conventional preparation.
- **Caspofungin:** rarely used for prophylaxis due to limited experience, but has fewer side-effects than azoles or amphotericin, and offers protection against *Candida* and *Aspergillus* (but not rarer organisms including *Fusarium* and *Mucor*).

Viral infections

Antiviral prophylaxis usually includes:

- **Aciclovir:** provides protection against cytomegalovirus (CMV), herpes simplex virus (HSV) and varicella/herpes zoster virus (VZV/HZV)
- **Intravenous immunoglobulin** (IVIg): theoretically offers protection against many common viruses that may potentially cause severe infections post-HSCT (including CMV, adenovirus, herpes viruses and respiratory viruses), although many HSCT units use IVIg prophylaxis (especially in children at high risk of viral infection or reactivation), there is no convincing evidence that IVIg reduces infectious morbidity or survival, and a lack of consensus about optimal dosing schedules. Currently, the *routine* use of post-HSCT prophylactic IVIg is not recommended by the UK Department of Health Clinical Guidelines for Immunoglobulin Use.

- **Blood product transfusion strategies:** traditionally CMV antibody-negative recipients have been transfused with CMV-negative blood products. However, all blood products transfused in the UK are now leucodepleted, which greatly reduces the risk of CMV transmission, but many HSCT units still prefer to use blood products from CMV-negative donors.

Gut decontamination

Gut decontamination (e.g. with ciprofloxacin and metronidazole) is commonly, but not universally employed. As well as reducing the risk of potentially life-threatening gut-derived Gram –ve bacterial sepsis, it may reduce the frequency and severity of acute GvHD by reducing endotoxin production (and, hence, cytokine release) associated with translocation of gastrointestinal bacteria.

Complications

Although the complications of HSCT may be helpfully classified according to their timing and cause, there may be considerable variability in the time of onset (e.g. a clinical picture resembling acute GvHD may occur after day +100) and interaction between more than one potential cause (e.g. early pulmonary toxicity may be due to infection, immune-mediated 'inflammatory' pneumonitis or chemotherapy/radiotherapy toxicity, and two or more of these may contribute to the clinical picture in any individual patient).

Timing

- **Early:** generally related to consequences of RRT and/or acute GvHD.
- **Late:** generally related to later onset RRT and/or chronic GvHD.
- The distinction between early and late is somewhat arbitrary (more so in HSCT than after non-HSCT treatment), but most early complications will develop within the first 100 days post-transplant, whilst the onset of most late complications occurs ≥6–12 months post-HSCT (with a 'grey period' in between where both early and late complications may be seen).

Cause

- **RRT:** due to the direct effects of chemotherapy, radiotherapy, and/or serotherapy, or the secondary consequences of these (e.g. infection due to chemotherapy-induced neutropenia).
- **Immune-mediated complications:** GvHD (both acute and chronic), other inflammatory events often occurring in tandem with GvHD (e.g. pneumonitis), other immune-mediated events (e.g. haematological cytopenias).
- **Other drug toxicity:** particularly common in HSCT recipients due to the large number of potentially toxic drugs required for their post-transplant supportive care (especially anti-infective and immunosuppressive agents).

The range of complications that may occur after HSCT is very wide, and their nature varied (see Table 15.1). Many early (e.g. infection, emesis, mucositis) and late (e.g. cataracts, endocrinopathy) post-HSCT complications are common in children treated for malignancy without HSCT and are described elsewhere (Oncological emergencies 📖 pp.93–128, Other aspects of supportive care 📖 pp.253–292, Long-term follow-up 📖 pp.293–314). Only those aspects of toxicity that are commoner, more serious, or more specifically related to HSCT are described in Table 15.1 (indicated with asterisks).

Table 15.1 Timing and nature of complications of HSCT

Early	Early or late	Late
Alopecia	Infection	Impaired quality of life
Emesis*	Immune-mediated	Secondary malignancy
Infection*	haematological	Immune-mediated haemato-
Mucositis*	cytopenias*	logical cytopenias*
Organ toxicity	Organ toxicity	Immunological*
• Neurological	• CNS	Chronic GVHD and sequelae*
(central nervous	• Cardiac	Visual
system, CNS)*	• Pulmonary	Auditory
• Cardiac*	• Hepatic	Craniofacial/dental
• Pulmonary*	• Renal	Oral
• Gastrointestinal*	GvHD (acute or	Gonadal/reproductive
• Hepatic (especially	chronic)*	Neurological
veno-occlusive	Endocrine	Neuropsychological
disease)*		Cardiovascular
• Renal*		Respiratory
• Haemorrhagic cystitis*		Renal
Acute GvHD*		Lower urinary tract
		Musculoskeletal
		Skin

* Described in the text. Those complications not marked by an asterisk are described elsewhere (Other aspects of supportive care 📖 pp.253–290, Long-term follow-up 📖 pp.293–212, Chemotherapy 📖 pp.131–147).

Infection

Although the major types, sites, and causes of infection in HSCT patients have much in common with those seen in other immunosupressed patients (who have not undergone HSCT; Infection 📖 pp.207–230), viral and fungal infections are proportionately commoner and more serious. The spectrum of disease caused by infection in recipients of HSCT is very wide and frequently unexpected, necessitating an aggressive approach to investigation, often involving invasive procedures to obtain fluid or tissue samples for microbiological, virological, or histological diagnosis.

In allogeneic HSCT, three post-transplant phases have been identified, each with characteristic patterns of infection (Table 15.2):

Table 15.2 Patterns of infection after HSCT

	Aplastic (pre-engraftment) phase	Early post-engraftment phase	Late post-engraftment phase
Timing (approximate)	0 – engraftment (typically by day +30)	day +30–+100	after day +100
Major determinants of immunosuppression	Neutropenia (note role of mucositis in allowing bacterial entry)	Immunosuppression 2° to both HSCT and treatment of acute GvHD	Immunosuppression 2° to chronic GvHD and its treatment
Commoner infections	Bacterial Fungal (especially *Aspergillus*) HSV	Viral (especially CMV) Fungal	Encapsulated bacterial Viral (VZV, late CMV)

However, the increasing use of non-myeloablative HSCT has reduced the duration and severity of neutropenia, albeit often at the cost of increased immunosuppression. Likewise, the increasing use of mismatched (especially haploidentical) donors has increased the duration and severity of immunosuppression, and led to an increase in the frequency of viral infections (e.g. adenoviral) and the risk period (exemplified by an increase in late CMV infection).

Specific infections are described elsewhere (Infection 📖 pp.207–230). It is important to note that the range of micro-organisms that may cause disease in an extremely immunosuppressed HSCT recipient is very wide, and that even organisms usually regarded as having low or no virulence may cause severe infection in these patients.

⚠ It is vital to have a very high index of suspicion of infection in HSCT patients and a very low threshold for investigation and treatment.

Other early complications

Neurological

Several early post-HSCT neurological complications may occur, with a variety of causes.

Infection

- **Encephalitis/meningitis:**
  - *viruses* (e.g. HSV, CMV, adenovirus, enteroviruses, HHV6) – account for most cases, often severe;
  - rarely due to bacterial and fungal infections in early post-HSCT period;

- **Focal infection:**
  - *fungal* (e.g. *Aspergillus*) – high mortality despite aggressive treatment;
  - *CNS toxoplasmosis* – very difficult to confirm diagnosis ante-mortem, requires prolonged (≥6 weeks) treatment with pyrimethamine and sulfadiazine;
  - bacterial abscesses rare.

Drug toxicity
- Usually → encephalopathy/fits or sedation (Seizures 📖 pp.110–111).
- Ciclosporin or (less commonly) tacrolimus may cause reversible posterior leucoencephalopathy syndrome → headache, hypertension, visual disturbance (occasionally cortical blindness), convulsions, varying degrees of encephalopathy → wide variety of manifestations; usually fully reversible, but occasional reports exist of irreversible or even fatal toxicity.
- Other potential causes of drug-induced acute neurotoxicity include:
  - *Chemotherapy* –
    - *seizures* – busulfan (prophylactic anticonvulsants usually given during busulfan conditioning), methotrexate;
    - *encephalopathy* – methotrexate, cytosine arabinoside (high dose), ifosfamide;
  - *Anti-infectives* – encephalopathy – aciclovir/ganciclovir, amphotericin B.
  - *Other supportive care drugs* – sedation – opiates, benzodiazepines, anticonvulsants.

Cerebrovascular events
- Haemorrhage related to severe thrombocytopenia +/– hypertension (usually drug-induced).
- Thromboembolic events rare in children – consider underlying CNS infection or endocarditis.

Biochemical/metabolic derangements
- **Electrolyte disturbances:** (Other aspects of supportive care 📖 pp.253–292, Acute biochemical abnormalities 📖 pp.116–119).
- **Metabolic:** hyperammonaemia (very rare, but potentially reversible).

Transplant-associated thrombotic microangiopathy (TA-TMA)
- Often referred to as thrombotic thrombocytopenic purpura (TTP), but unclear if they represent the same or different entities.
- Results from endothelial cell damage.
- Reported frequency very variable (up to 10% in some series), probably reflecting differences in diagnostic stringency (especially of microangiopathy).
- Numerous risk factors described, including URD or mismatched transplants, ciclosporin, infection.
- Presents with microangiopathy (red cell fragmentation), fever, thrombocytopenia, anaemia, renal impairment, variable and often subtle CNS symptoms/signs.

- **Management difficult:** potential causative factors should be treated or withdrawn, preliminary reports of defibrotide or rituximab suggest possible efficacy, but no proven beneficial treatment. Conventional treatments for TTP (e.g. plasmapheresis) is seldom effective.
- High mortality.

Cardiac

- Often multifactorial including important contribution from previous anthracycline chemotherapy.
- Rarely, acute cardiac failure may occur after high-dose cyclophosphamide, which may also cause haemorrhagic pericarditis/pericardial effusion.
- Pericarditis is uncommon, but well described.

Pulmonary

- Early pulmonary toxicity is common and occurs in up to 50% of patients in adult or mixed series. It accounts for at least 10% of all deaths after HSCT.
- Usually presents with:
  - cough (often dry in children);
  - tachypnoea, dyspnoea;
  - hypoxia, which may progress to acute respiratory failure;
  - +/– fever and other features of infection;
  - occasionally haemoptysis;
  - CXR may show diffuse or focal infiltrates/consolidation, or diffuse interstitial shadowing.
- Much commoner after allogeneic than after autologous HSCT.

Numerous disease processes can cause this clinical picture, but it is often very hard to identify clearly a single major factor despite extensive efforts:

Infection

Early identification and treatment is vital:

- **Bacterial pneumonia:** numerous potential organisms; important to consider 'atypical bacterial pneumonias' (e.g. caused by *Legionella*, *Mycobacteria*, or *Mycoplasma*), although they are relatively uncommon post-HSCT.
- **Fungal pneumonia:** most commonly due to *Aspergillus*, associated with very high mortality.
- **Viral pneumonia:** numerous respiratory viruses may cause pneumonia post-HSCT, including respiratory syncytial virus (RSV), para-influenza virus, influenza virus A or B, adenovirus, human metapneumovirus (HMPV), measles, herpes viruses (including CMV, HHV6, HSV, VZV); these infections are usually more serious than in non-HSCT patients and lower respiratory tract involvement is a sinister development.
- *Pneumocystis jiroveci.*

- **Pneumonitis:** may be due to:
  - chemotherapy toxicity, e.g. busulfan;
  - radiotherapy (TBI) toxicity;
  - inflammatory reaction, often occurring in tandem with acute GvHD, especially (but not always) in the presence of pre-existing or current respiratory infection (often viral);
  - although pneumonitis may be the major component of respiratory failure early post-HSCT, it is always desirable and often vital to exclude infectious causes by microbiological/virological/histological investigation of respiratory secretions (including bronchoalveolar lavage, BAL) or biopsy specimens.

Isolation precautions are important to minimize the risk of pneumonia in early post-HSCT patients.

Investigation:
- Possible infective causes should be sought vigorously (as above).
- **Imaging:** although CXR usually performed initially, CT chest is much more sensitive and may reveal findings strongly suggestive evidence of fungal pneumonia (e.g. cavities, 'halo' sign).
- Helpful to involve the Paediatric Respiratory team at early stage to faciltate investigation.

Treatment
- Early and aggressive anti-infective treatment is essential, initially providing broad cover against bacteria and fungi as a minimum.
- Antiviral treatment and cover for atypical bacterial infections often added in severe illness or if no improvement to initial treatment.
- Nebulized and/or systemic corticosteroids usually given as initial anti-inflammatory treatment for pneumonitis.
- Pneumonitis associated with GvHD is usually also treated with additional systemic immunosuppressive treatment.
- Close and early liaison with Paediatric Intensive Care Unit is desirable – early non-invasive intervention may avoid need for invasive respiratory support.

Prognosis depends on the cause and severity, but invasive fungal pneumonia and any cause of respiratory failure requiring ventilation has a very poor outlook in a post-HSCT patient.

Gastrointestinal
Mucositis
- Due to chemotherapy and/or radiotherapy (TBI), but may be aggravated by superadded infection especially with *Candida* and/or HSV.
- May affect any part of gastrointestinal mucosa, most commonly:
  - oropharyngeal;
  - oesophageal;
  - small bowel.
- Presents with mucosal ulceration and pain (oropharyngeal pain frequently very severe, necessitating intravenous opiate infusion), and diarrhoea.
- Duration and severity increased by post-transplant methotrexate.

- Severity very variable between patients, but usually worse after myeloablative conditioning, especially with TBI.
- Often reduces or prevents oral intake of food, drugs, and even fluids, necessitating intravenous treatment (including parenteral nutrition).
- Prevention is difficult, but several strategies employed to reduce duration and severity:
  - use of ice lollipops/cubes to reduce oral mucosal blood flow and hence vulnerability during short-duration conditioning chemotherapy (e.g. melphalan);
  - vigorous mouth care from start of conditioning may reduce symptoms and aid recovery, but there is a paucity of good evidence that it reduces post-HSCT mucositis;
  - maintenance of at least some enteral intake (nasogastric feeding is usually necessary) is believed to reduce the duration and severity of mucositis.
- **Typhlitis (neutropenic enterocolitis):**
  - due to bacterial (rarely fungal) invasion of ulcerated mucosa;
  - commonest in ileocaecal region;
  - presents with abdominal pain, diarrhoea and fever;
  - managed conservatively (due to high surgical risks) unless complicated by major haemorrhage or perforation.

Other early gastrointestinal complications
- **Nausea and vomiting:**
  - prevention and treatment strategies as for post-chemotherapy emesis (Other aspects of supportive care 📖 pp.253–292, Nausea and vomiting 📖 pp.256–263), but often prolonged post-HSCT (due to mucositis, acute GvHD, numerous potentially emetogenic drugs);
  - frequently requires aggressive and lengthy combination anti-emetic treatment.
- **Diarrhoea:** often multifactorial due to acute chemoradiotherapy toxicity, mucositis, infection, drug toxicity, enteral feeds, and acute GvHD.

Hepatic veno-occlusive disease (HVOD)
- Recently renamed as sinusoidal obstruction syndrome (SOS), a histopathologically more descriptive term, but not yet widely used.
- Reported incidence very variable depending on patient population and conditioning regimen, but can range up to 40%.
- Risk factors include pre-existing liver disease (may be manifest by ↑ ALT pre-HSCT), intensive conditioning regimens (especially including alkylating agents, e.g. busulfan, or hepatic radiotherapy including TBI), prior or concurrent use of other hepatotoxins e.g. methotrexate.
- Commoner after allogeneic HSCT (compared with autologous).
- Clinical features:
  - *jaundice* – classical diagnostic criteria;
  - *painful hepatomegaly* – classical diagnostic criteria;
  - *weight gain +/– ascites* – classical diagnostic criteria;
  - *other features include* –
    - increased platelet consumption;
    - coagulopathy → bleeding;
    - multi-organ failure (MOF; renal ± pulmonary ± cardiac).

Investigation
- FBC, coagulation profile, biochemical profile (including LFTs).
- Exclusion of other causes of liver disease.
- Abdominal ultrasound (ascites, hepatomegaly) with Doppler studies of hepatic venous portal flow (looking for reversed flow, but failure to demonstrate this does not exclude HVOD).
- Liver biopsy risky (often → severe bleeding), rarely performed.
- Increased serum concentrations of several marker proteins may be seen (e.g. plasminogen activator inhibitor-1 [PAI-1]), but are of little clinical value.

Differential diagnosis of post-HSCT liver disease includes acute hepatic GvHD, viral hepatitis, bacterial or fungal infections, drug and TPN toxicity; therefore, a definite diagnosis of HVOD requires careful exclusion of these other causes.

Prevention
- Several strategies are used despite a paucity of evidence that they reduce the incidence of severe HVOD and, hence, reduce mortality.
  - ursodeoxycholic acid;
  - *low dose heparin* – may reduce the risk of HVOD, but not clear if it prevents severe disease, and may increase risk of bleeding; some preliminary evidence of safety and possible efficacy of low molecular weight heparin;
  - *defibrotide* – increasing evidence of efficacy.

Treatment
- **Intensive supportive care:**
  - reduction of extracellular fluid retention by careful fluid management (judicious fluid restriction and diuretic use);
  - *conservation of renal function* - trying to minimize pre-renal impairment despite fluid restriction, but dialysis or haemofiltration may be necessary;
  - management of coagulopathy;
  - organ support as indicated with the emergence of MOF.
- **Specific treatment:** many agents tried with limited success, but current management is based on defibrotide. There are numerous modes of action including fibrinolytic and antithrombotic action, but without systemic anticoagulant effect. Recent studies have confirmed efficacy in severe HVOD. Recombinant tissue plasminogen activator (rtPA) is effective, but there is a significant risk of major systemic haemorrhage. Therefore, it is now usually reserved for patients where defibrotide has failed.

Prognosis of established severe HVOD is grave, but early treatment and the increasing use of defibrotide has improved the outlook greatly.

Renal

Acute renal failure early post-HSCT is frequently multifactorial. The most important factors include:

- **Drug toxicity:** numerous drugs used in HSCT may be nephrotoxic, including:
  - *chemotherapy* – e.g. melphalan;
  - *anti-infectives* – e.g. aminoglycosides, amphotericin, high dose IV acyclovir;
  - *immunosuppressives* – e.g. ciclosporin, tacrolimus.
- Severe sepsis causing hypovolaemic shock.
- Other causes of hypovolaemia, including major bleeding, severe diarrhoea, HVOD.

Haemorrhagic cystitis (HC)

- Occurs in 5–25% of paediatric HSCTs.
- Aetiology of post-HSCT HC:
  - probably multifactorial in many patients;
  - conditioning treatment:
    - cyclophosphamide;
    - bladder radiotherapy (usually as TBI);
  - urinary tract infection, especially viral:
    - BK papovavirus is the commonest identified infecting agent, but the extent of its role in the pathogenesis of HC is unclear;
    - adenovirus, CMV, and bacterial infection may be implicated in some patients;
  - ?presence of acute GVHD – HC is commoner after allogeneic HSCT than autologous.
- **Clinical features:** wide range of severity, including:
  - *very mild* – asymptomatic microscopic haematuria;
  - *severe* – macroscopic haematuria with blood clots, urinary frequency, dysuria, painful bladder spasms, clot retention, urinary tract obstruction;
  - life-threatening due to acute blood loss.
- **Prevention:**
  - hyperhydration and mesna during cyclophosphamide administration;
  - maintenance of good urine output.
- **Investigation:**
  - *urine culture* – virology (including electron microscopy for papovavirus), bacteriology;
  - *abdominal ultrasound* – urinary tract obstruction, bladder size, wall thickness, and clots.
- **Management:**
  - Maintenance of high urine flow rate to reduce formation of bladder clots and reduce risk of urethral obstruction;
  - Aggressive transfusion support (keep platelets >50 × 10^9/L);
  - Treatment of associated infection. Consider cidofovir in severe virus-associated HC, but toxicity (especially nephrotoxicty) may limit treatment;
  - Analgesia;
  - Antispasmodics (oxybutynin).

- *Very difficult in severe cases* – close collaboration with Paediatric Surgery colleagues is essential:
  - urethral catheterization if severe dysuria, frequency, urgency, or clot retention;
  - consider bladder washout and continuous bladder irrigation by large-bore suprapubic catheter inserted surgically;
  - consider bladder installations (e.g. prostaglandin PGE_2, which promotes mucosal vasoconstriction, alum, or formalin, which 'coagulates' exposed mucosal vessels), but little evidence for consistent benefit and rarely used in children since very painful.
- High dose oral conjugated oestrogen (e.g. Premarin) has been used to facilitate mucosal healing, but case reports describe improvement only after several weeks treatment, and convincing evidence is lacking. Potential side effects include hepatotoxicty and gynaecomastia.
- Intravenous factor VII reduces severity of bleeding, but its use may be complicated by thromboembolic events.
- **Prognosis:** generally self-limiting, but may take several weeks or even months to improve, but severe bleeding may be life-threatening:
  - late bladder dysfunction may occur (uncommon);
  - risk of late bladder neoplasms (perform regular urine cytology).

Graft-versus-host disease (GvHD)

GvHD is the commonest severe complication of HSCT. Historically, it has been associated with a high frequency of serious morbidity and a significant risk of death, especially in unrelated donor HSCT. Treatment by immunosuppression, which often needs to be intensive and/or prolonged, contributes greatly to infectious morbidity and mortality. Improved HLA-typing techniques that allow optimal donor selection and more effective GvHD prophylaxis strategies have reduced the frequency and severity of GvHD after conventional HSCTs, but these developments have also led to more higher risk HSCTs being performed, with a consequent resurgence in the occurrence of GvHD.

Furthermore, since conventional chemotherapy approaches are now able to cure most children with leukaemia, there is increasing recognition of the potential role of using HSCT to harness GvL as a possibly curative treatment modality for some of the remainder. However, despite advances in understanding the biology of GvHD and GvL, this strategy still carries an appreciable risk of potentially severe GvHD.

Therefore, despite major improvements in prophylactic and therapeutic management options, GvHD remains one of the most important factors determining the success or otherwise of HSCT in children.

Acute GvHD
Acute GvHD occurs in up to 80% of all patients undergoing HSCT (depending on many factors including age, donor type and match, and GvHD prophylactic regimen), although it is less frequent in children. A recent registry-based study of HSCT in children and adolescents reported incidences of 28% for grades II–IV and 11% for grades III–IV acute GvHD.

Pathogenesis

Acute GvHD occurs due to interaction (alloreactivity) between recipient (host) antigen-presenting cells (APrCs) and donor T-cells, leading to target organ damage. A three-phase model of acute GvHD is now generally accepted:

- **Conditioning toxicity:** tissue damage (epithelial calls, APrCs) → release of cytokines (including IL-1), adhesion molecules, lipopolysac-charides, and GIT-derived endotoxins, which gain vascular access due to disruption of GIT mucosal integrity.
- **T-cell activation:** mediated by cytokine-amplified (especially via IL-2 and γ-interferon) donor T-cell recognition of and response to recipient APrCs.
- **Effector phase** ('cytokine storm'): cellular and inflammatory responses promoted by TNF-α and IL-1, and mediated via cytotoxic T-cells and NK cells.

Prevention

See Preparation for haemopoietic stem cell transplantation, Graft versus host disease prophylaxis 📖 p.176.

Clinical features

Acute GvHD typically develops soon (few days) after engraftment, but may occur weeks later (e.g. in RIC HSCT). Occasionally, it may precede engraftment. Although, by definition, acute GvHD occurs within the first 100 days post-HSCT, a similar picture may occur later (e.g. during reduc-tion/after withdrawal of immunosuppression).

It primarily involves epithelial surfaces, classically affecting:

- Skin → rash:
  - typically itchy/painful, maculopapular, erythematosus;
  - may involve any part of body;
  - often starting with palmar or plantar erythema;
  - may progress to extensive erythroderma with bullae and desquama-tion.
- Gastrointestinal tract → diarrhoea, abdominal pain (lower GIT):
  - diarrhoea is typically secretory – watery, often green, sometimes bloody; may be profuse leading to severe fluid/electrolyte loss;
  - may be associated with ileus;
  - upper GIT acute GvHD is less common in children, but increases in frequency during adolescence → nausea, vomiting, and anorexia.
- Hepatic → jaundice:
  - intrahepatic cholestasis → conjugated hyperbilirubinaemia, usually with elevated alkaline phosphatase (ALP) and γ-glutamyl transpepti-dase (GGT), but little rise in transaminases (ALT, AST);
  - hepatomegaly – not usually painful (unlike HVOD);
  - hepatitic variant described – usually later onset (up to 1 year post-HSCT), marked rise in ALT, but other LFT abnormalities less promi-nent, negative viral studies;
  - Δ may be difficult, including HVOD, drug toxicity (including TPN), infections (hepatic and systemic) and haemolysis.
- Frequency of involvement – skin > GIT > liver.

- Other less common epithelial manifestations include:
  - pneumonitis;
  - conjunctival injection.
- Additional features include:
  - fever (common);
  - bone marrow involvement → thrombocytopenia usually more prominent than neutropenia.

Risk factors
- **Donor factors:**
  - *HLA disparity* – affecting either major HLA antigens (HLA-A*, B*, Cw*, DRB1*, DQB1*, DPB1*) or minor histocompatibility antigens (mHAgs; cellular antigens coded by polymorphic genes separate to the HLA system). Degree of mismatch likely to be greater in unrelated donor HSCTs.
  - *Sex mismatch* – mediated via gender-specific mHAgs (e.g. HY antigen on Y chromosome). Parous ♀ donors → higher risk acute GvHD in male recipients due to increased likelihood of prior allosensitization from foetal antigens.
  - Older age.
  - *Stem cell source* – risk highest with PBSC > BM > UCB.
  - *Stem cell dose* – some evidence that higher CD34 cell doses associated with a higher risk of chronic GvHD in PBSCT.
  - *CMV seropositivity* – increased risk in CMV-negative recipients.
- **Recipient factors:**
  - Older age.
  - Underlying advanced stage disease.
  - *Conditioning regimen* – increased intensity → higher risk acute GvHD.
  - Efficacy of GvHD prophylaxis regimen.
  - Presence of infection during pre- and peri-engraftment phases (cytokine-mediated effect?).
  - *Genetic predisposition* – related to cytokine gene polymorphisms (e.g. IFN-γ, IL-6, IL-10, TNF-α).

Diagnosis
Suspicion and initial clinical diagnosis are based on characteristic clinical features, but confirmatory biopsy is often desirable before committing the patient to immunosuppressive treatment (with its attendant toxicity).
- Benefits of biopsy include:
  - confirmation of diagnosis;
  - grading of (pathological) severity (**NB.** not necessarily clearly related to clinical severity/grading);
  - exclusion of other potential diagnoses, e.g. viral infection → rash, diarrhoea;
  - important in clinical studies/trials of e.g. new conditioning regimens or GvHD prophylaxis strategies.
- Disadvantages of biopsy include:
  - may be misleading, especially when performed for skin rash;
  - potentially serious risks include bleeding, especially with liver and/or GIT biopsies in thrombocytopenic early post-HSCT patients.

- Although the decision whether or not to perform biopsy may be difficult, general principles include:
  - clinical diagnosis alone may be justified in low stage skin acute GvHD;
  - suspicion of GIT acute GvHD usually merits biopsy – upper GIT biopsy is increasingly used in addition to lower GIT;
  - liver biopsy is usually performed only when severe liver acute GvHD is suspected or in presence of isolated liver GvHD (i.e. if diagnosis of GvHD cannot be confirmed by other means).
- The characteristic pathological features of acute GvHD are 2° to epithelial cell apoptosis, often occurring in vicinity of lymphocytic infiltration → 'satellite cell necrosis', typically seen in:
  - *skin* – basal layer keratinocytes;
  - *GIT* – basal crypt cells;
  - *liver* – biliary tracts, with lymphocytic infiltration of portal tracts.

Grading (Tables 15.3 and 15.4).

Table 15.3 Staging of acute GvHD

Stage	Skin	GIT	Liver
1	Maculopapular rash <25% BSA	Persistent nausea +/or diarrhoea 10–19.9mL/kg/day	Bilirubin 34–50µmol/L
2	Maculopapular rash 25–50% BSA	Diarrhoea 20–30mL/kg/day	Bilirubin 51–100µmol/L
3	Generalized erythema	Diarrhoea >30mL/kg/day	Bilirubin 101–255µmol/L
4	Desquamation bullae	Abdominal pain +/or paralytic ileus	Bilirubin ≥256µmol/L

BSA = body surface area.

Table 15.4 Grading of acute GvHD

Grade	Skin	GIT	Liver
0 (none)	0	0	0
I (mild)	1–2	0	0
II (moderate)	1–3	1	1
III (severe)	2–3	2–3	2–3
IV (life-threatening)	2–4	2–4	2–4

Management
Depends on grade and, to a lesser degree, site. Policies vary between centres, especially with respect to steroid doses and second line treatments. Patients are usually already on prophylactic ciclosporin (or tacrolimus) and/or other prophylactic immunosuppressive agent(s) at the onset of acute GvHD.

- **Grade I (skin only):**
  - may resolve spontaneously without needing treatment;
  - if treatment required, topical treatment (steroids, tacrolimus) often suffices;
  - if no sustained response to topical treatment → systemic treatment, usually 'low' dose steroids (typically 2mg/kg/day IV methylprednisolone), with tapering of dose once GvHD controlled (typically after 5–7 days).
- **Grade II:**
  - *Steroids* – IV methylprednisolone usually preferred, although different units may prefer different doses and durations, e.g.
    - low dose as above;
    - 'moderate' (e.g. 5mg/kg/day) or 'high' dose (500mg/m^2/day) IV methylprednisolone for 3 consecutive days, followed by continued weaning dose (e.g. halving dose every 2–3 days initially, with slower final taper);
    - although individual patients may appear to respond better to higher steroid doses, a randomized controlled trial of low (2mg/kg/day) vs. high dose (10mg/kg/day) IV methylprednisolone showed similar response and survival rates.
  - Usually with intention to give between 4 and 8 weeks of steroids.
  - Usually converted from IV methylprednisolone to oral prednisolone after about a week (if responding).
  - Treatment is often tailored according to needs of individual patients. Duration of treatment, timing of conversion to oral, speed of weaning may be modified according to severity and acuteness of onset, and to a lesser degree on timing of onset (later onset acute GvHD is often more indolent and may be treated satisfactorily with lower doses and shorter durations).
  - *Steroid-refractoriness* – defined by:
    - no response after 7 days of steroids;
    - incomplete response after 14 days of steroids;
    - progression after 3 days of steroids;
    - necessitates additional/alternative immunosuppressive treatment (see Grade III below);
    - implies a poorer survival prognosis and greater likelihood of developing chronic GvHD.
- **Grade III:** as for Grade II, but usually using moderate or high dose IV methylprednisolone, often with addition of further immunosuppressive treatment, e.g. infliximab (TNF-α antagonist), mycophenolate mofetil (MMF), extracorporeal photopheresis (ECP), pentostatin. These treatments may also have a steroid-sparing effect.
- **Grade IV:** As for Grade III, but usually with the addition of extra immunosuppressive agents, sometimes including serotherapy (e.g. ATG or CAMPATH).
- Ciclosporin (or tacrolimus) is usually continued during the management of acute GvHD. It may be possible to improve their use, e.g. by ensuring that optimum trough serum concentrations are achieved.
- Patients on prophylactic ciclosporin who develop severe hepatic acute GvHD are often switched to tacrolimus.

- In the event of Grade III or IV acute GvHD, total treatment duration of steroids may be for much longer (e.g. 3–6 months, sometimes longer) and the duration of ciclosporin may be much longer still (e.g. 9–12 months or even longer). There are no exact stopping rules, since treatment duration depends on speed, quality and durability of response.
- Supportive treatment includes:
  - prevention and treatment of infections (commonest cause of death in acute GvHD);
  - *acute GIT GvHD* – analgesia, nutritional support, replacement of fluid and electrolyte losses, octeotride and/or bowel rest in severe cases.

Outcome
- Depends on:
- Severity (grade) and, to lesser extent, site – better in lower grade acute GvHD, and in skin compared to GIT or liver acute GvHD.
- Speed and quality of response to treatment (most important determinant).

Chronic GvHD

Pathogenesis

Chronic GvHD occurs in up to 50% of post-HSCT patients, but is less common in children (5–15%). It results from the later consequences of alloreactivity, usually (but not always) following the earlier occurrence of acute GvHD. It has characteristic clinical and histological features, many of which are reminiscent of auto-immune diseases.

Clinical features

The onset of chronic GvHD classically occurs after day +100, although rarely it may commence earlier. It is unusual for chronic GvHD to arise *de novo* more than 2 years post-HSCT.

Although chronic GvHD may affect one organ system only (most commonly skin), it has numerous possible manifestations and may progress to multi-system disease.

- **Mode of onset:**
  - *progressive* – evolving directly from acute GvHD;
  - *quiescent* – arising in the context of previous acute GvHD, which responded to treatment;
  - *de novo* – occurring without any previous evidence of acute GvHD.
- **Skin:** erythema, hypo-, and/or hyperpigmentation, dystrophic nails, poikiloderma, alopecia, lichenoid lesions, progressing to sclerodermatous skin involvement with joint contractures in severe disease.
- **Mucosa:**
  - oral (xerostomia, lichenoid and/or atrophic lesions, ulcers);
  - female genital tract (dryness, atrophy, stenosis → dyspareunia).
- **Eye:** keratoconjunctivitis sicca.
- **Lung:** typically obstructive airways disease → cough, wheeze, dyspnoea.

- **Liver:** cholestasis → abnormal LFTs (especially ALP, GGT), jaundice, rarely cirrhosis.
- **GIT:** nausea, vomiting, dysphagia (oesophageal stenosis), abdominal pain, diarrhorea, malabsorption, weight loss.
- **Renal:** proteinuria, nephrotic syndrome.
- **Musculoskeletal:** arthralgia, cramps, polymyositis, sclerodermatous joint contractures.
- **Peripheral nervous system:** myasthenia gravis, peripheral neuropathy.
- **Serosal:** pericardial, pleural and/or peritoneal effusions.
- **Haematological:** immune-mediated cytopenias.
- **Immunological:** delayed immune reconstitution, increased risk of late infections.
- **Autoimmunity:** hypo- and hyperthyroidism.
- **Secondary malignancies:** possible association with squamous carcinoma of buccal cavity and skin.
- **Adverse effects of immunosuppressive treatment:**
  - increased risk of infections;
  - nephrotoxicity (ciclosporin, tacrolimus);
  - steroid toxicities.

Risk factors
- Previous acute GvHD is the most important risk factor for the later development of chronic GvHD.
- Other factors include:
  - *Donor factors* – alloimmune female donor for male recipient;
  - *Recipient factors* – age – chronic GvHD much commoner in older (>10 years) recipients.
  - *Transplant factors* –
    - stem cell source – ↑ risk with PBSC and T-cell replete BM;
    - inadequate prophylaxis;
    - use of DLI post-transplant.

Diagnosis
- Suspicion usually raised by constellation of clinical symptoms/signs (as above), but important to confirm clinical diagnosis by biopsy when feasible and appropriate (in view of toxicity of prolonged and intensive immunosuppressive treatment).
- Characteristic pathological findings on biopsy include presence of excess collagen, as well as lymphocytic reaction:
  - *skin* – prominent lymphocytic infiltrate in upper dermis and dermo-epidermal junction (lichenoid chronic GvHD), collagen deposition in upper dermis (sclerotic chronic GvHD);
  - *liver* – chronic lymphocytic infiltrate accompanied by atrophy and destruction of biliary duct epithelial cells ('vanishing bile ducts' syndrome).

Staging

Traditionally, chronic GvHD has been graded as either limited or extensive.

- **Limited chronic GvHD:** either or both
  - localized skin involvement;
  - hepatic dysfunction due to chronic GvHD (without aggressive histology).
- **Extensive chronic GvHD:** either
  - generalized skin involvement; or
  - localized skin involvement and/or hepatic dysfunction due to chronic GvHD; and
  - *liver histology* – chronic aggressive hepatitis, bridging necrosis, cirrhosis; or
  - involvement of eyes; or
  - involvement of minor salivary glands or oral mucosa on labial biopsy; or
  - involvement of any other target organ.

Subclinical chronic GvHD is also described, characterized by histological changes of GvHD in screening or incidental biopsies in the absence of clinical symptoms or signs of chronic GvHD.

Recently, a newer system has been proposed based on the number of organs/sites involved, and the severity of disease at each site, allowing grading as either mild, moderate, or severe chronic GvHD.

Management

- **Limited:**
  - topical emollients;
  - topical steroids or tacrolimus;
  - oral prednisolone 0.25–1.0mg/kg/day may be necessary if topical treatment does not achieve complete control – sometimes given on an alternate day basis to reduce toxicity;
  - continue oral ciclosporin/tacrolimus, optimizing trough levels.
- **Extensive:** occasionally as above for limited chronic GvHD, but nearly all patients will need:
  - oral prednisolone 1–2mg/kg/day for at least 2 weeks, followed by very slow taper according to speed and durability of clinical response – typically continued for at least 6–12 months;
  - continued ciclosporin/tacrolimus, optimizing levels, but consider changing ciclosporin to tacrolimus in appropriate cases (e.g. liver GvHD) – start tapering dose very slowly (over at least 6 months) once GvHD control has been maintained for 3–6 months after steroids withdrawn;
  - addition of other immunosuppressive/immunomodulatory agents (e.g. MMF, infliximab, thalidomide, azathioprine, etc.) may be required – in these cases, drugs are weaned/stopped in a stepwise manner, but the order in which this is done may depend on previous response and on toxicity.
- Consider PUVA (psoralen-enhanced ultraviolet A irradiation) or ECP in patients with severe/refractory cutaneous (or oral) acute or chronic GvHD.

- Total duration of treatment of chronic GvHD (limited or extensive) varies considerably, but is usually at least 6-9 months, and often much longer
- Supportive treatment includes:
  - Prevention and treatment of infections:
    - infection is commonest cause of death in chronic GVHD;
    - penicillin (prophylaxis against encapsulated gram-positive bacteria);
    - antifungal prophylaxis, e.g. oral azole;
    - antiviral prophylaxis – aciclovir, with regular viral PCR surveillance;
    - anti-pneumocystis – cotrimoxazole;
    - consider IVIg – decision may be guided by serum immunoglobulin concentrations;
    - immunization – consider use of non-live vaccines in patients not on IVIg, but response may be suboptimal; live vaccines should be avoided until off all immunosuppression for at least 12 months and no evidence of active GvHD.
  - Ursodeoxycholic acid improves biliary flow in hepatic chronic GvHD.
  - Artificial tears and saliva relieve symptoms of keratoconjunctivitis sicca and xerostomia.
  - Maintenance of good nutritional status.

Outcome

Historically poor. Prognosis may be improving with introduction of newer immunosuppressive treatments, although published evidence of improved survival is not yet available.

Graft versus leukaemia effect

This was initially suspected after early studies, which demonstrated a reduced relapse risk in transplanted leukaemic patients with acute or chronic GvHD (compared with patients who did not develop GvHD). However, this effect was not translated into improved overall survival due to the increased mortality associated with GvHD. Subsequent experience with DLI (Post-haemopoietic stem cell transplant relapse 🕮 p.198), especially in CML, has clearly demonstrated the anti-leukaemic potential of GvL. Nevertheless, the occurrence and efficacy of GvL is difficult to predict – clinically significant GvL may occur without apparent GvHD, whilst the occurrence of GvHD is not a guarantee of GvL or of leukaemia-free survival.

Clinical separation of GvL from GvHD

There is increasing interest in the potential for achieving clinically effective GvL without significant GvHD in HSCT for AML by deliberately seeking a mismatch between the donor NK cell inhibitory receptor (KIR) and the recipient KIR ligand present on haemopoietic cells.

Post-haemopoietic stem cell transplant relapse

The commonest cause of failure of HSCT performed for malignancy. Although relapse is greatly feared post-HSCT, cure may still be possible in a minority of patients.

Prognosis depends on:
• Site of relapse (isolated extramedullary better).
• Timing of relapse (outlook very poor if within 12 months of HSCT).
• Conditioning treatment for, and occurrence (or not) of GvHD after, 1st HSCT (influences ability to perform, and likelihood of achieving any benefit from, a 2nd transplant).

Potential management strategies may still vary widely, including:
• Secondary HSCT may occasionally be appropriate if late relapse (>12 months), no/only mild GvHD (or occurrence of autologous reconstitution) after 1st transplant, especially in malignancies where GvL may have an important role (e.g. AML) – conditioning strategies dictated by regimen used for 1st HSCT, but usually involve RIC approach.
• DLI may be curative (without need for further chemotherapy or 2nd transplant) in CML especially when performed early (i.e. molecular or cytogenetic relapse, rather than overt haematological). Potential complications include GvHD or graft failure.
• Further chemotherapy may be offered in an attempt to control leukaemia for a period of time (usually months, occasionally longer) and, hence, keep patient 'as well as possible for as long as possible', but often limited by, or refused due to, poor tolerance:
  • possible treatments may include Phase I investigational agents;
  • several conventional agents may be feasible in ALL with relatively little toxicity (e.g. vincristine, steroids) until cumulative toxicity and/or refractory leukaemia supervene;
  • few conventional options in AML – hydroxyurea or low dose cytosine arabinoside sometimes offered.
• Symptom control/palliative care (Other aspects of supportive care pp.253–292, Palliative care pp.280–285).

Prophylaxis of other serious complications

Bleeding

- Prophylactic platelet transfusions are typically given to keep the platelet count >20 × 10^9/L, or raise it to higher levels prior to surgery or biopsy.
- Clotting factors are usually given in the presence of significant coagulopathy, especially in the context of severe clinical complications associated with increased risk of haemorrhage (e.g. HVOD), or to normalize abnormal clotting times prior to invasive procedures, e.g. biopsy.
- Norethisterone is commonly used to suppress menstrual bleeding during HSCT.

Late complications and long-term follow-up

Late adverse effects of HSCT are very frequent, diverse, and often severe due to the additive effects of chemotherapy or radiotherapy given months/years before transplant, and in the conditioning regimen, as well as the consequences of chronic GvHD. Some late effects are specific to HSCT:

- Delayed immune reconstitution:
  - post-HSCT lymphocyte (especially T cell) reconstitution much slower than neutrophil recovery;
  - may → ↑ risk of potentially severe late infections (Infection 📖 pp.207–219).
- Immune dysregulation occasionally → autoimmunity (especially in context of chronic GvHD):
  - immune-mediated cytopenias;
  - myasthenia gravis;
  - diabetes mellitus;
  - hepatitis.

Results of haemopoietic stem cell transplantation

The results of clinical studies of HSCT are often very hard to interpret due to low patient numbers in single or limited centre reports, multiple underlying diagnoses, and/or co-variables in registry reports, confounding factors (e.g. prior treatments, historical controls, or comparative treatments with cohort influences, such as supportive care). Most fundamentally, since HSCT is a very rapidly changing and advancing field, the published literature often does not reflect 'state of the art' treatment.

Therefore, it is perhaps more meaningful to view the results of HSCT by comparison with alternative/conventional treatments:

- Results of conventional treatment offer some limited prospect of cure (≤50%), and HSCT is performed in the anticipation that it will improve outcome, but without definite evidence that this is the case, e.g. ALL in CR2.
- Results of conventional treatment very poor (≤10–25%), whilst non-comparative data suggests that HSCT improves prognosis, e.g. Ph+ and other high risk ALL.
- HSCT represents only known curative strategy, e.g. constitutional bone marrow failure, SCID.
- Conventional treatment allows prolonged survival, but successful HSCT may offer improved quality of life, e.g. thalassaemia.

The future

The role of HSCT will probably become more refined in the next decade as improved risk stratification allows the development of more appropriate criteria for the use of either conventional treatment or transplantation. Refinements in conditioning chemoradiotherapy, especially protocols with specific activity against certain diseases and in GvHD prophylaxis, allied to improvements in supportive care, may reduce relapse rates (in malignancy) and TRM, and hence improve survival rates.

New developments that may increase the success of HSCT include:

- Mesenchymal stem cells (MSCs) may facilitate stem cell engraftment and subsequent immune reconstitution by improving bone marrow stromal recovery. The use of MSCs in the treatment of the refractory acute GvHD is under investigation following preliminary results demonstrating suppressed proliferation of activated graft lymphocytes in a non-HLA-restricted manner.
- Stem cell engineering is a rapidly developing field with many potential applications, such as cytotoxic antiviral T cells (e.g. EBV, CMV) or prevention/reduction of GvHD, ideally with preservation of GvL.
- Gene therapy, despite much hype, is not yet of proven benefit, although it is likely to be of considerable future benefit for many genetic haematological or immunological diseases (e.g. thalassaemia, FA, X-linked SCID).

Clinical trials

A clinical trial is a research study involving human subjects, designed to evaluate the safety and effectiveness of new diagnostic strategies, or (more commonly) new drugs or treatment approaches.

There are three types of clinical trial in paediatric oncology:
- Phase I.
- Phase II.
- Phase III.

Phase I

Primary objective
Determine the maximum tolerated dose (MTD).

Secondary objectives
- Define dose limiting toxicities (DLTs).
- Often mandatory pharmacokinetic and pharmacogenetic profiling of drug.
- Evaluate efficacy.

Patient population
- Patients who have failed first and second line therapy.
- No therapy of higher curative potential available.
- Typically not disease specific.

Trial design
- Paediatric Phase I trials start at a defined percentage of the adult phase I MTD (commonly 60–75%).
- Cohort of three patients at each dose level.
- Defined evaluation period for each patient.
- Dose escalation to next cohort only after the third patient has been evaluated and no DLT seen.
- If a DLT is experienced in a cohort of three patients a further three patients will be recruited at the same dose level.
- The MTD is the dose level immediately below that in which two patients out of six experience a DLT.

Phase II

Primary objective
Determine efficacy.

Secondary objectives
- Assess duration of response.
- Document overall survival.
- Assess time to progression.
- Further define or assess toxicity.
- Pharmacokinetic and pharmacogenetic profiling of drug (but not compulsory).

Patient population
- As for Phase I.
- Often disease(s) specific.

Trial design
- Use defined MTD from phase I trial.
- Defined time points for disease re-evaluation.
- Defined response criteria for trial continuation.
- Defined stopping rules.

Phase III
Primary objective
To compare the currently best available or standard treatment with new treatments in a randomized trial. This may involve using different doses or schedules of standard treatment, often in combination with new drugs to improve outcome.

Secondary objectives
- Assess and document toxicity.
- Assess duration of response.
- Document event-free survival and overall survival.
- Use results of study to develop subsequent trial.

Patient population
Disease specific.

Trial design
- Large, multi-centre, international.
- Treatment stratified according to stage of disease at presentation.
- Disease re-assessment at specific time points to inform randomization.
- Continuous data collection and central review.
- Close post-treatment follow-up and late effects monitoring.

Points to remember
Paediatric oncology clinical trials differ from adult oncology trials in several ways:
- Smaller patient population.
- Most children are registered onto a clinical trial.
- Rare and diverse disease groups need international trials to recruit enough patients to achieve the trial's aims.
- National, European, and international collaboration and protocols.
- Multiple randomizations are commoner.
- Lengthy recruitment period required to achieve required patient numbers.
- Much smaller proportion of paediatric clinical trials are commercially sponsored trials due to lack of commercial viability.
- Parental consent necessary if child <16 years old.

Administration/legislation

In the UK clinical trials are predominantly performed in 21 regional Paediatric Oncology Principal Treatment Centres, with central organization of trial co-ordination, data collection, and analysis undertaken by Children's Cancer and Leukaemia Group (CCLG). All clinical trials are conducted in accordance with the European Union Directive (EUD) and Good Clinical Practice (GCP) and are subject to:

• National and local ethical approval.
• NHS Trust approval (R&D).
• Inspection by the Medicines and Healthcare Regulatory Agency (MHRA).
• NHS Trust Audit.

Section 5
Supportive care

Infection

Historical perspective

Empirical antibiotic treatment

The high mortality rate in febrile neutropenia became apparent following the pioneering early experience with chemotherapy in the treatment of childhood malignancies [e.g. acute lymphoblastic leukaemia (ALL), Wilms' tumour) in the late 1950s and 1960s. Subsequently, during the 1970s this mortality was reduced by the early use of empirical antibiotic treatment in any febrile neutropenic child, even in the absence of any additional clinical (e.g. signs of systemic sepsis or focal infection) or microbiological evidence of infection. Numerous different empirical protocols have been developed, usually guided by a knowledge of local bacterial and antibiotic resistance patterns.

Empirical antifungal treatment

Improved chemotherapy regimens in the 1970s and 1980s increased response rates and survival from malignancy, but were associated with the emergence of fungal infections as a major cause of infective mortality in the context of prolonged periods of severe neutropenia. In view of the recognition that it was and, indeed, remains very hard to diagnose fungal infections with confidence until advanced infection was present, at which stage the prognosis (even with antifungal treatment) was very poor, empirical antifungal policies were introduced, whereby IV amphotericin B was started if the child remained febrile despite the use of empirical antibacterial treatment for a defined period. Over the years empirical antifungal treatment has been added at progressively earlier time points, and many units now commence it after 72h of continued fever.

Recent trends

During and since the 1980s, the widespread use of more aggressive empirical antibiotic policies and the availability of newer more potent and broader spectrum antibiotics has reduced the mortality of febrile neutropenia to <1% in children with malignancy. Subsequently, during the 1990s and 2000s, many paediatric oncology/haematology units have introduced more aggressive antifungal prophylaxis and empirical treatment policies, and adopted more intensive investigation strategies in an attempt to permit earlier diagnosis of fungal infections. However, there is no conclusive published evidence that empirical antifungal treatment has reduced the mortality from fungal infection in neutropenic patients.

The 2000s have also been characterized by increasing levels of concern about the emergence of antibiotic and antifungal resistant organisms [e.g. extended spectrum beta-lactamase (ESBL) producing bacteria, vancomycin-resistant enterococci (VRE), teicoplanin-resistant coagulase negative *Staphylococci*, many *Pseudomonas* family bacteria, and some *Candida* species), although methicillin-resistant *Staphylococcus aureus* (MRSA) is fortunately relatively uncommon in most UK paediatric units.

The continued use of increasingly intensive chemotherapy and immuno-suppressive treatment regimens is generating an expanding population of children at greatly increased risk of potentially fatal infections. In addition to those treated for malignancy, this population includes children with a wide range of primary immunodeficiencies and numerous other condi-tions treated with immunosuppressive therapy, e.g. auto-immune or inflammatory disorders, recipients of solid organ transplants.

Epidemiology

Incidence

- Infection is very common in children with or undergoing treatment for malignancy, but:
  - published information about the overall frequency and types of infections is patchy, and has mostly been derived from treatment centres or clinical trials, rather than population-based studies;
  - individual centre reports vary considerably, probably due to differences in patient populations, e.g. in underlying malignant diagnosis, cytotoxic treatment received, presence of other risk factors (Pathogenesis and risk factors 🛍 p.212);
  - profile of infection (type, severity, outcome) varies greatly due to the nature and intensity of chemotherapy, with highest rates of infection (especially viral and fungal) in recipients of haemopoietic stem cell transplantation (HSCT).
- Overall infection rates of ~1 per 100 patient days have been described for patients with active malignant disease and ~0.4–0.6 for those with disease in remission. Rates are usually higher in patients with haematological malignancies, when compared with solid tumours.

Patterns of infection

- Immunosuppressed patients are at increased risk of both:
  - infections with recognised pathogens that occur relatively commonly in healthy individuals (e.g. viral respiratory and gastrointestinal infections, bacterial urinary tract infections); and
  - opportunistic infections that occur only very rarely in immunocompetent individuals (e.g. pneumonia due to *Legionella* or *Pneumocystis*).
- Although poorly documented in overall terms, clinical experience, and numerous published case reports and series indicate that morbidity and mortality rates of most infections are higher in immunosuppressed patients than in healthy individuals:
  - some infections are notorious for high mortality rates in immunosuppressed patients, e.g. measles, Gram –ve septicaemia, invasive fungal infections;
  - other infections that rarely cause mortality in immunocompetent individuals have increased mortality rates in immunosuppressed patients, e.g. varicella, Gram +ve bacterial infections.
- Although Gram –ve organisms (e.g. *Pseudomonas*) were the commonest cause of bacterial infections in the 1960s and 1970s, since the 1980s Gram +ve organisms (especially *Staphylococci* in central venous access device [CVAD] associated infections) have become the commonest bacterial isolates.
- Viral infections are diagnosed increasingly frequently, at least in part due to greater use of and improvements in viral diagnostic investigations.

- Fungal infections are documented more frequently, largely due to the increasing use of highly myelosuppressive chemotherapy and HSCT (especially in haematological malignancies), but probably also partly due to improvements in diagnostic awareness and investigations. Filamentous fungi (moulds, e.g. *Aspergillus*) have taken over from yeasts (predominantly *Candida*) as the commonest fungal pathogens in immunosuppressed patients, but an array of rarer fungi (e.g. *Scedosporium*) is recognized increasingly.

Pathogenesis and risk factors

Infection is associated with the severity and duration of neutropenia, prolonged lymphopenia and/or hypogammaglobulinaemia. T cell defects or underlying immune deficiencies will also increase the risk of bacterial, fungal and viral infections.

Numerous contributing factors include:

- **Neutropenia:** severity and duration of neutropenia very important, as well as quality of subsequent neutrophil recovery. Chemotherapy and steroids decrease phagocytic activity, chemotaxis, and migration.
- **Duration:** risk of bacterial infection increases significantly when severe neutropenia (<0.5 × 10⁹/L) persists beyond 1 week.
- Alterations in innate, cellular, and humoral defences (e.g. lymphopenia, hypogammaglobulinaemia, decreased specific antibody responses) due to chemotherapy, steroids and radiotherapy.
- Intensity and nature of chemotherapy regimen used:
  - Intensity ranges from low (e.g. low stage Wilms' tumour) to high-intensity [e.g. acute myeloid leukaemia (AML), neuroblastoma].
  - Low-intensity chemotherapy may cause very little myelo- or lymphosuppression.
  - High-intensity chemotherapy likely to cause severe and prolonged myelosuppression, including neutropenia and prolonged lymphopenia.
- **Radiotherapy:** irradiation of large volumes of bone marrow (e.g. spinal or pelvic fields) may cause neutropenia.
- Damage or breach of mucosal barriers (e.g. mucositis, oesophagitis).
- Mechanical, structural, or functional damage caused by the malignancy (e.g. urinary tract obstruction or damage due to rhabdomyosarcoma, impaired gag reflex in brain stem glioma), which may predispose to infection.
- Presence of foreign bodies (e.g. CVADs).
- Hyposplenism due to surgery, radiotherapy or disease infiltration, leading to impaired polysaccharide specific antibody responses.
- Malnutrition,
- Previous latent infection (CMV, EBV),
- Bacterial colonization (coagulase negative *Staphylococci*, aerobic Gram –ves, e.g. *E. coli*, *Pseudomonas* spp., *Klebsiella* spp.).
- Extensive antibiotic use resulting in alterations in endogenous flora (mainly bacterial, also *Candida*) and resistant organisms (ESBL, *Staph. epidermidis*, enterococcus).
- Underlying immune deficiency.
- Hygiene (e.g. GI viruses and bacteria spread by faecal/oral route, respiratory virus).
- **Haemopoietic stem cell transplant** (HSCT): usually intensely myelo- and immunosuppressive, but recently developed reduced intensity conditioning (RIC) protocols may be non-myeloablative (thereby shortening duration of neutropenia), yet still very lymphosuppressive.

Prevention of infection

Prevention is always better than treatment and includes the following:

Hygiene

Hand hygiene is the single most important procedure to prevent spread of infection. This should be emphasized to parents, visitors, and patients. Personal hygiene is also essential and, where possible, daily baths/showers with a suitable body wash should be attempted.

Isolation procedures

Contact should be avoided with individuals who may have transmissible infections (especially measles, other respiratory viruses, and VZV). On the hospital ward, gloves, aprons, and barrier nursing should be used for patients with potential infections (especially gastrointestinal, e.g. rotavirus). In more severely immunocompromised patients, gowns, masks, and full reverse barrier nursing in isolation rooms with positive pressure ventilation may be practised in some units. However, most bacterial infections in neutropenic children are caused by the patient's own endogenous bowel or skin flora, and are not prevented by isolation measures. Therefore, few units routinely practice strict isolation precautions except in the context of allogeneic HSCT. High efficiency particulate air (HEPA) filtered rooms or laminar air flow (LAF) units or rooms are used in allogeneic HSCT units.

General mouth care

The aim of mouth care is to reduce the frequency and severity of oral complications, which occur commonly during and after chemotherapy and/or radiotherapy. These may include:
- *Candida* infection: best treated with an azole that is absorbed from the GIT, e.g. fluconazole.
- **Herpes simplex infection:** treated with acyclovir.

The mainstay of basic mouth care is thorough tooth brushing twice daily with fluoride toothpaste and a soft toothbrush, or if this is not possible, oral cleaning with sponges moistened with water or diluted chlorhexidine antibacterial solution.

Antibacterial prophylaxis

Cotrimoxazole covers bacteria, *Pneumocystis jiroveci* (previously *Pneumocystis carinii* [PCP]) and toxoplasma. It is useful where there is a high risk of PCP infection with high intensity regimens producing prolonged lymphopenia (e.g. HSCT, ALL, AML, some solid tumour chemotherapy protocols). In significantly immunocompromised patients, oral ciprofloxacin, and metronidazole may be used as bacterial gut decontamination; although this is not routinely used it may be more useful where there is pre-existing or anticipated gastrointestinal damage, e.g. from viral pathogens or HSCT conditioning treatment.

Antifungal prophylaxis

For chemotherapy regimens that produce prolonged periods of neutro-penia (e.g. AML protocols, intensification blocks in ALL) systemic oral imi-dazole compounds (usually itraconazole, fluconazole, or voriconazole) are usually used to prevent systemic fungal infection. Itraconazole provides a reasonable range of antifungal cover. Liquid or capsules are most usefully given with fizzy drinks, such as cola, to aid absorption, but can be unpalat-able and it may be difficult to achieve therapeutic drug levels. Fluconazole, only prevents *Candida*, and has no mould cover against, e.g. *Aspergillus*). Voriconazole has effective mould and yeast activity (see Table 17.1) and, although, there is little published evidence, its use in prophylaxis has been increasingly adopted.

Antiviral prophylaxis

Aciclovir prevents reactivation of herpes simplex virus (HSV) and CMV. Where tablets can be swallowed, valaciclovir has superior absorption and provides more reliable aciclovir levels in blood.

Augmentation of host defences

G-CSF stimulates progenitor cells in the bone marrow to produce neu-trophils, and may be used either prophylactically or to encourage more rapid neutrophil recovery in the context of severe established infection.

Antimycobacterial prophylaxis

Treatment with isoniazid alone, or the combination of isoniazid and rifampicin may be considered where there is a history of previous infec-tion with tuberculosis as evidenced by a positive Mantoux or interferon gamma release assay. Pyridoxine is not usually necessary in children, but may be considered depending on the chemotherapy regimen and nutri-tional status of the child.

Splenectomized patient

Where there is actual or functional splenectomy, lifelong penicillin V or amoxycillin prophylaxis should be given as there is a significant risk of infection from encapsulated bacteria (*Streptococcus pneumonia*, *Haemophilus influenzae*, and *Neisseria meningitidis*). It is important to provide additional protection by immunization with pneumococcal polysaccharide (Pneumovax) and conjugate (Prevenar) vaccine, as well as *Haemophilus influenzae* type b (Hib) and meningococcal C vaccines; these are best given pre-operatively when splenectomy is performed electively (Immunization 📖 pp.270–275).

Febrile neutropenia

Fever in a neutropenic child should be regarded seriously and assessed urgently. There is no universally accepted definition for febrile neutropenia and different units use different cut-offs ranging from:

- **Fever:** a single spike of fever >38.5°C to two spikes of >37.5°C.
- **Neutrophils:** <0.5 to <1.0 × 10^9/L.

Empirical antibiotic treatment should be started when the local definitions of fever and neutropenia are reached (as per local protocol) or when there are symptoms and signs of sepsis even in the absence of fever.

Prompt administration of empirical broad spectrum antibacterial agents to this group of patients has been shown to reduce mortality and is considered a standard of care.

Initial clinical assessment

- Look for signs of septic shock, hypotension, tachycardia.
- Search for a focus of infection with particular attention to intravascular catheter sites, mouth, perianal region.
- Digital rectal examination should be avoided due to the risk of infection secondary to damage of the rectal mucosa.
- Full examination including pulse oximetry.

Initial investigations

Should include:

- **Blood cultures:** from each lumen of the CVAD, and if possible, peripheral blood.
- Full blood count, serum C-reactive protein (CRP).
- Chest X-ray.
- Biochemical profile including U&Es.
- Cultures of urine, sputum, or nasopharyngeal aspirate, faeces, throat swab. CVAD exit site swab as clinically indicated.

Assessment of the risk of bacterial or fungal infection in children with febrile neutropenia

Although the evidence base in paediatrics is still scanty, initial assessment and treatment is increasingly approached within a risk stratification strategy, e.g.

- Identification of low and high-risk groups. In addition to clinical condition at presentation, criteria for risk stratification may include patient age, chemotherapy protocol, presence of comorbidity, and evidence of a significant source of infection
- Typical low-risk treatment strategies include reduced intensity (e.g. switch to oral after 48 h) or reduced total duration antibiotic policies.
- Typical high-risk treatment strategies comprise aggressive empirical treatment policies with early introduction of additional or alternative antibiotics, and of antifungal agents, in patients with continued fever.

Initial empirical treatment

Rapid administration of broad spectrum antibiotics is essential. Each unit should have an agreed, and regularly reviewed, antibiotic regimen depending upon local infection rates and antibiotic resistance profiles. The antibiotics used need to cover both Gram +ve and –ve organisms, e.g.

- Ceftazidime + aminoglycoside (most commonly gentamicin).
- Piperacillin/tazobactam (Tazocin) + aminoglycoside.
- Meropenem +/– aminoglycoside.

Teicoplanin or vancomycin may be added if there are clear signs of a CVAD infection.

Subsequent management

Good clinical response

- **Positive culture:** continue the appropriate antibiotic for 5–14 days depending on the organism, clinical severity of initial presentation, expected duration, and severity of neutropenia.
- **No positive culture or obvious focus of infection:** if fever resolves continue for at least 48 hours on initial antibiotic regimen. If no other evidence of active infection (CRP low or falling) antibiotic therapy may be discontinued. Assess each child individually.

Persistent fever or poor clinical response

Close monitoring and repeated examination is necessary, specifically looking for localizing signs of focal infection. Regular measurement of inflammatory markers (e.g. CRP and ESR) may reveal helpful trends. Consider appropriate modification of antibiotics in the light of positive cultures.

- **Empirical antibiotics:** second and third line agents vary with unit policies. Most would consider a change after 48–72 h with addition of teicoplanin or vancomycin if not already used. Additional antibacterials, such as ciproflxacin and amikacin may be useful at this stage. Treatment may need to be continued until neutrophil recovery occurs (neutrophils >0.5 × 10^9/L).
- **Empirical antifungals:** absence of response after 72 h usually warrants the addition of an empirical antifungal agent, guided by local policy, and knowledge of yeast and mould patterns. Amphotericin B or its lipo-somal derivatives have traditionally been used as first line antifungals, although increasingly voriconazole is being used. Symptoms or signs, such as haemoptysis, epistaxis, pleural pain, maxillary tenderness, peri-orbital swelling, nodular skin lesions, pleural rub, meningism, or focal neurological signs may suggest invasive fungal infection.
- **Colony stimulating factors:** G-CSF may hasten neutrophil recovery and contribute to clinical improvement in selected patients with severe bacterial or fungal infection, but there is no evidence that routine use is beneficial.

- IVIg may be a useful adjunct in the significantly immunosuppressed with severe viral infection where additional specific antibody is important in disease control, e.g. RSV, CMV. The DOH Clinical Guidelines for Immunoglobulin Use agree that IVIg in conjunction with ganciclovir is the treatment of choice for CMV-induced pneumonitis. However, routine use of IVIg to prevent infection following allogeneic BMT or HSCT is listed as having insufficient evidence for a recommendation, despite widespread use in many paediatric HSCT units.
- Granulocyte transfusions are used very rarely, but may be considered as an adjunct to antibacterial/antifungal treatment in patients with life-threatening bacterial or fungal infection occurring in the context of prolonged severe, but potentially reversible neutropenia. However, their use requires careful assessment of the balance of potential benefit vs. the risk from side effects such as allosensitization and respiratory complications.

System specific infections

Central venous access device (CVAD) associated infections

Indwelling central venous catheters, including tunnelled Hickman or Broviac catheters and portacaths, are very commonly used. CVAD infections can be considered as either:

- CVAD ('line') infection.
- Exit site infection: in tunnelled catheters.
- Tunnel infection: in tunnelled catheters.

Exit site infections present with erythema/exudate around the catheter exit site. Tunnel infections are characterized by erythema or tenderness along the subcutaneous tunnel track.

CVAD infection is suggested by:

- Fever and/or rigors with or after CVAD use.
- Pathogen from a blood culture from the line (first pull of blood), but not from blood taken simultaneously from a peripheral vein.

In practice, peripheral cultures are difficult to take in children and so when organisms are cultured from any in-dwelling venous cathether, a repeat blood culture should be taken and empirical treatment commenced, whilst awaiting results. If the repeat cultures taken before starting the antibiotics are negative and the child is well with no fever, antibiotics may be stopped.

Pathogens

- **Frequent:** coagulase negative *Staphylococci*, corynebacteria, *Streptococcus* spp.
- **Less frequent:** other *Staphylococci*, Gram −ve bacteria, and yeasts.

Management

CVAD removal is warranted in the presence of:

- **Rigors and/or haemodynamic instability and/or sepsis:** urgent and rapid removal indicated after stabilization. ▶▶ Medical emergency. Stop using CVAD (requires insertion of other route of temporary venous access, whilst awaiting CVAD removal).
- Infection not responding to antimicrobial therapy.
- Repeated infections with the same organism.
- Infection with *Candida*, some Gram −ve bacteria (*Pseudomonas*, *Stenotrophomonas*), *Staphylococcus aureus*, and non-tuberculous mycobacteria (NTM).
- New CVAD should be inserted only after the initial CVAD-associated infection has been adequately treated. In practice, this means at least 48 h after CVAD removal, and (usually) resolution of fever and other signs of infection.

Antibiotic treatment without CVAD removal is appropriate for:

- Coagulase negative *Staphylococci* or other skin organisms. A systemic glycopeptide (vancomycin or teicoplanin) is given for 5–14 days (depending on unit policy and clinical scenario), sometimes combined with an antibiotic lock (usually vancomycin). Locks are left *in situ* for at least two hours (sometimes up to 48 h), and then removed and discarded prior to re-using the line.

- Other locks sometimes used include taurolidine (antiseptic), alcohol, or hydrochloric acid (according to unit policy).
- Avoid glycopeptide locks in situations where VRE is a frequently isolated pathogen in the unit.
- Rarely medical treatment of CVAD-associated infection with some Gram −ve bacteria (e.g. *E. coli*) may be attempted if the child is haemo-dynamically stable, using systemic antibiotics plus antibiotic locks (gentamicin or amikacin).

Upper respiratory tract infections

Otitis media

Presents with ear pain, fever, aural discharge. Tympanic erythema may be minimal in neutropenia. Both Gram +ve and Gram −ve bacteria are possible pathogens; hence, antibiotic treatment should reflect this, e.g. amoxicillin and ciprofloxacin.

Otitis externa

Topical treatment is usually effective (e.g. gentamicin ear drops). However, 'malignant otitis externa' with *Pseudomonas aeruginosa* infection extending through the petrous bone into the brain requires aggressive systemic treatment with good CNS penetration (e.g. meropenem).

Sinusitis

- Presents with headache and facial pain, with or without fever. Usually due to anaerobic streptococci, *Streptococcus pneumoniae* or *Haemophilus* and other Gram −ve bacteria. Broad spectrum antibiotics should include anaerobic cover, e.g. cefotaxime or meropenem or Tazocin, and metronidazole.
- Crusting or eschar of nares, palate or turbinates suggests fungal infection. Consider *Aspergillus*, *Fusarium*, or *Zygomycetes*. These moulds may lead to rapid erosion across tissue planes and into orbit, cavernous sinus and brain. ▶▶ Life-threatening invasive disease requiring urgent treatment.
- Urgent CT and/or MRI needed to assess extent.
- Surgery with extensive debridement may be required, along with aggressive antifungal therapy (Table 17.1). Zygomycoses have a poor prognosis and respond poorly to antifungal therapy. Recent reports suggest improved outcomes with posaconazole. G-CSF may be indicated to hasten neutrophil recovery.

Lower respiratory tract infections

Presentation

Any clinical picture is possible – pneumonia, bronchiolitis, pneumonitis.
- ↑ Respiratory rate:
  - >60 in children <1 year;
  - >50 in children 1–2 years;
  - >40 in children >2 years.
- Use of accessory muscles, nasal flare, tracheal tug, dyspnoea.
- Cough, wheeze.
- Oxygen requirement; SaO_2 <92% in air.
- Auscultation → crackles or wheeze, which may be widespread or focal.

Investigations
- **Chest X-ray:** initial bilateral interstitial pattern may imply viral infection, whilst 'honeycombing' or bilateral patchy changes may suggest PCP. However, CXR changes do not reliably indicate particular pathogens.
- Ultrasound if any pleural effusion.
- **CT scan:** request if any suspicion of fungal infection. CXR, especially early in the disease may be normal or non specific, high resolution CT scan may show specific changes. Discuss with radiologist.
- FBC, CRP, blood gas analysis.
- Blood culture.
- Nasopharyngeal secretions (NPS) or sputum for viral detection [either immunofluorescence (IF) or increasingly polymerase chain reaction (PCR)] and, if available, culture. These should include, where possible; respiratory syncytial virus (RSV), para-influenza virus 1–4, influenza A/B, cytomegalovirus (CMV), adenovirus, human metapneumovirus (HMPV), bocavirus, coronavirus. Some laboratories do not routinely look for para-influenza 4.
- NPS or sputum for bacterial and fungal culture. Increasingly, bacterial PCR is available including *Bordetella pertussis*, mycoplasma, chlamydia.

Further investigations
Should be guided by clinical condition, CXR changes, response to initial treatment. Where clinical response poor:
- Repeat CXR.
- **Bronchalveolar lavage:** microscopy and culture, PCP (detected by IF or PCR), viral investigations as above.
- Blood for CMV PCR, adenovirus, PCR, pneumococcal PCR.
- Blood for fungal/aspergillus PCR, galactomannan (antigen from *Aspergillus* cell wall) and mannan (antigen from *Candida* cell wall) and 1,3-B-D-glucan (common fungal cell wall antigen). These non-culture techniques may be useful when used consecutively as two or more sequential positives are constitute a more reliable indicator of fungal infection, especially with galactomannan and fungal PCRs.
- Pleural fluid culture.
- **Lung biopsy:** bacterial, fungal, viral culture, viral IF, or PCR, histology. Consider in unexplained, severe or deteriorating respiratory disease.

Pathogens
- **Viral:** RSV, CMV, adenovirus, para-influenza 1–4, influenza A/B, HMPV.
- **Bacterial:** *Strep. pneumoniae*, *H. influenzae*, *M. catharralis*, *Pseudomonas* spp., *Klebsiella* spp., mycoplasma, *Chlamydia pneumoniae*, *Nocardia*.
- **Fungal:** PCP; moulds, e.g. *Aspergillus* spp., Fusarium, Mucor; yeasts, e.g. *Candida* spp., *Cryptococcus neoformans*.

Management
Initial empirical treatment:
Initial choice must cover likely bacterial pathogens, as well as *Pneumocystis*, if there is any suggestion of or risk for this. Local bacterial patterns and resistances should be considered. Treatment should include streptococcal and *Pseudomonas* cover, as well as mycoplasma and Chlamydia, especially in those over 3 years old. This may incorporate meropenem, ceftazidime, or Tazocin, a macrolide ± high dose IV cotrimoxazole.

Further empirical management in the event of deterioration
- Add high dose IV cotrimoxazole if not already started.
- Add voriconazole or amphotericin.
- Further investigations as above.

Specific treatment;
RSV

Ribavirin: nebulized or IV.
- IVIg 0.4g/kg once weekly.
- There is anecdotal and minimal literature on the use of palivizumab (humanized monoclonal antibody directed against RSV) as treatment. In the severely immunocompromised child with significant disease this may be a potential option.

CMV
- Ganciclovir: IV 6mg/kg bd
- IVIg: 0.4 g/kg twice weekly
- Foscarnet or cidofovir are alternatives if no there is improvement or if use of ganciclovir is precluded due to concern about bone marrow suppression:
  - foscarnet requires careful administration to avoid renal dysfunction. Prolonged infusion over 18h, rather than standard tds dosing can help reduce this;
  - cidofovir is given with probenecid and requires careful fluid management to prevent renal dysfunction.
- Oral valganciclovir is a realistic alternative to IV ganciclovir in older children (>5 years) who are able to swallow tablets, as the blood levels achieved are equivalent to those with IV ganciclovir. Valganciclovir suspension will be commercially available in the near future. Some pharmacies are able to manufacture solutions locally, although the pharmacokinetics of these are uncertain.

NB. If poor response on ganciclovir (or valganciclovir), blood levels should be measured to ensure therapeutic dosing has been achieved.

Adenovirus
- Ribavirin (nebulized or IV) or cidofovir.
- IVIg 0.4g/kg twice weekly.
- Adenovirus type can guide initial therapy. *In vitro*, only subtype C is sensitive to both ribavirin and cidofovir (all other subtypes are resistant to ribavirin).
- Overwhelming adenoviral infection is extremely difficult to treat and outcome is poor.

Influenza
- Oral oseltamivir for 10 days.
- Cover for secondary bacterial infection.

Para-influenza
No effective antiviral treatment. Although a few case reports describe use of ribavirin, there is no *in vitro* evidence to support this.

Pneumocytis
Typically presents with unexpectedly low oxygen saturation.
- IV cotrimoxazole 180mg/kg tds for 14–21 days.
- IV methylprednisolone 1mg/kg for 14 days.

- Alternative (or 2nd line) anti-*Pneumocystis* treatments include:
  - clindamycin and primaquine;
  - pentamidine;
  - dapsone;
  - atovaquone (oral);
  - important side effects include methaemaglobinaemia with primaquine and dapsone.

Nocardia

IV cotrimoxazole: a high rate of relapse and late metastatic disease necessitates long-term treatment, with 3–4 months for minor infection and up to 1 year for systemic disease. Although primary infection is most frequently pulmonary, blood vessel erosion may lead to disseminated disease, especially in CNS.

Aspergillus

- **IV amphotericin:** *Aspergillus* invades blood vessels and airways causing haemorrhagic infarction, haemoptysis, haematogenous spread, and pneumonia, abscess, and cavity formation. Paranasal sinuses are often also involved.
- Alternatives include:
  - voriconazole (available in IV and oral preparations);
  - caspofungin (IV).
- Most experience is with amphotericin, usually given in liposomal form as 1st line treatment in children. AmBisome and Abelcet are both widely used. Initial AmBisone treatment dose 1–3mg/kg daily, increasing to 5–6mg/kg/day when required.
- Voriconazole is increasingly used as a first line antifungal agent for empiric and specific treatment.
- Surgical resection may be necessary for localized lung lesions.
- Treatment is usually for 3–4 weeks, but is usually tailored according to response and neutrophil count recovery.

Mucormycosis

This includes infections with species in the class *Zygomycetes*. A slowly progressive, insidious, pneumonia with angio-invasion, and frequent dissemination, especially to the CNS. Traditionally, these infections have been difficult to treat with variable clinical response to amphotericin and high mortality. Recent evidence suggests that posaconazole may have promising activity.

Candida

Isolated respiratory disease is unusual:
- fluconazole;
- voriconazole.

Combination antifungal treatment

No evidence yet to suggest that combinations of antifungals are more effective than monotherapy. However, combination treatment is increasingly used, and some *in vitro* data suggests a synergistic effect of caspofungin and voriconzole, each of which acts via a different mechanism.

Orointestinal infections

Mucositis due to chemotherapy or radiotherapy (Mucositis 📖 pp.254–255) leads to breakdown of mucosal protection and is a major potential route of infection in immunocompromised children.

Local infection around gums, buccal mucosa, and pharynx may be caused by oral anaerobes (gingivitis), *Candida*, or HSV. Oral candidiasis may respond to oral nystatin, miconazole, or require systemic treatment with either fluconazole, voriconazole, or amphotericin. Oral HSV requires oral (if mild) or more commonly IV aciclovir.

Oesophagitis
Pain on swallowing. May be difficult to detect clinically in the young child. Diagnosis is suggested by barium swallow or endoscopy, although a swab or biopsy is required for identification of pathogen. Treatment is often therefore empirical. *Candida*, HSV, and bacteria (Gram +ve) are the likeliest pathogens.

Typhlitis (neutropenic enterocolitis)
- Inflammatory necrotizing cellulitis of caecum, associated historically with Gram −ve organisms and a high mortality rate.
- Subacute or acute right lower quadrant abdominal pain becoming generalized.
- Fever, diarrhoea, bleeding with circulatory collapse.
- Ultrasound shows bowel wall thickening, ascites.
- Treat with antibiotics to cover Gram −ves (e.g. meropenem, Tazocin).
- **Surgery:** resection may be necessary, but only if significant bleeding or signs of perforation.

Table 17.1

Organism	Ampho	Vori	Posa	Caspo	Flucon	Itra
Asp.fumigatus	S	S	S	S	R	S Occ R
Asp.flavus	S	S	S	S	R	S
Asp.terreus	Often R	S	S	S	R	S
Zygomycetes	S Occ R	R	S	R	R	R
C.guilliermondii	S	S	S	S Occ I	S Often R	S Occ R
C.albicans	S	S	S	S	S	S
C.glabrata	S	S Occ I or R	S	S	Often I or R	Often I or R
C.krusei	S	S	S	S	I or R	Often I Occ R
C.parapsilosis	S	S	S	I or R Occ S	S	S
C.lusitanea	S	S	S	S Occ R	S	S
Rhodotorola	S	Often I or R	S	R	R	I or R
Scedosporium	Often R	S Occ R	S	R Occ S	R	S Occ I or R
Trichosporon spp.	S Occ R	S	S	R	S	S Occ I
Cryptococcus neoformans	S Occ R	S	S	S	S Occ I	Often I

S, sensitive; I, intermediate resistance; R, resistant; Occ, occasionally; Ampho, amphotericin; Vori, voriconazole; Posa, posaconazole; Caspo, caspofungin; Flucon, fluconazole; Itra, itraconazole.

Gastrointestinal infections

Presentation
- Acute or chronic diarrhoea.
- Prolonged, profuse diarrhoea; subsequent malnutrition, malabsorption, failure to thrive, abdominal pain, fever.
- Diarrhoea either caused by persistence of an enteropathogen or by damage to gastrointestinal mucosa from a pathogen.
- Pain.

Pathogens
- **Fungus:** *Candida, Aspergillus.*
- **Virus:** rotavirus, norovirus (small round structured virus [SRSV]), adenovirus, CMV, HSV.
- **Bacteria:** *Salmonella, Campylobacter, Yersinia, Listeria, Mycobacterium avium,* Gram –ve bacilli.
- **Protozoa:** *Giardia, Cryptosporidia,* microsporidia.
- **Toxin:** *Clostridium difficile.*

Investigations
It is very important to know what tests your microbiology/virology laboratory use and which pathogens are routinely tested for. Norovirus and *Cryptosporidia* may not be tested for unless specifically requested.
- **Stool culture:** bacteria, viruses.
- Stool electron microscopy (EM).
- **Stool enzyme immunoassay (EIA):** rotavirus, *C. difficile* toxin.
- **Microscopy:** *Giardia, Cryptosporidia.*
- PCR (norovirus, *Cryptosporidia*).

Further investigations
- Endoscopy and colonoscopy.
- **Bowel biopsy:** histology, microscopy, culture, EM, EIA, PCR.
- **Blood PCR:** CMV, adenovirus.

Management
Should be directed at pathogen. Empirical treatment is difficult.
- Pay careful attention to fluid replacement, electrolyte balance, and nutrition.
- **Rotavirus, norovirus:** supportive management only. No specific therapy available.
- **Adenovirus, CMV:** treatment not always necessary. May be required in disseminated, symptomatic disease.
- *Campylobacter:* transmission occurs by food or water. Presents with bloody diarrhoea. Increased incidence in lymphopenic patients (especially with low CD4 counts in HIV) and may cause severe disease in hypogammaglobulinaemia. Treat with ciprofloxacin or erythromycin.
- *C. difficile:* environmental colonization very common, symptoms occur only when toxins are produced, causing mucosal damage and inflammation. Risk factors include cytotoxic chemotherapy and antibiotics. Presents with watery diarrhoea, hypoalbuminaemia, and in severe

disease, toxic megacolon. However, young children often have toxin present, which is not necessarily pathogenic. Treat with oral metronidazole preferentially or vancomycin.

- **Salmonella:** more frequent in sickle cell disease, HIV infection and in defects of IL-12/γ-IFN pathways. Fulminant disease (e.g. in HIV) results in entercolitis, bacteraemia, and death.
- **Yersinia:** disease spectrum ranges from mild enterocolitis to systemic infection with disseminated disease and abscess formation (e.g. liver, spleen). Iron overload increases risk of Yersinia infection. Cefotaxime, cotrimoxazole and aminoglycosides are usually effective.
- **Giardia:** treat with oral metronidazole.
- **Cryptosporidia:** macrolides, especially azithromycin, may have some effect. Nitazoxonide has been shown to speed resolution of cryptosporidial diarrhoea in the immunocompetent patient.

Central nervous system infections

CNS infections are relatively infrequent. Important to consider differential diagnosis, since neurological symptoms and signs may be caused by drug-induced toxicity (e.g. methotrexate, cyclosporin A), or progression of malignant disease. Symptoms include gradual or rapid alteration in mental status, confusion, headache, cranial nerve palsies (e.g. VI), signs of raised intracranial pressure, proptosis, seizures, meningism, focal neurological signs, such as hemiparesis, visual fields defects. Infection may be focal or meningoencephalitis/meningitis.

Pathogens

- **Aspergillus:** presents with multifocal cerebral abscesses, rather than cerebellar or brain stem lesions, and may be associated with tissue infarction as a result of angio-invasive disease. Commonly occurs in association with another focus of infection; most often in the respiratory tract.
- **Candida:** typically presents with multiple small lesions located in the grey or deep white matter.
- **Zygomycetes:** classically infects the rhino-facial-cranial area, with blood vessel invasion causing tissue embolization and necrosis, and secondary, suppurative pyogenic infections. Cavernous sinus and internal carotid artery thrombosis may complicate the clinical picture.
- **Bacteria:** Klebsiella, Pseudomonas aeruginosa, and Staphylococcus aureus are often implicated in both cerebral abscesses and meningitis. Anaerobic streptococci are also seen in abscesses, whilst meningitis may be caused by Streptococcus pneumoniae, Haemophilus influenzae, or rarely Listeria.
- Toxoplasma has a predilection for the CNS and causes infection either by local invasion or haematogenous spread to the brain. Cysts may form with surrounding calcification in the brain, giving typical CT changes. Prognosis is often poor, with published mortality rates of 40–66%.
- **Nocardia:** usually secondary to pulmonary disease.

- **Viral infections:** CMV, adenovirus, parvovirus, HSV, HHV6. HHV6 is associated with febrile seizures in immunocompetent children and in the severely immunocompromised it can be a rare CNS pathogen.
- *Cryptococcus:* most often presenting as meningitis, with gradual onset of symptoms and headache. Primary infection may be mild pulmonary disease.
- *JC virus:* a human polyoma virus causing a usually fatal, progressive, demyelinating disease throughout the CNS, presenting as progressive multifocal leucoencephalopathy (PML).

Investigations

- **Radiology:** CT scan and/or MRI scan with contrast. May demonstrate:
  - single or multiple abscesses;
  - *location* – periventricular, grey, or white matter;
  - ring enhancing lesions (*Toxoplasma*, tuberculosis);
  - hydrocephalus;
  - meningeal enhancement.
- The respiratory tract should be imaged to look for evidence of fungal infection in any patient found to have a brain abscess.
- **Biopsy:** either brain lesion itself or a lung lesion if present. Send for histology and culture (including fungal and mycobacterial). Histology of biopsied areas may be suggestive, whilst tissue and CSF cultures are diagnostic, but not sensitive. Look for *Toxoplasma* and JC virus with PCR.
- **CSF:** microscopy, India ink staining (*Cryptococcus*), protein, glucose, cell count, cryptococcal antigen, viral, and bacterial culture. PCR for CMV, HSV, HHV6, adenovirus, *Toxoplasma*, *Streptococcus pneumoniae*, meningococcus where necessary.
- **Blood:** PCR for *Streptococcus pneumoniae*, meningococcus, CMV, adenovirus, *Aspergillus*.

Management

- **Yeast or fungal:** amphotericin B or liposomal derivatives. Voriconazole penetrates the brain and CSF, and is likely to be useful in treatment of most CNS mould and yeast infections.
- **Zygomycoses:** posaconazole has potential in the treatment of zygomycoses. Given the very high mortality associated with fungal brain abscesses and rhino-cerebral mould infection, many clinicians currently utilize a combination of antifungal agents.
- *Toxoplasma:* pyrimethamine and sulphadiazine, with clindamycin and pyrimethamine as an alternative. Folinic acid should also be added. Steroids may be useful to prevent intracranial pressure effects. Treatment should be continued for at least 6 weeks and maintenance considered whilst immunosuppression continues.
- *Cryptococcus:* combination of amphotericin and either fluconazole or flucytosine for 2 weeks, or until CSF is sterile, followed by at least 10 weeks further treatment with amphotericin B or fluconazole.
- **Bacterial:** standard broad spectrum empirical antibacterial treatment often includes a combination of 3rd generation cephalosporin, metronidazole and amoxicillin.
- **Viral:** directed at pathogen.

Skin and soft tissue infections

- Skin is often compromised by indwelling CVADs, biopsy needles, or mucositis. Frequent antibiotic courses encourage *Candida* skin colonization. Folliculitis is also relatively common, often much more extensive than that seen in immunocompetent individuals.
- Rashes are frequently viral. Reflect usual childhood pathogens, though disease may be more severe.

Pathogens

- **Virus:** HHV6, HHV7, HSV, VZV, enterovirus, adenovirus, measles, rubella, parovirus B19, molluscum.
- VZV may cause an overwhelming systemic disease with pneumonitis.
- **Parvovirus:** as well as typical slapped cheek rash may cause red cell aplasia and severe chronic anaemia.
- *Staphylococci* and *Streptococci* are common, but Gram –ve organisms, such as *E. coli*, *Klebsiella*, and *Pseudomonas* less so.
- Fungal skin infections (e.g. intertrigo, nappy rash) occur commonly. Superficial fungal infection are usually due to *Candida* or other yeasts (e.g. *Saccharomyces*) and should be treated with topical agents in the first instance, after sending appropriate swabs or skin scrapings to the microbiology laboratory. *Candida* spp. and other yeasts may be responsible and sensitivity, especially to azoles, cannot be predicted. Rarely skin lesions are due to disseminated yeast infection (*Candida* or *Cryptococcus*). Mould infections of skin, other than dermatophytes, are usually as a result of invasion from a deep-seated invasive infections.
- Ecthema gangrenosum is a skin disorder specific to neutropenic patients, which occurs as a result of infection within deep subcutaneous veins.
  - Most often due to bacteria such as *Pseudomonas aeruginosa*, but can also occur 2° to fungal infection, such as aspergillosis or mucormycosis.
  - Clinically, the lesions are painful, well circumscribed, bright red, and usually just palpable with a ring or surrounding pallor. Over a relatively short time (24h) the centre becomes darker and may be raised into a bulla. Eventually, the sharply demarcated central portion becomes black.
  - Treatment of these lesions is best guided by identification of the responsible organism. Biopsies may be necessary.

Investigation

- Blood culture.
- Blood PCR for herpes virus, enterovirus, parvovirus.
- **Skin swab, scraping:** microscopy and culture for bacteria and fungi. PCR for herpes virus, enterovirus, parvovirus. EM for virus and molluscum.

Management

- Antibiotic therapy may be chosen empirically, particularly if the patient is profoundly neutropenic, but treatment should be guided by cultures of the particular lesions.
- **HSV, VZV:** aciclovir.
- **Parvovirus:** IVIg.

Urinary tract infection

Risk increased where obstruction is present, e.g. related to tumour, catheterization, neurological damage, or local effects of surgery or radiotherapy.

Pathogens
- Gram −ve bacilli.
- Entercococci.

Diagnosis and investigation
- Symptoms, e.g. dysuria, urgency, frequency, fever.
- Urine dipstick and microscopy: if positive, send for culture.
- Pyuria may not be present if neutropenic.

Management
- IV empirical broad spectrum antibiotic therapy may be chosen initially, following local guidelines, particularly if the patient is profoundly neutropenic. It may be appropriate, initially, to use oral antibiotics in afebrile and asymptomatic patients, especially if non-neutropenic, whilst awaiting confirmation of culture results and sensitivities.
- Colonization with *Candida* is seen in catheterized patients, especially in presence of concomitant broad spectrum antimicrobial treatment. Two or more persistently positive cultures with fever should be treated.
- Prophylaxis should be commenced and subsequent appropriate imaging performed, depending on age and local guidelines.

Blood transfusion

Introduction

Patients with malignant disease frequently have potentially dangerous cytopenias or coagulation disturbances as a result of their disease and its treatment. The ability to support patients with appropriate blood component transfusion has made a major contribution to improved survival. Knowledge of the availability of a wide range of blood components and how they are produced, stored, selected, and administered under carefully quality controlled conditions is fundamental to oncological practice.

Safe transfusion practice

Even with the most rigorous quality control, no blood product transfusion is without risks from various types of allergic or immunological reaction, volume overload, or the transmission of infection. Blood product transfusion must not be undertaken unless appropriately indicated and in the absence of alternatives (e.g. correction of haematinic deficiency).

Careful donor selection is undertaken by transfusion services in order to minimize the risks of transmissible infections. Potential donors with lifestyle risk factors for HIV and hepatitis infection are excluded, and time-sensitive geographical exclusions are applied to minimize the risk of malaria and other tropical zoonoses. Because of the theoretical, but unquantifiable risk of new variant CJD prion transmission, potential donors who have received blood transfusion in countries (such as the UK) at times when bovine spongiform encephalitis has been endemic in cattle are excluded, and plasma for many blood products is sourced from countries where BSE has not been endemic.

UK donor blood is tested for antibody and antigen evidence of hepatitis A and B, HIV 1 and 2 infection, and for serological evidence of syphilis infection. A proportion of products is screened for serological evidence of CMV infection, so that CMV antibody negative products can be made available to immunosuppressed recipients at risk of this complication. For some plasma products, viral inactivation with detergent or heat treatment can provide additional safety. Since 1999, cellular blood products for transfusion in the UK have been leucodepleted.

Patient, specimen, and product identification and recording

Cellular blood products and fresh frozen plasma for transfusion need to be blood group compatible with the recipient. It is critically important that blood group specimen identification is accurate and specific. Three points of reference (e.g. name, date of birth, hospital number) are required on the specimen tube. Prelabelled tubes and preprinted labels have been identified as a major risk factor for mislabelling, and in the UK handwritten specimen tube labelling immediately after collection is required. Most hospital blood banks operate a 'zero tolerance' approach to breaches of labelling protocol because of the potentially dangerous consequences.

Cellular products are issued from blood banks specifically labelled for the individual recipient. Checking of the product label against patient identification and blood group record by more than one appropriately qualified member of staff is important. The unit numbers of all transfused products must be recorded in the recipient's notes.

Storage, expiry dates, and usage

Products must be used within their stated expiry dates. Products requiring refrigeration must only be stored in appropriated designated and monitored blood bank fridges, and transfused within appropriate timescales following removal. Products should be checked for bag damage, unusual appearance, or discoloration that might herald contamination or infection. Any warming of products must only be undertaken with appropriately certified equipment.

Risks of blood transfusion

Allergic reactions

Minor pyrexial reactions to blood product transfusions due to recipient anti-HLA antibodies are less common since the introduction of leucodepletion of blood components and can usually be managed by slowing the rate of transfusion and/or administration of an antipyretic (e.g. paracetamol).

Immediate-type hypersensitivity reactions may manifest as an urticarial or maculopapular rash or as generalized erythema. The transfusion should be interrupted. Administration of an antihistamine (e.g. chorphenamine) and steroid (hydrocortisone) may be considered. More severe anaphylactic reactions with bronchospasm and/or hypotension are rare. Intravenous colloid and/or adrenaline administration may be necessary.

Haemolytic transfusion reactions

Haemolysis is caused by recipient antibody against donor red cells.

Acute

Immediate intravascular haemolysis is almost always due to anti-A or anti-B antibodies due to ABO incompatibility. This implies an error in the identification of the patient either at the time of the collection of the compatibility testing sample or at the time of administration. Suspicion of this complication should prompt an immediate review of patient and component identity paperwork. A rapid temperature rise to >40°C should prompt immediate cessation of the transfusion. Other symptoms and signs of this complication include:

- **Patient agitation/anxiety:** 'a feeling of impending doom'.
- Abdominal, flank or chest pain, pain at infusion site.
- Nausea, vomiting, diarrhoea.
- Fever, hypotension.
- Bleeding from venepuncture sites/wounds.
- Haemoglobinuria/haemoglobinaemia.

Management of a suspected acute haemolytic reaction

- Stop the transfusion, recheck all identity paperwork, inform transfusion laboratory.
- Change giving set, maintain IV fluid.
- Monitor urine output accurately (catheterization may be necessary).
- Appropriate IV colloid support to maintain urine output (consider CVP monitoring).
- Consult senior medical staff for advice.

Delayed

Previous sensitization due to transfusion (or pregnancy) may stimulate antibodies to red cell antigens, which then fall to a low level undetectable at compatibility testing. Re-exposure to the same antigen by subsequent transfusion may then restimulate antibody production. Haemolysis may manifest as anaemia, jaundice and sometimes haemoglobinuria occurring 7–10 days after the transfusion. A direct antiglobulin test (DAT) is positive, and the antibody will be detectable in the serum. Further transfusion with appropriate antigen-negative blood may be necessary.

Post-transfusion purpura

This is a rare, but potentially dangerous delayed transfusion reaction causing profound thrombocytopenia 5–10 days after red cell or platelet component transfusion. It is caused when an individual negative for the HPA-1a platelet antigen (<2% of the population) has been previously sensitized to HPA-1a (by transfusion or pregnancy). Anti-HPA-1a antibody stimulated by the subsequent transfusion complexes with antigen and is adsorbed on to the recipient's HPA-1a negative platelets resulting in immune destruction. Management includes administration of IVIg and platelet support. Plasmapheresis may be considered.

Alloimmunization

Red cell (and platelet) component transfusion may stimulate antibody production against cell surface antigens not possessed by the recipient. This is fortunately relatively rare in the oncology patient population, partly perhaps because of the immunosuppressive effects of therapy. It is more common in the context of haemoglobinopathy (e.g. sickle cell disease and thalassaemia), where in addition to the frequency of transfusion and the absence of immunosuppression, ethnic differences between donor and recipient populations may play a part. In these patients more extensive red cell genotyping is undertaken, allowing selection of donor red cells matched for Rhesus and Kell antigen status.

Transfusion related acute lung injury (TRALI)

This fortunately rare reaction is characterized by acute respiratory distress with hypoxia and pulmonary shadowing on chest X-ray despite normal central venous pressure, and occurs within 1–6h of the administration of plasma-containing blood products. It is thought to be due to the effects of donor anti-HLA antibodies on granulocytes in susceptible individuals. The incidence has been reduced by the exclusion of multiparous donors as a source of fresh frozen plasma (FFP) and platelet products. Management includes intensive respiratory support with oxygen and if necessary mechanical ventilation. High dose steroid therapy may be effective.

Transfusion-associated graft-versus-host disease (TA-GvHD)

Cellular blood products may contain small numbers of circulating stem cells. Individuals with marked T-cell immunosuppression are at risk of engraftment of these stem cells, with the effect of achieving an HLA unselected stem cell transplant. The consequent graft-versus-host disease (GvHD) in this situation is life-threatening. Gamma irradiation (to prevent subsequent cell division) of cellular blood products prior to transfusion is therefore mandatory for recipients at risk of this complication. Leucodepletion also provides some protection.

Transfusion transmitted infection

Bacterial contamination

This is rare, but dangerous and sometimes fatal, particularly with Gram −ve organisms. Sudden onset of marked fever, rigors, collapse, hypotension, oliguria, and disseminated intravascular coagulation (DIC) occur soon after the start of transfusion. Differential diagnosis is acute haemolytic transfusion reaction and TRALI. Discontinuation of transfusion, IV fluid resuscitation and broad spectrum IV antibiotics are required pending microbiological investigation of the product bag and patient culture specimens.

Other transfusion transmissible infections

- Hepatitis viruses C, B, G, E.
- Human immunodeficiency viruses (HIV 1 and 2).
- CMV.
- CJD and new variant CJD.
- West Nile virus.
- *Plasmodia*, Trypanosomes, and *Babesia*.

Iron overload

An adult red cell unit contains 250mg elemental iron. There is no physiological mechanism for excreting excess iron. Iron from red cell transfusions is accumulated in the body. This is more of a problem for patients with a long-term transfusion requirement (e.g. homozygous beta-thalassaemia, unresponsive Diamond Blackfan anaemia) than in oncological practice, when the duration of a transfusion requirement is often limited to a finite period of time on chemotherapy. If the serum ferritin rises significantly above 1000µg/l in the context of an ongoing red cell transfusion requirement, consideration should be given to chelation therapy with parenteral desferrioxamine.

Special requirements

CMV antibody-negative and irradiated donor material

CMV

Certain categories of immunosuppressed patient and low birth weight (LBW) infants are at risk of new or reactivated CMV infection after transfusion. CMV is harboured in white blood cells. The risk of transmission is considerably reduced by leucodepletion, and there is evidence that this may be as effective as CMV antibody-negative donor selection as a prevention strategy.

Indications for CMV antibody negative donor material are:
- Neonatal (and intrauterine) transfusion.
- Bone marrow and solid organ transplants who are CMV antibody-negative.
- Severe aplastic anaemia.
- GvHD on immunosuppressive therapy.
- Congenital cellular immunodeficiency syndromes.

Irradiation

Gamma irradiation (25Gy) of cellular blood products for transfusion is indicated to prevent the risk of TA-GvHD in the following recipients:
- Congenital cellular immunodeficiency syndromes.
- Intrauterine transfusion (IUT) or top-up transfusions in previous IUT recipients.
- LBW neonates.
- Recipients of autologous or allogeneic BMT.
- Any patient with Hodgkin disease.
- Recipients of HLA-matched cellular components (e.g. platelet transfusion).
- Recipients of blood products from family members.
- Recipients of granulocyte transfusions.
- Patients treated intensively with purine analogues (e.g. fludarabine) or other specific T-cell suppressants.

ABO compatibility

Within the first four months of life, cellular blood products need to be ABO compatible with the recipient <u>and</u> with the mother's serum. In older children, ABO compatibility selection is as shown in Table 18.1.

Table 18.1 ABO compatibility selection

Patient ABO group		Red cells	Platelets	FFP
O	1st choice	O	O	O
	2nd choice	No alternative	A	A, B, or AB
A	1st choice	A	A	A or AB
	2nd choice	O	O	No alternative
B	1st choice	B	B	B or AB
	2nd choice	O	A or O	No alternative
AB	1st choice	AB	AB	AB
	2nd choice	A or B	A	A
	3rd choice	O		

Group O products given to non-group O recipients should have been demonstrated to have low titres of anti-A and anti-B antibodies.

Special considerations apply to recipients of ABO-incompatible haemopoietic stem cell transplants:

- **Red cells:** Group O cells should be given until ABO antibodies to the donor ABO type are undetectable and DAT is negative. Thereafter, select donor group.
- **Platelets:** platelets of recipient group are given until there is conversion to donor group and antibodies to donor ABO group are undetectable. Thereafter select donor group.

Red cells

Preparations
In the UK, red cells for transfusion are supplied in units that are plasma depleted. The red cells are suspended in an anticoagulant additive solution with an average haematocrit of 0.65, a volume of about 280mL, and have a shelf life of 35 days at 4°C.

Compatibility testing
Red cells for transfusion should be ABO and RhD group compatible, and it must be established with a fresh recipient specimen that the recipient has no antibodies against any antigens which may be present on the proposed donor unit(s). In the UK, whenever a potential recipient 'Group and Screen' specimen is received by a hospital blood bank, the ABO group is determined by direct and reverse techniques (cells and plasma) and the RhD group established. The plasma is subjected to a sensitive antibody screen against a panel of cells which between them express all of the clinically significant red cell antigens against which antibodies might represent a clinically significant problem. The results are recorded against the patient's details in the blood bank computer.

The 'electronic cross-match'
If there is a previously documented result in the blood bank computer with the same ABO and RhD group (providing some evidence against the possibility of a mislabelled specimen), and the antibody screen is negative, then ABO and RhD compatible blood may be safely labelled for the recipient and issued without the need for further direct cross-match testing.

Cross-matching and further antibody testing
If a previous result is not available, direct cross-matching of cells from potential donor units against recipient plasma is undertaken.

If the antibody screen is positive, then identification of the specificity of the antibody is sought and appropriate antigen-negative blood selected. Direct cross-matching is then undertaken to confirm compatibility.

Indications for red cell transfusion

Red cell transfusion is undertaken in order to replace oxygen carrying capacity in anaemia due to acute blood loss, haemolysis unresponsive to therapy or marrow failure. Transfusion should not be used to correct chronic anaemia due to haematinic deficiency unless there is an urgent requirement to correct oxygen carrying capacity. There is no particular threshold haemoglobin (Hb) concentration, which indicates the need for transfusion. Multiple factors including symptomatology, oxygen delivery, and volume status need to be considered.

How much to transfuse?

For standard red cell concentrate transfusions the volume required may be calculated using the formula:

$$\text{Transfusion volume (mL)} = [\text{Desired Hb (g/dL)} - \text{Actual Hb}] \times \text{Body weight (kg)} \times 3$$

In practice, for routine 'top-up' transfusions, a dose of 10–15mL/kg will raise the Hb level by 2–3g/dL.

Rate of transfusion

For 'top-up' transfusions, where the recipient has no volume deficit an administration rate of 5mL/kg/h is appropriate. Faster infusions may be indicated if the recipient is hypovolaemic or tolerant of additional volume load. Slower rates ± consideration of diuretic therapy may be necessary if there is volume overload or cardiac compromise. Material from individual red cell units should be transfused within 4h of refrigeration for microbiological safety.

Massive transfusion

Replacement of more than a recipient's total blood volume in less than 24h is likely to result in dilution of plasma coagulation factors and platelets. Regular monitoring of the platelet count and plasma coagulation profile will enable logical component replacement (Platelets, 📖 p.241; Plasma components 📖 pp.242–243) aiming to maintain the platelet count above 50×10^9/L and the fibrinogen level above 1.0g/L if there is ongoing bleeding.

Platelets

Platelet concentrates are prepared either by separation from donated blood units, which are then pooled into a single bag or by donor apheresis into a single bag. Platelets for transfusion have a shelf life of 5 days. They are kept at room temperature rather than refrigerated, and require gentle agitation during storage. An adult platelet pool or apheresis unit will typically contain around 1.5×10^9 platelets/mL in 200–300mL plasma. Platelets for transfusion should be ABO and RhD compatible (see Table 18.1), but do not require individual compatibility testing.

Indications

Platelet transfusion support may be required for treatment of active bleeding, or to cover surgery or invasive procedures in patients with thrombocytopenia due to marrow failure or increased platelet destruction, or in patients with platelet dysfunction. Platelet transfusion is also indicated prophylactically for patients with marrow failure in order to prevent bleeding complications.

Prophylaxis

For paediatric oncology patients with reduced platelet production, the following guideline thresholds are appropriate:
- Platelet count $<10 \times 10^9$/L, no additional risk factors for bleeding.
- Platelet count $<20 \times 10^9$/L and high temperature/sepsis, severe mucositis, additional plasma coagulation abnormality.
- Platelet count $<50 \times 10^9$/L and active bleeding or impending invasive/ surgical procedure.

Dose and administration

- Children <15kg: 15ml/kg.
- Children >15kg: one adult platelet pool.

Platelet transfusions are given over 30min. Pyrexial reactions are not unusual in multiply transfused patients, and prophylactic IV chlorphenamine may be appropriate in selected patients.

Platelet refractoriness

An incremental increase in platelet count lasting at least 24h usually follows platelet transfusion. Increased consumption due to hypersplenism, DIC, or medication (e.g. amphotericin, anti-thymocyte globulin [ATG]) may abrogate this. Some multiply transfused patients develop anti-HLA antibodies, which cause destruction of randomly selected donor platelets. If a patient is demonstrated to have no numerical increment to platelet transfusion and has anti-HLA antibodies, HLA-compatible apheresis donor platelets may be available from the transfusion services.

Granulocytes

Granulocyte concentrates may be prepared by 'buffy coat' separation from donor blood units, or by donor apheresis. With modern antibiotic therapy and the availability of granulocyte colony stimulating factor (G-CSF), granulocyte transfusion is now very rarely used. HLA-sensitization is an obvious complication.

Granulocyte transfusion may be considered in the management of a patient with severe neutropenia with a documented severe bacterial or fungal infection not responding to therapy with antibiotics to which *in vitro* sensitivity has been demonstrated. Granulocytes for transfusion must be irradiated to prevent TA-GvHD.

Plasma components

Fresh frozen plasma

FFP provides volume and coagulation factor replacement. It is not indicated for volume replacement alone. FFP for children in the UK is currently sourced from US (minimizing new variant CJD risk) male (minimizing TRALI risk) donors, and subjected to viral inactivation with methylene blue and light. Solvent detergent-treated frozen plasma is an alternative equivalent product.

Indications

Treatment or prevention of bleeding in the context of multiple coagulation factor deficiency or single factor deficiency, where no specific coagulation factor preparation is available. Common situations include:
- Liver disease (**NB.** Vitamin K supplementation is also important).
- DIC.
- Massive blood transfusion.
- Replacement therapy following plasmapheresis.

Dosage and administration

FFP must be ABO compatible (see Table 18.1), but does not require individual compatibility testing. The RhD group is not relevant. A dose of 15mL/kg will provide haemostatic levels of coagulation factors. Once thawed it should be given as rapidly as volume tolerance permits.

Cryoprecipitate

This product is a rich source of fibrinogen and factor VIII in a small volume. It is no longer used in the treatment of haemophilia and von Willebrand disease (VWD) because of the availability of specific factor concentrates.

Indication

Maintenance of fibrinogen levels above 1.0g/L in DIC and massive transfusion, particularly if poor volume tolerance compromises the use of FFP.

Dose

I unit/5–10kg of recipient weight. The thawed pooled product should be administered as quickly as volume tolerance permits. Units should be ABO compatible (as for FFP).

Human albumin solution

This is available in the UK in 2 concentrations – 4.5% (physiological) in saline, and 20% in water ('salt-poor'). The use of human albumin solution (HAS) as a volume expander has been largely replaced by crystalloid and synthetic colloid preparations. It should not be used for the treatment of mild nutritional hypoalbuminaemia, but may be useful in the management of nephrotic syndrome resistant to diuretics and after large volume paracentesis.

Coagulation factor concentrates

Specific factor concentrates are available for the treatment of inherited deficiencies:

- Fibrinogen (cryoprecipitate also useful).
- Factor VIII.
- Factor IX.
- Factor XI.
- Factor XIII.
- Prothrombin complex concentrates (factors II, VII, IX, and X) are used in addition to vitamin K for the management of bleeding in the context of warfarin over-anticoagulation.
- Factor VIII inhibitor by-pass agent (FEIBA) and recombinant factor VIIa are used in the management of clinical problems due to factor VIII inhibitors.
- Recombinant factor VIIa may also be used in the context of life-threatening haemorrhage unresponsive to appropriate component replacement in discussion with a senior haematologist.

Pain

Pain

Pain is a common symptom and a major problem for children during the different phases of cancer treatment. The type and severity of pain experienced by children with cancer varies:
- Pain due to organ or tissue infiltration by the tumour.
- Treatment-related, e.g. side effects of chemotherapy and/or radiation treatment.
- Procedure-related pain, e.g. lumbar puncture (LP), bone marrow aspiration (BMA) and post-operative pain.
- Progressive chronic pain associated with disease progression.

Pain associated with cancer treatment is often the most overriding concern for children and their families.
- Ineffective management of pain interferes with sleep, and leads to fatigue and a sense of helplessness.
- Experience and interpretation of pain is strongly influenced by the child's maturity, cognitive development, and degree of dependence. Children are not simply little adults.
- In identifying and treating pain in children with cancer, one must keep in mind the complexity of pain as a physiological, psychological, and social phenomenon.

Types of pain

There are two main types of pain:
- **Nociceptive:** somatic and visceral pain transmitted through normal intact nociceptors and neurones. This includes organ, bone, and other non-neuropathic pain.
- Neuropathic pain: occurs when the normal pathway of nerve conduction is interrupted by nerve compression or destruction giving rise to abnormal pain conduction. Frequently due to tumour compression or infiltration, but nerves can also be damaged by surgery, chemotherapy, or radiotherapy. May be related to peripheral nerve injury, central spinal or brain lesions. Usually described as a burning or stabbing sensation, which is not adequately relieved by opiates.

Assessment of pain

Before pain can be successfully managed or controlled, it must first be assessed. In assessing pain, the healthcare professional should always assume that the child's report of pain is valid. Assessment should be an integrated process within pain management. A validated assessment tool should be selected based upon age, developmental stage, and clinical condition of the child. It is important that continuity is maintained by using the same tool throughout the child's pain experience.

One can use a number of strategies to assess pain:

• Visual analogue scale.
• Faces pain scale.
• Pain diary.
• Observation.

Drugs are the mainstay of pain management. Accurate and timely pain assessments lead to appropriate administration of the appropriate drug at the time of need. Assessment should be a continuous process at appropriate time intervals, especially after analgesia has been administered. It is important to ensure ongoing evaluation and to monitor the appropriateness, efficacy and side effects of management.

Management

The principles of pain management include:
- The application of the WHO analgesic ladder (Fig. 19.1), appropriate drug dose escalation, the use of adjuvant analgesics, and the use of non pharmacological methods of pain control. Note that in the WHO publications recommendations are based on expert opinion, rather than evidence; little research has focused on pain control in paediatric oncology.
- Effective pain management is essential in children, and there should be ready access to specialist multidisciplinary pain services available for advice and support in complex pain management.

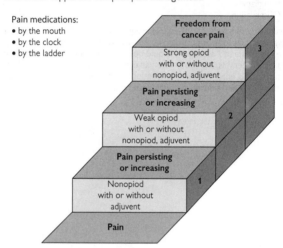

Pain medications:
- by the mouth
- by the clock
- by the ladder

Freedom from cancer pain

Strong opiod with or without nonopiod, adjuvent 3

Pain persisting or increasing

Weak opiod with or without nonopiod, adjuvent 2

Pain persisting or increasing

Nonopiod with or without adjuvent 1

Pain

Fig. 19.1 WHO Pain Ladder. Source: www.who,int/cancer/palliative/painladder/en

Pharmacological interventions

Initial drug doses should be individualized on the basis of age, weight, disease status, and previous or current analgesic exposure. The need for drug therapy is frequent and doses required for the child can be as high or higher as those used in adults.

It needs first to be established whether the pain is nociceptive or neuropathic in nature or a combination of both.

It is often necessary in severe pain to establish whether the pain is opiod sensitive by using escalating doses of opiods. If the pain is sensitive to opiods then the correct dose of short-acting opiods should first be used before calculating the dose of longer acting opiods, e.g. use sevredol/ oramorph to start with then use MST/fenatnyl patch). Breakthrough pain should be controlled with boosts of short acting opiods. The same principles apply if using IV morphine. Breakthrough pain for morphine/diamorphine infusions are in the form of boosts via the infusion pumps.

The severity of the pain determines the type of analgesia used but care should be taken when prescribing antipyretic analgesia as it may mask underlying infection in immunocompromised children. Caution should also be used when prescribing non-steroidal anti-inflammatories as they may affect platelet function especially in thrombocytopaenic patients.

Analgesics for mild to moderate pain
- Non opioids, e.g. paracetamol.
- Opioids, e.g. codeine phosphate, dihydrocodeine.

Analgesics for moderate to severe pain
Opioids, e.g. morphine, diamorphine, oxycodone, hydromorphone, fentanyl. Most common side-effects of opioids are:
- Excessive sedation.
- Respiratory depression.
- Nausea and vomiting.
- Pruritis.
- Constipation.
- Urinary retention.

Co-analgesics
Non-steroidal anti-inflammatory drugs
- Diclofenac, ibuprofen, celecoxib.
- Corticosteroids.
- Dexamethasone.

Treatment of neuropathic pain

- Imipramine, amitriptyline.
- Sodium valproate.
- Gabapentin.
- Carbamazepine.

Pain should be treated by regularly prescribed administration of medication sufficient to control pain with closely monitored titration of the medications in response to the child's needs.

Non-pharmacological interventions

It is important to recognize the importance of non-pharmacological intervention. This should not be regarded as a substitute for analgesics, but rather as a means to increase the effectiveness of the pharmacological management. Play and the use of play techniques enhance coping skills. Play specialists and activity co-ordinators are able to facilitate, and assist in preparation for painful procedures utilizing strategies dependent on age and cognitive development.

Strategies can be divided into:
- Physical, e.g. heat, cold stimulation, acupuncture, and massage.
- Behavioural, e.g. relaxation, art/play therapy, distraction.
- Cognitive, e.g. distraction, imagery, play therapy, music therapy, hypnosis.

Routes of administration

Analgesia should be administered to children by the simplest safest most effective and least painful route. The oral route of administration is therefore the first choice.

Indications for alternatives are:
- Persistent vomiting.
- 'Nil by mouth'.
- Bowel obstruction.
- Patient too weak to take oral preparations.
- Unsatisfactory response to oral medication.
- Child's dislike of oral medication.

Alternatives to the oral route of administration are:
- Intravenous.
- Subcutaneous.
- Intramuscular (not indicated in paediatrics).
- Rectal.
- Epidural/intrathecal.
- Transdermal.
- Buccal.

The route of administration of the drug may be determined by the choice of drug and the indication for its use.

Conclusion

Diagnosis of the cause and treatment of pain are crucial components in the care of children with cancer. Pain control and treatment can be improved by:
- Increased education.
- Regular use of pain analysis.
- Pain intensity measurement.
- Regular contact with pain specialists.

Giving information to children and parents about pain and pain treatment will significantly enhance communication about pain.

The challenge of pain management in children with cancer can only be met if the goal of pain control is associated with an acceptable side effect profile, and an improvement in function and quality of life.

Other aspects of supportive care

Mucositis

Mucositis is painful inflammation and ulceration of the mucosal membranes. The mouth is affected most commonly, but any part of the gastrointestinal tract (GIT) may be involved. Other mucous membranes (e.g. larynx) may be affected, but less commonly.

Epidemiology

Mucositis is one of the commonest complications of treatment for childhood malignancy, affecting 35–75% of patients depending on the nature of the treatment. Its severity varies from mild to very severe, but the most extreme form (neutropenic enterocolitis, typhlitis) is rare (2–3% of patients, usually during induction treatment for acute leukaemia).

Diagnosis

Mucositis is diagnosed clinically, in the presence of:
- **Gastro-intestinal tract pain:** severity should be assessed by a Pain Score scale.
- **Mucosal ulceration:** often → reduced oral intake and impaired nutrition.
- **Diarrhoea:** not always present.

▶ Remember to consider, diagnose (swabs → microbiology and virology), and treat concomitant or superadded infection of the ulcerated mucosa.

Typhlitis is characterized by severe abdominal pain and tenderness, often with fever and paralytic ileus, and may be complicated by haemorrhage or bowel perforation. Abdominal ultrasound or CT scan findings may support the diagnosis, and exclude other intra-abdominal pathology.

Causes

Mucositis may be caused by:
- **Chemotherapy:** especially anthracyclines, high dose methotrexate, etoposide, high dose alkylating agents.
- **Radiotherapy:** especially head and neck, abdominal or total body irradiation (TBI).

It may also be exacerbated by infection, e.g. *Candida*, *Herpes simplex*.

Management

Prevention is important:
- Maintenance of regular routine dental check-ups should reduce the potential for intra-oral infection.
- Vigorous mouth care is often employed in an effort to prevent or reduce the severity of mucositis and/or infection, although clear evidence of efficacy is lacking.
- Mouth washes are used to keep oral mucosa moist and local analgesic preparations (e.g. Difflam) may reduce pain.
- Dental brushing should be continued with soft toothbrushes.
- Lips should be protected to reduce cracking.

Treatment of established mucositis comprises:
- **Removal of pain:** often needs parenteral opioids.
- Maintenance of hydration and nutritional status.
- Treatment of concomitant or superadded infection:
  - *oral candidiasis* – systemically absorbed antifungal agent, e.g. fluconazole;
  - *herpetic gingivostomatitis* – acyclovir.

Anti-diarrhoeal agents are seldom used in children with mucositis, although loperamide (and/or an octreotide infusion) may reduce severe diarrhoea due to irinotecan or HSCT.

Typhlitis can usually be managed successfully by using a similar conservative non-surgical approach, reserving operations only for ill children with evidence of perforation, gut necrosis, or bleeding refractory to medical treatment.

Outcome

Whilst rarely life-threatening (except in typhlitis), mucositis causes considerable pain, diarrhoea, weight loss, and impaired quality of life, and has been associated with an increased risk of severe infection.

Non-operative management of typhlitis is generally effective with only a small mortality rate (≤5%).

Long-term sequelae of mucositis are rare.

Nausea and vomiting

Nausea and vomiting are considered to be amongst the most distressing side effects of cancer treatment with approximately 70–80% of patients receiving chemotherapy experiencing these symptoms. They may lead to significant physical consequences, such as dehydration, electrolyte imbalance, anorexia, weight loss, and increased susceptibility to infection. Psychological morbidity is also a significant problem, often resulting in non-compliance with chemotherapy, thereby compromising the delivery of optimal treatment.

Nausea and vomiting can be classified as follows:
- **Acute:** occurring within 24h of therapy.
- **Delayed:** occurring >24h after initiation of therapy and persisting for up to 7 days after completion of treatment.
- **Anticipatory:** occurring prior to commencement of therapy. This commonly results from previous adverse experience of nausea/vomiting.
- **Breakthrough:** occurring despite anti-emetic prophylaxis, requiring the use of rescue medication.
- **Refractory:** occurring during subsequent treatment cycles, when anti-emetic treatment was ineffective in earlier cycles.

The effective management of these distressing symptoms is integral to the patient's ongoing physical and psychological well-being.

Pathophysiology of nausea and vomiting

The mechanism of chemotherapy-induced nausea and vomiting is complex.
- It arises from an interaction between neurotransmitters and receptors in the central and peripheral nervous system.
- The process is initiated by stimulation of dopamine, opiate, histamine, acetylcholine, neurokinin 1 (NK_1) or serotonin receptors. The most common mechanism is thought to be stimulation of the chemoreceptor trigger zone (CTZ) located in the area postrema in the floor of the 4th ventricle.

Although the precise mechanism is unclear, it is thought that the CTZ is activated via neurotransmitters released into blood or cerebrospinal fluid which stimulate the vomiting centre. Damage to the GI mucosa also results in release of neurotransmitters, which stimulate the vomiting centre via vagal afferents.

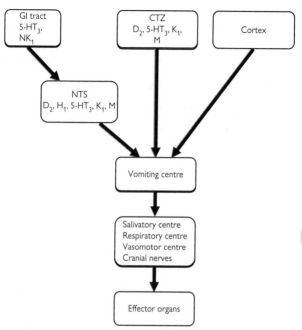

Fig. 20.1 Pathways and neurotransmitter receptors in chemotherapy induced nausea and vomiting. GI, gastrointestinal; CTZ, chemoreceptor trigger zone; NTS, nuclear tractus solitarius; D_2, dopamine type 2 receptor; 5HT-3, serotonin type 3 receptor; M, muscarinic receptor; H_1, histamine type 1 receptor; NK_1, tachykinin neurokinin type 1 receptor.

Management of nausea and vomiting

It is essential to understand the degree of emetogenicity of different drugs in order to provide effective pharmacological management. The emetogenic potential of chemotherapy agents may be categorized as high, moderate, low, or minimal. For most chemotherapy agents, higher doses are more emetogenic than lower doses (see Table 20.2).

When considering anti-emetic drug regimens it is important to take into account:

- Type, dose, and schedule of chemotherapy.
- Timing of symptoms (acute or delayed).
- Frequency and severity of nausea and vomiting.
- Anticipated adverse effects of anti-emetic therapy.
- Outcome of previous anti-emetic therapy.
- Patient preference of anti-emetic therapy.

The goals of anti-emetic therapy are to maintain and enhance the patient's quality of life by providing appropriate care, which can, in turn, reduce the number of visits to the hospital to adjust ant-emetic treatment.

Currently in the UK there are no national guidelines for the management of nausea and vomiting. Most centres will have local policies and protocols in place incorporating the above factors. The anti-emetics generally considered to be most effective in the management of chemotherapy-induced nausea and vomiting (CINV) are as follows:

- Type 3 serotonin (5-HT$_3$) antagonists, e.g. ondansetron.
- Corticosteroids.
- **Benzamides (e.g. metoclopramide):** dopamine antagonist (however, its use is limited in children and young adults by the risk of extrapyradmidal reactions).
- **Other dopamine antagonists:** e.g. levopromazine, phenothiazines, domperidone.
- Cannaboids, e.g. nabilone.
- **NK$_1$ receptor antagonists:** aprepitant. Recent evidence suggests that this agent may be particularly effective in delayed CINV; however, despite some reports of its use in adolescents, there is very little experience in children).
- Antihistamines may be useful in the prevention and treatment of delayed CINV e.g. cyclizine.
- Benzodiazepines are useful in anticipatory nausea, e.g. Lorazepam.

The exact mode of action of corticosteroids is unknown, but when given with a 5-HT$_3$ antagonist, the overall anti-emetic efficacy is greatly increased.

General principles of prescribing include:
- Anti-emetic regimens should be based on the most emetogenic drug of the chemotherapy treatment.
- When chemotherapy regimens include two drugs of the same emetogenicity, prophylaxis should be based on the next level, i.e. where two moderately emetogenic drugs are used, the anti-emetic therapy should be based on *highly* emetogenic chemotherapy.
- Oral anti-emetics should be used whenever possible. Evidence suggests that the oral route is as efficacious as intravenous therapy when used appropriately.
- Corticosteroids should be used concurrently with 5-HT$_3$ antagonist, but discontinued on the last day of the most emetogenic drug unless otherwise indicated.
- Consider previous successful regimens for subsequent courses.
- Antihistamines, dopamine antagonists and cannabinoids are useful in the prevention and treatment of delayed CINV.
- Benzodiazepines are useful in anticipatory nausea.

Table 20.1 provides a classification of drugs and their mode of action and Table 20.2 classifies the emetogenicity of different chemotherapy drugs.

Table 20.1 Antiemetic drugs: classification, mechanism of action, and adverse effects

Anti-emetic agents	Mechanism of action	Adverse effects
Serotonin 5HT$_3$ antagonists, e.g. ondansetron, granisetron, tropisetron, dolasetron	5-HT$_3$ antagonist	Headache, constipation
Corticosteroid: dexamethasone	Unknown	If prolonged use, increased appetite, weight gain, hypertension, fluid retention, electrolyte disorders, hyperglycaemia, proximal myopathy, mood disturbances, adrenal suppression, occasionally avascular necrosis, cataracts
Phenothiazines, e.g. prochlorperazine, perphenazine, trifluoperazine, chlorpromazine	Dopamine antagonist	Extrapyramidal symptoms, hypotension, neuroleptic malignant syndrome, drowsiness, sedation, antimuscarinic effects (e.g. dry mouth), photosensitivity, rash
Butyrophenones, e.g. haloperidol, levomepromazine	Dopamine antagonist	Extrapyramidal symptoms, hypotension, neuroleptic malignant syndrome, drowsiness, agitation, excitement, insomnia, antimuscarinic effects, impaired liver function, bronchospasm
Benzamides, e.g. metoclopramide	Dopamine antagonist	Extrapyramidal symptoms, anxiety, sedation, antimuscarinic effects, diarrhoea, urinary frequency
Domperidone	Dopamine antagonist	Acute dystonic reactions (less commonly than with metoclopramide)
Antihistamines, e.g. cyclizine, diphenhydramine	Histamine antagonist	Sedation, antimuscarinic effects, urinary retention, blur vision
Cannabinoid (synthetic) nabilone	Complex CNS effects	Drowsiness, dizziness, dissociative reactions, hallucinations, dysphoria, hypotension
Benzodiazepines, e.g. lorazepam	CNS depressant	Sedation, blurred vision, visual hallucination, delirium
Neurokinin 1 antagonist aprepitant	NK$_1$ antagonist	Uncommon (headache, dizziness, tinnitus, taste perversion, phargyngitis)

Table 20.2 Emetogenic potential of commonly used chemotherapy agents (incidence of emesis when given without anti-emetics)

Minimal (<10%)	Low (10-30%)	Moderate (30-90%)	High (>90%)
Asparaginase	Cyclophosphamide (<300 mg/m^2)	Amsacrine	Actinomycin D
Bevacizumab	Cytarabine (<1g/m^2 or IT)	Carboplatin	Carmustine
Bleomycin	Docetaxel	Cyclophosphamide (<1500mg/m^2)	Cisplatin
Busulphan (oral low dose)	Etoposide	Cytarabine (>1g/m^2)	Cyclophosphamide (>1500mg/m^2)
Chlorambucil	Fluorouracil	Daunorubicin	Dacarbazine
Fludarabine	Gemcitabine	Doxorubicin	Melphalan (≥100mg/m^2)
Mercaptopurine	Methotrexate (<1g/m^2)	Epirubicin	
Methotrexate (<50 mg/m^2 or IT)	Mitoxantrone	Idarubicin	
Rituximab	Paclitaxel	Ifosfamide	
Thioguanine	Procarbazine	Irinotecan	
Vinblastine	Topotecan	Lomustine	
Vincristine		Methotrexate (>1g/m2)	
Vinorelbine		Oxaliplatin	
		Temozolomide	

IT, intrathecal.

Non-pharmacological management of nausea and vomiting

Non-pharmacological management of nausea and vomiting is useful when used as an adjunct to pharmacological strategies. Non-pharmacological strategies may include progressive muscle relaxation, guided imagery, self-hypnosis, acupressure and acupuncture, TENS, cognitive feedback, and music therapy.

Such interventions are likely to be useful because:

- They can reduce feelings of distress and decrease affective and psychological arousal.
- Redirect attention from a conditioned stimulus by acting as a cognitive distractor.
- Allow the patient to gain control and reduce feelings of helplessness through self-help.
- Methods can be easily learned and used with minimal side effects or risks.

Non-pharmacological methods are under-used by health care professionals in everyday practice, possibly because of the lack of evidence surrounding specific techniques. They do not usually form part of clinical guidance for the management of nausea and vomiting, but a holistic approach to care can be beneficial, both to the patient and professionals involved.

Conclusion

Nausea and vomiting are very distressing symptoms. Appropriate management is based on an understanding of the pathophysiology of nausea and vomiting, the emetogenic potential of cytotoxic drug treatment and the mechanism of action of anti-emetic drugs. Non-pharmacological management should also be incorporated into clinical practice, not only when pharmacological methods are unsuccessful, but also as an adjunct to drug treatment before this stage. Protocols for management should be evidence-based and standardized. However, treatments should be individualized and incorporate a holistic approach, centred on the patient and their family.

Constipation

Constipation in paediatric oncology

Constipation is a subjective symptom that is difficult to define. Inter-individual differences in bowel habits may lead to misinterpretation regarding the presence or severity of constipation.

A widely used definition is 'the 'passage of small hard faeces infrequently and with difficulty'.

Constipation is a common problem encountered by many children and young people during treatment for cancer. It is possible to categorize constipation into three distinct types:

- **Primary constipation** related to extrinsic/lifestyle changes: ↓ exercise, ↓ mobility, poor diet, lack of privacy, and emotional change.
- **Secondary constipation** related to intrinsic/disease-related factors: bowel obstruction, spinal cord damage, dehydration, electrolyte imbalance.
- **Iatrogenic constipation** caused by medical intervention or pharmacological factors, e.g. radiotherapy, chemotherapy (especially vinca alkaloids), opiates, anti-emetics, anticonvulsants.

Constipation is a subjective symptom that can be distressing and have a significant impact on 'quality of life' for the child, young person, and subsequently their family. Associated symptoms and signs may include:

- Anorexia.
- Nausea and vomiting.
- Abdominal pain.
- Abdominal distension.
- Lethargy/malaise.
- Localized (perianal) trauma (e.g. fissures).
- Diarrhoea (overflow).
- Urinary retention.
- Distress.

Constipation can be prevented, but there is a real need to recognize individuals at risk and institute pro-active management.

Assessment

Assessing constipation is essential to determine the cause and to facilitate development of an effective management strategy.

A baseline assessment should reflect the individual's:
- Previous bowel pattern: character, amount, and frequency.
- Current medications.
- Disease site.
- Disease treatment (including surgery).
- Dietary changes.
- Fluid and electrolyte status.
- Degree of mobility.
- Emotional status.
- Physical examination.

Assessment provides the health professional with the opportunity to determine and define what constipation means to the individual, so preventing confusion, misinterpretation, and mismanagement.

The information gained is of use to professionals, patients, and parents by identifying deviation from the individual's normal bowel habit enabling early and appropriate intervention.

Intervention

Therapy should involve treating the cause, as well as restoring bowel function. Intervention needs to highly individualized because its success depends entirely on the patient's willingness to accept the treatment.

Non-pharmacological interventions should be promoted where achievable:
- ↑ Activity.
- ↑ Oral fluids.
- ↑ Fibre-rich diet.
- Promote suitably sensitive environment and facilities.

Pharmacological interventions are categorized according to their mode of action. Knowledge of these basic mechanisms ensures appropriate prescription.

Three principle groups
- Predominantly softening.
- Predominantly peristalsis-stimulating.
- Combination of both.

Softeners
These soften hard faeces and include:
- **Surfactant laxatives:** acting as detergents, thereby allowing ↑ water penetration into the stool, e.g. docusate. They take 24–48h to work and may cause abdominal cramps.
- **Osmotic laxatives:** attract water into the bowel or retain the administration fluid, preventing dry/hard stools, e.g. lactulose, Movicol. Take up to 48h to work, may cause flatulence, abdominal discomfort, and nausea.
- **Bulking agents:** increase faecal mass, considered to be stool normalizers, rather than laxatives, e.g. Bran, Fybogel. Take 12–24h to work, may cause flatulence and abdominal distension, which is difficult for children and young people with cancer to tolerate.

Stimulants
Increase peristalsis/rectal motility, e.g. senna, dantron, bisacodyl, sodium picosulfate. Take 6–12h to work, may cause abdominal cramps. Danthron is only licensed in palliative care setting since it may be carcinogenic, and should be avoided in incontinent patients due to severe skin irritation/burning.

Combination therapy

Combine softening and stimulating properties, which may be useful in opiate induced constipation, e.g. Co-danthrusate (docusate + dantron), Co-danthramer (poloxamer + dantron).

Rectal measures

Seldom used in the paediatric oncology setting due to inconvenience, as well as concerns about risks (infection in neutropenia, bleeding in thrombocytopenia) and invasive nature, which may impact negatively on the child's quality of life. Decision-making frequently falls to the consultant medical staff.

However, rectal administration of laxatives is more frequently used in the palliative setting. Prior to administration it is important to establish:

- Is the rectum full?
- Is the stool hard or soft?
- Is the rectum empty, but the colon full?
- Are both colon and rectum full?
- Is there any rectal sensation?
- Is anal tone normal?
- Any there are spinal cord involvement? If so, at what level?

The information yielded will determine the intervention:

- **Bisacodyl suppository** (stimulant): evacuates stools from rectum.
- **Glycerine suppository** (softener): softens stools in rectum.
- **Phosphate enema** (osmotic): evacuates stool from lower bowel.
- **Arachis oil enema** (softener): softens hard impacted stool, often given overnight.

For patients with a neuropathic bowel where anal tone is absent, a combination of glycerine and bisacodyl will be effective. Otherwise, where rectal laxatives are required, an appropriate oral laxative should be prescribed concurrently at an effective dose.

Further evaluation/advice

- Continue regular review of bowel movements noting character, amount, and frequency. Encourage the use of a 'bowel diary' and constipation assessment tool if available.
- Anticipate the problem and prescribe prophylactically, e.g. after vincristine or when starting opiate analgesia.
- Administer laxatives regularly, rather than 'as required' (PRN) for efficacy.
- Start gently with a stool softener and assess. If this is not effective, add a stimulant laxative. Combination therapy will often be effective.
- Doses should be titrated against response.
- Avoid using two agents with similar mode of action.
- Consider use of topical anaesthetic (lignocaine gel) prior to bowel movement in the case of localized trauma (e.g. anal fissure) and/or pain on passing faeces.

Nutrition

Definitions

- **Protein energy malnutrition** (PEM): present when there is insufficient protein, carbohydrate, and fat (macronutrient) intake to meet metabolic requirements.
- **Cachexia:** state of severe malnutrition with
  - Anorexia.
  - Weight loss.
  - Muscle wasting.
  - Anaemia.
  - Metabolic derangements which may include:
    - hypoalbuminaemia;
    - hypoglycaemia;
    - lactic acidosis;
    - glucose intolerance;
    - insulin resistance.

Aetiology

Reduced oral intake is very common in children with malignancy due to:
- Physical factors, e.g. mucositis, pain, nausea/vomiting, constipation, lethargy.
- Psychological factors, e.g. anorexia, impaired taste, psychological dysfunction.
- Social factors, e.g. lack of opportunity due to disruption of routine by repeated hospitalization or by medical procedures ('nil by mouth').

Cachexia is usually multifactorial, due to effects of:
- Malignancy itself (may be mediated in part by cytokines, e.g. TNFα).
- Treatment and complications (e.g. infection, which may increase metabolic rate).
- Reduced intake.

Epidemiology

- The prevalence of PEM at diagnosis is low (6–8%) in children with ALL, but higher in those with solid tumours.
- PEM is commoner during treatment.

Importance of treating malnutrition

Effective management of PEM may:
- Restore lost weight.
- Permit delivery of cytotoxic treatment with fewer delays and complications.
- Improve immune response (but no proof that this ↓ risk of infection).

Evaluation of malnutrition

Initial evaluation should include assessment of baseline nutritional status, which may itself indicate the need for nutritional supplementation, and identification of those patients whose future treatment will place them at greater risk of developing PEM.

Assessment of baseline nutritional status should include:
- Dietary history.
- Anthropometric measurements, including:
  - Weight, height (plotted on centile charts).
  - *And* (if trained personnel can measure them):
    - mid-upper arm circumference;
    - triceps skin-fold thickness;
    - ideally, lean body mass should be measured with DXA (dual-energy X-ray absorptiometry) scanning or bioelectrical impedance, very rarely achieved in clinical practice.
- Biochemical measurements:
  - Often based on serum albumin concentration:
    - appropriate for evaluation of long-term malnutrition (due to its long half-life), but insensitive to acute malnutrition;
    - hypoalbuminaemia may also be caused by reduced hepatic synthesis or increased renal loss;
  - Serum prealbumin concentration may be preferable for early detection of acute malnutrition due to its much shorter half-life.

Treatment of malnutrition

Nutritional interventions are usually performed in a stepwise manner, but there is considerable inter-centre variation in practice due to a lack of clear evidence.

Nutritional support
- General nutritional advice for all.
- When predefined anthropometric criteria are reached (e.g. ≥5% weight loss from baseline) or nutritional intake is significantly reduced for a prolonged period of time (e.g. <75% of required intake for >1 week):
  - improve nutritional content of regular intake with high calorie foods;
  - add calorie or nutritionally complete supplements (but compliance is often poor);
  - role of specific nutritional supplements (e.g. glutamine) is not well established;
  - actual predefined criteria used vary greatly between centres.
- If there is further weight loss or intake is still poor, commence enteral nutrition via one of following routes:
  - nasogastric tube;
  - gastrostomy (often inserted by percutaneous endoscopic method, PEG);
  - jejunostomy (rarely used).
- Parenteral nutrition (PN) may be indicated in the presence of:
  - severe weight loss;
  - inability to deliver effective enteral feeding due to gastrointestinal symptoms (e.g. in severe enteritis, post-HSCT);
  - use of PN may be complicated by CVAD-associated infection, electrolyte imbalance or hepatic dysfunction.

Immunization

Aim of immunization

- Ideally, the aim of immunization in children who are undergoing or have received cytotoxic treatment, or have undergone a haemopoietic stem cell transplant (HSCT), is to provide same degree of protection against vaccine-preventable infections as healthy immunized individuals.
- In general, immunizations that may benefit these patients should be given and not avoided, provided each vaccine being delivered is safe.
- The recommendations outlined below are based on the Best Practice Statement on Immunization of the Immunocompromised Child (published by the Royal College of Paediatrics and Child Health, 2002).

Types of immunization

Active immunization uses the individual's own immune system to generate a response to a vaccine:

- **Live (attenuated) vaccines:** e.g.
  - measles, mumps, rubella (MMR);
  - varicella zoster virus (VZV);
  - BCG;
  - yellow fever.
- **Non-live vaccines:**
  - Inactivated bacteria or viruses, e.g.
    - inactivated poliomyelitis virus (IPV);
    - *Haemophilus influenzae* type b (Hib);
    - pertussis (P), acellular pertussis (aP);
    - meningococcal group C (MenC);
    - pneumococcal polysaccharide vaccine (PPSV);
    - pneumococcal conjugate vaccine (PCV).
  - Toxoids (inactivated toxins acting as antigens), e.g.
    - diphtheria (D);
    - tetanus (T).

Passive immunization relies on the transfer of antibodies (and hence protection) from immune individuals.

- Intravenous immunoglobulin (IVIg).
- Varicella zoster immunoglobulin (VZIG).
- Human normal immunoglobulin (HNIG).

Standard chemotherapy

Standard chemotherapy is defined as that which is not followed by HSCT. The severity and nature of immunocompromise during and after cytotoxic treatment is determined predominantly by the nature of the treatment received.

General principle

▶ *Avoid all live vaccines* during and for 6 months after completion of treatment.

Recommended schedule
During treatment and until 6 months after completion
Consider giving *non-live vaccines* when scheduled in the universal child-hood immunization schedule (e.g. pre-school boosters), provided the child's general condition is stable (i.e. free from infection and major organ toxicity) and expected to stay so for 3 weeks from immunization.

- It is likely that responses will be suboptimal, but some patients may achieve protective antibody levels.
- May be important, e.g. if at higher than usual risk of tetanus exposure.
- Influenza vaccine recommended annually in autumn.

Six months and later after completion of treatment
- Administer additional booster of DT, aP, IPV, Hib, MenC, PCV, and MMR vaccines 6 months following treatment completion.
- If the patient has previously been given BCG and is in a high risk group for tuberculosis, check tuberculin test and, if negative, revaccinate. If patient has not previously had BCG, immunize according to local policy.
- Ensure primary health care team informed.

Varicella zoster vaccine: routine administration rarely practised in UK. It has been given to susceptible (VZV seronegative) children during ALL maintenance chemotherapy in some other countries (e.g. Japan, USA), with strict precautions, e.g.

- Leukaemia in continued and stable remission, *and*
- Lymphocyte count >0.7 × 10^9/l, *and*
- Immunosuppressive therapy withheld for 1 week prior to and 1 week after the first dose, *and*
- No steroids given for the following 2 weeks.

Passive immunization
Required for all patients on or within 6 months of completion of standard chemotherapy.

Measles
- Contact requires action regardless of antibody status.
- Children in significant contact (play or direct contact for >15min, on ward or in household) with virologically confirmed measles during infectious period (from 5 days before to 4 days after onset of rash) require passive immunization. Try to confirm measles diagnosis in index case.

If <14 days (most effective when <72h) from contact, give either IM HNIg or (especially if thrombocytopenic) IVIg. Protection lasts ~4 weeks.
- **HNIG dose:**
  - *<1 year age* – 250mg;
  - *1–2 years age* – 500mg;
  - *>2 years age* – 750mg.
- **IVIg (standard dose):** 0.4g/kg.

Varicella zoster
- History of past infection should be recorded and current antibody status checked before giving any blood products and starting chemotherapy.
- Significant contact with an individual with chickenpox (defined as for measles, see above) during the infectious period (from 2 days before onset of rash, until crusting of all vesicles), or with herpes zoster virus (HZV; direct contact with exposed lesions only) requires prophylaxis with either aciclovir/valaciclovir or VZIG in VZV-antibody negative patients.
- Consider IV high dose aciclovir if any suspicious skin lesions develop within incubation period after contact with VZV /HZV (conventionally up to 21 days, but may be longer in immunocompromised patients).

Either:
- High dose oral aciclovir/valaciclovir from 7 to 21 days following the initial contact. Widely used for prophylaxis, although no clinical literature for immunocompromised patients.
- Aciclovir dose:
  - *<2 years age* – 200mg qds;
  - *2–6 years age* – 400mg qds;
  - *>6 years age* – 800mg qds.
- Valaciclovir is a pro-drug of aciclovir and is more completely absorbed from gastrointestinal tract than aciclovir. Therefore, it can be given in a TDS regimen.

Or:
- IM VZIG if <72h from contact (may attenuate infection if administered up to 10 days post-exposure) *or* (especially if thrombocytopenic) IVIg. Protection lasts ~4 weeks.
- VZIG dose:
  - *<5 years age* – 250mg;
  - *5–10 years age* – 500mg;
  - *>10 years age* – 750mg.

Haemopoietic stem cell transplantation
General principles
All allogeneic HSCT patients are at high risk of losing immunity against a wide variety of potentially preventable infectious diseases, and the likelihood and speed of donor immune reconstitution is uncertain.

Loss of immunity is less common and severe after autologous HSCT in comparison with allogeneic HSCT, but many patients still lose antibody protection against, e.g. tetanus.
- All recipients of autologous or allogeneic HSCT in childhood should be considered for a re-immunization programme.
- Live vaccines are potentially dangerous until the patient has been off all immunosuppressive treatment for at least 12 months and has no evidence of active chronic GvHD.

- Chronic GVHD and its treatment both cause considerable and often prolonged immunosuppression. Such patients respond poorly to immunization and live vaccines are potentially dangerous. Replacement IVIg treatment is often given to these patients. However, in view of the high risk of infectious complications of prolonged immunosuppression, non-live vaccines are recommended if the patient is not receiving IVIg, even acknowledging that response may be suboptimal.

Recommended schedule

Re-immunization should commence:
- 12 months after:
  - autologous HSCT;
  - HLA-identical sibling donor allogeneic or syngeneic HSCT.
- 18 months after any other allogeneic HSCT (e.g. mismatched related donor, any unrelated donor).
- Providing that:
  - no evidence of active chronic GVHD; and
  - patient off all immunosuppressive treatment for ≥6 months (≥12 months before administering any live vaccines); and
  - patient off IVIg for ≥3 months.

Autologous, HLA-identical sibling donor allogeneic or syngeneic HSCTs
- **12 months post-HSCT:** 3 doses at monthly intervals of:
  - DT, aP;
  - IPV;
  - Hib;
  - MenC.
- **15 months post-HSCT:**
  - *Pneumococcal vaccine –*
    - PCV initially (3 doses if <24 months age, 2 doses if ≥24 months);
    - followed by PPSV at ≥24 months post-HSCT (1 dose).
- **18 and 24 months post-HSCT:** MMR.
- Every autumn, administer influenza vaccine (for as long as the patient remains clinically immunocompromised or is considered to be at increased risk from influenza virus infection).

Any other allogeneic HSCT
Re-immunization schedule as above, but starting and continuing 6 months later (i.e. starting at 18 months post-HSCT).

Other points
- Avoid BCG immunization unless there is a clear case of need and good evidence of immune function recovery, with no evidence of chronic GvHD.
- Significant contact with measles or with VZV infection in any at risk recipient of HSCT (autologous or allogeneic) requires passive immunization regardless of antibody status pre-HSCT. (See Immunization, Siblings and other family members 🕮 p.274, for a definition of at risk HSCT recipients.)
- Recipients of total body irradiation (TBI) are likely to have functional hyposplenism. Life-long antibiotic prophylaxis (usually phenoxymethyl-penicillin) is recommended.

Siblings and other family members

Avoid administration of live vaccines (except MMR and BCG) in siblings or other close family contacts of at risk patients, as defined by:
   • On or ≤6 months of completion of chemotherapy.
   • ≤1 year of HSCT (≤18 months for mismatched or unrelated allogeneic donor transplants):
      • ≤12 months of stopping immunosuppressive treatment;
      • presence of active chronic GvHD.
 • However, MMR can be given because transmission of these vaccine viruses has not been reported, and should be strongly recommended to reduce patient's risk of exposure to wild measles.
 • Consider using VZV vaccine in seronegative family members to provide indirect protection for at risk patient.

Further information

Royal College of Paediatrics and Child Health. (2002) Best Practice Statement on Immunization of the Immunocompromised Child. Available at: http://www.rcpch.ac.uk/Publications/Publications-list-by-date#2002 (accessed 1 April 2009).

Breaking bad news

When breaking bad news, a number of factors have to be considered. Children and young people are recognized as different both in terms of their needs and the disorders they experience. Depending on the age, maturity, and cultural and spiritual background of the individuals whose needs are being addressed, very different issues may arise. Childhood and adolescence is a time of enormous change physically, psychologically, and socially, and this has to be borne in mind by doctors who are breaking bad new to these patients and their families.

There is no 'right' way to break bad news. It should not be seen as a 'one off' meeting, but as part of a series of discussions. Doctors need to consider that what is said will have both an immediate and a subsequent impact on the patient, the family, and the doctor him/herself. In order to improve skills and develop strategies to impart bad news, best practice dictates that a framework should be developed that is broken down into several stages:

- Preparation.
- *Beginning the session* – setting the scene.
- Sharing the information.
- Dealing with the patient's and family's reactions.
- Planning and support.
- Follow-up.

Preparation

It is important to find out whether departmental guidelines are available and who is most often involved. Breaking bad news can be a painful and difficult task, and support from colleagues can be very helpful. Talking to others can be a useful way of preparing oneself.

Breaking bad news should be done in a private setting with both parents present. If there is only one parent, it is important that the parent has the choice to have someone else present, i.e. a relative or friend. Depending on the age and level of understanding, the child should also be present. A young person aged 16 years and over should be offered the choice as to whom they want with them at the meetings. There should not be too many people in the room as this can be overwhelming for the patient and the parents. It is useful to have a nurse present as this can help with reinforcement and can alert the nursing staff to the needs of the family following the meeting. If English is not the family's first language, arrangements should be made to have an interpreter present. Ideally, this should not be a relative, as this can place an additional strain on the family and, in order to protect the family, the person acting as the interpreter may not have passed all of the information on. There may be occasions when it would be helpful to have a social worker present. Many families benefit from talking afterwards with someone who is not a member of the medical team, and who will be able to provide emotional and practical support.

Ideally, the meeting should take place away from the open ward to ensure privacy. Potential interruptions should be controlled, i.e. bleep turned off, ask colleagues not to disturb you and put a 'Do not disturb' notice on the door. Sufficient time should be allowed to answer any questions and to assess the patient's and parent/s' understanding of the information that has been given. Ensure that the surroundings are comfortable and that there is enough seating for everyone and that there are tissues available.

Know all the facts, i.e. what has happened before and what the management options are. The facts need to be given in a compassionate yet direct way that can help the patient and parents set realistic goals. It may be helpful to find out from members of the medical team how much the patient and the family already know and understand. Being aware of the family and social environment in which the patient and the family are living, knowing the educational background, job, and lifestyle can also help.

Beginning the session

Assess the patient's and parents' understanding first and what they already know, are thinking or have been told. It is also helpful to gauge how much information is wanted.

Sharing the information

Use appropriate language, and avoid jargon and medical terminology. Open communication is a prerequisite for success and it is essential that the information being given is understood, in particular what the treatment involves and any choices that there may be.

A simple, clear explanation can be the best way to deliver the bad news. As most patients and their parents will be in shock the content must be kept to the most important aspects. Most people will retain very little of the subsequent information once the bad news has been given. Therefore, having some written information to hand that they can refer to later is helpful. Many patients with cancer can recall in detail how the news was given, even if they remember little of the conversation that followed. How bad news is presented may affect the comprehension and adjustment to the news, as well as the satisfaction with the doctor.

Give the information in small manageable amounts, and stop and ask if clarification is needed or if there are any questions. Go at the pace of the patient and the parents. Rushing through the meeting heightens anxiety, causes confusion of the information being given, and gives the family a feeling of lack of self-worth. Repetition and clarification are helpful in enabling the information to be retained. Be honest, as a more respecting and professional relationship will be developed. Being sensitive to the situation enables the doctor to read non-verbal clues; face/body language, silence, and tears.

Dealing with the patient's and parent/s' reactions

When the shock has been absorbed, a variety of reactions may follow. It is not possible to predict the exact reaction of any individual, but denial, anger, fear, guilt, and/or blame are commonly experienced. It is important for the doctor to acknowledge these feelings. Allow for 'shut down' when it is evident that no more information is being taken in. Stop if there is an indication that the patient and/or parents are unable to take any more information on board, or that he/she/they want to bring the meeting to an end. Respond to feelings and predicaments with empathy and concern, and having identified any concerns, offer specific help by breaking down any overwhelming feelings into manageable concerns, prioritizing, and distinguishing between the fixable and unfixable. A doctor's own discomfort can have an impact on the therapeutic process especially if powerful feelings emerge such as fear or anger. It is important to stay calm and allow time for feelings to be thought through. Avoid trying to fill silence with more information. Wait for the patient or parent to say something or after a period of silence ask how they are feeling and if it is alright to carry on.

Planning and support

After receiving bad news, a sense of isolation and uncertainty may be experienced. A doctor can minimize some of the anxiety by summarizing the areas discussed, checking for comprehension, and formulating a strategy and follow-up plan. Give a broad time frame for what may lie ahead. It is helpful to identify what support systems are in place and what extra help may be needed. The patient and/or parents should be encouraged to be write any questions down so that these can be addressed at subsequent meetings.

It is important to offer availability for further meetings for several reasons:

- The details of the information are not remembered at first, rather the way the information was given.
- Emotional adjustment takes time.
- It is an opportunity to see other family members /support network.
- It provides an opportunity for the doctor to answer questions, as well as discuss any change of treatment plans/options.

Not only should further meetings be arranged be arranged, but also the offer of telephone contact. Be prepared to go over the same information that has previously been discussed.

Palliative care

Although childhood death remains a rare experience for many health care professionals, cancer remains a significant cause of death in children and young people.

Children's palliative care involves care of the child/young person from the time when treatment will no longer be given with a curative intent. The aim of palliative care is to maintain and improve the child's quality of life, not only in the terminal stages, but also in the weeks, months, and years beforehand.

Palliative care focuses on symptom relief, promotion of well-being, psychological and social support for the child and family. 'The goal is to add life to the child's years, not simply years to the child's life (Craft & Killen, 2007). It is vital that, when cure is no longer possible, families are given the means to make full and informed choices. These choices will be influenced by variation in local service provision.

Place of care/death

In the UK, treatment of children and young people with cancer is delivered at or directed under the guidance of one of 21 Principle Treatment Centres (PTCs). Although many of these centres have access to at least one children's hospice, several PTCs seldom or never use hospice facilities. Outside the UK, the uptake of hospice provision may be greater depending on the resources available and/or the capacity of families to provide care for the sick child.

In the UK, most PTCs believe that the family home should remain the centre of caring whenever possible (The ACT Charter for children who live with life-limiting of life-threatening illnesses and their families, 2004). Others argue that this is not possible or, indeed, desirable. Each family will have different beliefs and values. It is therefore imperative that children, young people, and their families are empowered to make an informed decision about their preferred place of care and eventually place of death.

Access to specialist paediatric palliative care expertise from the oncology team (medical or nursing) is essential (Fig. 20.2). (The type and amount of support available may influence families' decisions. Children's and young people's palliative care is often multidisciplinary, involving many healthcare professionals from both primary and secondary care sectors. Where community provision is limited, the parents/extended family may need to take a leading role in the care of the sick child.)

A 'key worker' is vital to ensure the co-ordination of care between all settings. This provides the child/young person and family with a named individual, who can be contacted about all aspects of their care, thus avoiding confusion and replication. The National Institute for Health and Clinical Excellence (NICE) Improving Outcomes Guidance (2005) implies that the Paediatric Oncology Outreach Nurse Specialist (POONS) role would provides an ideal 'key worker.' However, implementation of this role needs to be negotiated on an individual basis for each PTC, as different centres have different workload priorities.

Equally important is identification of the lead clinician, again preventing confusion and potential errors. Often, the consultant paediatric and adolescent oncologist leads the care, even in the community with the support and permission of the GP.

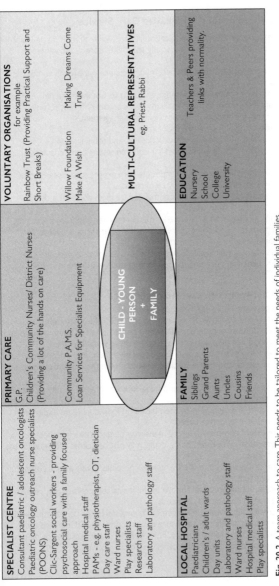

SPECIALIST CENTRE
Consultant paediatric / adolescent oncologists
Paediatric oncology outreach nurse specialists (POONS)
Clic-Sargent social workers - providing psychosocial care with a family focused approach
Hospital medical staff
PAMs - e.g. physiotherapist, OT, dietician
Day care staff
Ward nurses
Play specialists
Research staff
Laboratory and pathology staff

PRIMARY CARE
G.P.
Children's Community Nurses/ District Nurses (Providing a lot of the hands on care)

Community P.A.M.S.
Loan Services for Specialist Equipment

VOLUNTARY ORGANISATIONS
for example
Rainbow Trust (Providing Practical Support and Short Breaks)

Willow Foundation   Making Dreams Come
Make A Wish   True

CHILD - YOUNG PERSON + FAMILY

MULTI-CULTURAL REPRESENTATIVES
eg. Priest, Rabbi

LOCAL HOSPITAL
Paediatricians
Children's / adult wards
Day units
Laboratory and pathology staff
Ward nurses
Hospital medical staff
Play specialists

FAMILY
Siblings
Grand Parents
Aunts
Uncles
Cousins
Friends

EDUCATION
Nursery
School
College
University

Teachers & Peers providing links with normality.

Fig. 20.2 A team approach to care. This needs to be tailored to meet the needs of individual families.

Key elements of the Palliative Care Service

- Ensuring a robust communication strategy with all multidisciplinary team (MDT) members especially the child's consultant, general practitioner (GP), and family.
- Co-ordinating a collaborative, multidisciplinary approach to holistic care.
- Providing specialist knowledge and skills to optimize the delivery and management of complex palliative care across different settings.
- Providing complex symptom control management.
- Promoting empowerment of families.
- Providing information, education, skills, and training.
- Providing emotional support for children, young people, and their families.
- Enabling children and young people with progressive disease to be cared for and die in their place of choice.
- Enabling families to retain control of care even during the dying phase, if it is their wish.
- On call provision is variable across centres, ranging from a weekday service to a 24h on call service providing telephone advice and/or home visits.
- Maintaining relationships with other professionals across all disciplines and utilizing their skills, experience and resources.

Specific symptom care management

- Prepare the family for the onset of symptoms.
- Timely and sensitive discussions (including 'Do Not Attempt Resuscitation' orders, use of antibiotics, treatment of haemorrhage and seizures) can help parents cope when these situations arise.
- Allay fears of the unknown, and dispel myths and misconceptions.
- Offer explanations at a suitable level to match the child/young person and family's understanding.
- Suggest modifying lifestyle and behaviour to enhance quality of life.
- Set realistic goals.
- Symptom management is often based on individual/team experience, rather than evidence-based.
- The use of complex drug regimens may be necessary for effective management of symptoms. Some drugs may not be licensed for regular use in children.
- Oral drugs should be used whenever possible, taking into account individual preferences.
- Longer-acting preparations are useful if available, as they may reduce the number of tablets required.
- Occasionally, invasive management is required after consultation with the patient and family to ensure patient comfort, and improve the quality of their remaining life. For example, draining ascites or pleural effusions when the child is otherwise relatively well.

Consider the route and appropriateness of drug administration. Options may include:

- Spinal, intravenous, or subcutaneous analgesia.
- Chemotherapy.
- **Antibiotics:** these may be used to treat infections that are compromising quality of life. These should be given orally in the first instance in order to avoid hospitalization.
- **Blood product support:** blood and platelets may be used for symptomatic relief. The decision to use these products should be done on the basis of symptomatic relief, rather than looking at the absolute values. These may be given at home (easier for blood than platelets), although often a short stay (4–6h) in a day unit may be necessary.
- **Nutritional support:** this is vital for well-being and unless very close to death attention should be paid to ways of ensuring adequate nutrition, e.g. high calorie drinks, nasogastric (NG) feeds, gastrostomy feeds for those with gastrostomies already *in situ*.
- Complementary therapies.

Routes of administration
Oral, nasogastrically, gastrostomy, transdermal patch, buccal, rectal, intravenous, subcutaneous.

Symptom care pack
A symptom care pack enables symptoms to be treated timely and effectively with minimal disruption. Medications in such a pack usually include:
- Antibiotics.
- Analgesics.
- Anti-emetics.
- Aperients.
- Sedatives.
- Other medications specific to the child/young person's disease.

This will then be stored safely in the family's home until time of need.

Symptom management at home
- Symptoms can be complex and multifactorial.
- Careful assessment is essential.
- Need to formulate individualized treatment plans.
- Consider appropriate use of drug regimens and route(s).

Summary
- Palliative care is multidisciplinary and usually requires a combination of approaches.
- Symptoms can be managed effectively across different settings, including the home, with appropriate support, skill, knowledge, and resources.
- Working in partnership with the family reduces isolation and vulnerability, and engenders confidence, control and independence.
- The way that a child dies will remain in the memory of their parents forever.

Further information

Association for Children's Palliative Care (2004) *The ACT Charter for children who live with life-limiting of life-threatening illnesses and their families.* Available at: http://www.act.org.uk/index.php/about-act/charter.html (accessed 2 April 2009).

Craft, A.W., Killen, S. (2007) Palliative care services for children and young people in England: an independent review for the Secretary of State for Health. Available at: http://www.dh.gov.uk/en/Publicationsandstatistics/Publications/PublicationsPolicyAndGuidance/DH_074459 (accessed 2 April 2009).

National Institute for Health and Clinical Excellence (NICE) Improving Outcomes Guidance (2005).

Central venous access devices

A central venous access device (CVAD) is an indwelling intravascular device used for medium/long-term central venous access. There are two main types of CVAD:

- Tunnelled external (usually cuffed) central venous catheter (CVC), e.g. Hickman line (single, double or, occasionally, triple lumen versions are used, depending on anticipated intensity of usage), account for about 85% of CVAD insertions in UK (data from mid-1990s).
- Implantable subcutaneous port, e.g. Port-a-cath (single or double lumen), about 15% of CVAD insertions.

They are inserted at diagnosis, or soon after, in most children receiving chemotherapy.

Benefits of CVADs

- Reduce distress for the child by avoiding the need for frequent venepuncture for:
  - collection of blood samples;
  - administration of IV fluids, drugs, blood products, and parenteral nutrition.
- Reduce greatly the frequency of potentially devastating extravasation of vesicant chemotherapy (e.g. vincristine, anthracyclines).

Some centres avoid CVAD placement during induction treatment for ALL since it may be associated with an increased risk of venous thrombosis at the site of, or adjacent to, the CVAD (although this is not conclusively proven; see Complications of thrombosis in childhood, Venous thrombosis pp.122–123).

Some children receiving protocols that involve no or only infrequent use of vesicant chemotherapy do not require CVADs, e.g. some children during maintenance ALL treatment.

Complications of CVADs

A large prospective observational study revealed a complication rate (CR) of 2.2 per 1000 CVC days at risk in paediatric oncology patients.

At least one CVC-related complication occurred in 40% of patients.

- Complications commoner in patients with leukaemia or lymphoma.
- Infection (CVC-related bacteraemia, or less commonly tunnel or exit site infections) accounted for 40% of all complications, most commonly with coagulase-negative *staphylococci*, occasionally other Gram +ve or Gram –ve bacteria, or fungi. Commoner in double-lumen (CR 1.4) than single-lumen (CR 0.5) CVCs.
- Malfunction (failure to sample blood or allow infusion despite flushing) – 36%.
- Mechanical (malposition, cuff migration, rupture, dislodgement) – 20%.
- Thrombosis (right atrial, deep venous, pulmonary embolism) – 4%.

CVAD-related infection

Usually (but not always) characterized by fever temporally associated with accessing the CVAD, without another identified source.

- Most important investigation is collection of blood cultures drawn from the CVAD.
- Most units do not collect peripheral blood cultures, although they may provide additional helpful information and are often recommended in treatment guidelines.
- Treatment should be commenced with appropriate intravenous antibiotics directed at likely causative Gram-positive organisms and delivered via the CVAD. Antibiotic regimen may sometimes be modified subsequently based on blood culture results/sensitivities.
- Adjuvant treatments, such as antibiotic, taurolidine (an antibacterial and antifungal) or urokinase (to disrupt CVAD-related clots and biofilm) locks instilled into the CVAD lumens are used sometimes, but their efficacy is unproven.
- *Staphylococcus aureus*, *Pseudomonas*, and *Candida* infections are highly unlikely to be cured, and CVAD removal is strongly advised.

Infectious and mechanical problems are commoner in external (especially multiple lumen) CVCs than in port.

Outcome

Fatal CVAD-related complications are rare, but may result from:
- Overwhelming sepsis.
- Venous thromboembolism.

Prevention of complications is preferable to treating them:
- Scrupulous attention to sterile technique when accessing or flushing CVADs.
- Regular flushing with heparinized saline reduces failure and infection rates.
- Prompt investigation and treatment of CVAD-related thrombosis, which should be suspected in the presence of poor CVAD function or suspicious clinical signs (Complications of thrombosis in childhood, Venous thrombosis 📖 pp.122–123).

Haemopoietic growth factors

Tissue culture experiments in the 1960s and 1970s identified a family of glycoproteins which selectively stimulate the growth and proliferation of blood-forming cells. Subsequent recombinant technology has allowed the production of purified preparations of these individual compounds for further study and for clinical use.

The following recombinant growth factors are now routinely used in clinical practice:

- Erythropoietin (Epo).
- Granulocyte colony stimulating factor (G-CSF).
- Granulocyte-macrophage colony stimulating factor (GM-CSF).

Clinical trials are currently investigating roles for:

- Thrombopoietin (stimulation of platelet production).
- Interleukin-3 (stimulation of all haemopoietic cell lines).

Clinical uses

Recombinant growth factors are used in the following clinical areas:

- In combination with chemotherapy for treating leukaemia (recruitment to cell cycle to enhance cytotoxicity) – G-CSF.
- Transient bone marrow failure post-chemotherapy – G-CSF, GM-CSF, Epo.
- Mobilization of progenitor cells for haemopoietic stem cell transplantation – G-CSF.
- Inherited bone marrow failure syndromes – G-CSF.
- Myelodysplasia – G-CSF, Epo.
- Idiosyncratic agranulocytosis following drug exposure – G-CSF.
- Chronic anaemia (especially renal) – Epo.

Theoretical risk of effect on tumour cell growth

Initial concerns about a possible stimulatory effect of G-CSF on tumour cell growth in myeloid malignancies have not been borne out, and there is no evidence for such an effect. G-CSF is widely used in the management of patients with AML and MDS.

There is a theoretical risk of leukaemogenesis due to G-CSF in severe congenital neutropenia (Kostmann's syndrome), which is often associated with molecular abnormalities of the G-CSF receptor. However, G-CSF has been life-saving in the prevention of infection in this disorder and there is a background increased incidence of leukaemia without G-CSF. The contribution of the therapeutic use of G-CSF to the risk of leukaemia is unknown.

Epo has been found to be effective in the improvement of Hb levels in adults following chemotherapy for malignant disease, and can reduce the need for transfusion support and improve quality of life with respect to anaemia symptoms. Theoretical concerns about possible stimulatory effects on residual tumour growth have so far limited its uptake in paediatric oncology practice.

G-CSF

Selectively stimulates neutrophil production. It is given daily SC or IV until count recovery. Pegylated products are available with a longer half-life for less frequent administration. G-CSF dose varies slightly according to manufacturers' specifications, but is of the order of 5μg/kg/day for treating neutropenia, and 10μg/kg/day for progenitor cell mobilization. There is no dose limiting toxicity, but fever and bone pain (the latter due to marrow expansion) are commonly seen. Its use in the context of chemotherapy for malignant disease can be divided into the following categories.

Combination treatment for tumour therapy

For example, in combination with fludarabine and cytosine arabinoside (FLAG) in the treatment of AML and relapsed ALL.

Primary prophylaxis

Planned use of G-CSF to reduce severity and duration of neutropenia following chemotherapy, which is predictably severely myelosuppressive enough to justify this intervention.

Secondary prophylaxis

Use of G-CSF following chemotherapy on an individual basis for patients who have demonstrated significant episodes of neutropenic fever or greater than expected myelosuppression with previous courses of therapy not normally requiring growth factor support.

Rescue therapy

Use of G-CSF to reduce the severity and duration of neutropenia in patients who have developed serious episodes of neutropenic fever prior to anticipated neutrophil recovery post chemotherapy.

GM-CSF

GM-CSF has a less specific spectrum of stimulatory activity and will increase monoctye, other granulocyte and erythroctye production in addition to neutrophils. In children it has a much higher incidence of allergic side-effects and is much less used in practice. It may be considered in situations such as refractory fungal infection or mycobacterial infection where monocyte recovery may be important.

Erythropoietin (Epo)

Epo has been shown to reduce transfusion support requirements in patients receiving cytotoxic therapy. The effect has been most beneficial for patients with non-haematological malignancies receiving platinum-containing chemotherapy regimens, and its use has been recommended as an effective alternative to transfusion in this situation in adults. Recombinant human Epo (rHEpo)-α and -β are available for SC or IV administration. Pegylated forms with a longer half-life are available for less frequent administration. Dose ranges from 50–300U/kg three times weekly are used by SC administration. It is important to ensure that tissue iron stores are plentiful in order to maximize response. It is also important to prevent substantial rises in haemoglobin and haematocrit, which may be associated with hypertension and increased thrombotic risk.

Long-term
follow-up

Long-term follow-up

Improving survival rates and longevity of survival after childhood malignancy have created an increasing need for long-term follow-up (LTFU). Wide range of late side effects of treatment, which may lead to physical and psychosocial morbidity and even mortality in patients cured of their malignancy. Early detection of incipient or established toxicity allows timely treatment that may improve outcome. Careful documentation of the nature and prevalence of late adverse effects (LAEs) enables identification of risk factors for chronic toxicity and ultimately facilitates development of less toxic treatments.

Late adverse effects: general comments

Incidence

- ~75% of children with malignancy become long-term survivors with contemporary treatment (nearly all will be cured).
- ~1 in 715 young adults is a survivor of childhood malignancy.
- 60% of adult survivors of childhood malignancy have at least one chronic medical problem attributable to treatment.
- 30% have two or more problems.
- Particularly high risk of late adverse effects in survivors of:
  - CNS tumours;
  - haemopoietic stem cell transplantation (HSCT).

Causes

- **Radiotherapy (RT):** total body irradiation (TBI) given during HSCT conditioning has the potential to cause or contribute to most of the individual RT toxicities mentioned under Specific late adverse effects.
- Chemotherapy.
- Surgery.
- Other treatment (e.g. aminoglycoside antibiotics).
- Genetic factors may predispose some patients to greater toxicity.
- Additive effects (e.g. cisplatin and ifosfamide may both cause nephrotoxicity).

Risk factors

Numerous risk factors described. Many are specific to individual late effects. Individual cytotoxic drugs have characteristic LAE profiles, whilst RT has well defined risks for tissues within the treatment field. Pathogenesis of LAEs is variable, often poorly understood.

Commoner 'general' risk factors for development of LAEs include:

- Patient age at treatment (many, but not all, LAEs more severe in younger patients).
- Treatment dose (especially higher cumulative dose, e.g. anthracycline cardiotoxicity).
- Treatment schedule of RT or CT (e.g. unfractionated RT often associated with higher risk).
- Patient's pre-existing clinical status (e.g. presence of organ dysfunction).
- Previous or concurrent exposure to other toxic treatments.

Long-term follow-up clinics: general comments

Ideally, a specific and separate LTFU clinic should be arranged for LTFU patients. Most patients prefer not to be seen in busy treatment clinic.

Staff

Ideally should include:
- **Senior medical staff:**
  - paediatric oncologist(s)/haematologist(s) with specific expertise/ interest in LAEs, or other experienced medical staff with specific knowledge of range of LAEs experienced by survivors of childhood malignancy, ideally including medical staff with expertise in the care of adolescents;
  - adult specialist(s) with appropriate knowledge of LAEs;
  - other paediatric or adult specialist staff according to needs of the specific patient group attending the clinic and local resources/ expertise, e.g. endocrinologist, cardiologist, respiratory, ophthalmology, reproductive medicine;
  - access to other specialist medical/surgical staff may be required on separate *ad hoc* basis.
- Specialist nursing staff with specific expertise in LAEs.
- Psychologist.
- Social worker.
- Access to other staff (e.g. physiotherapist) as required.

Locations and models of care

Clinics have been developed in a variety of locations, including:
- Paediatric oncology/haematology unit that provided initial treatment.
- Associated adult oncology and/or haematology unit.
- Other hospital-based adult specialist unit.
- Specific transitional clinic (covering changeover from paediatric to adult-led care) in either paediatric or adult setting.
- Community clinic.

These have been associated with many different models of care, e.g.
- **Surgery, low risk chemotherapy:** postal or telephone follow-up only.
- **Standard chemotherapy, low risk radiotherapy:** specialist nurse or primary care led follow-up in hospital or community.
- **Intensive chemotherapy, radiotherapy:** specialist medically supervised LTFU clinic in hospital.

Each location/model of care has specific advantages and disadvantages, but important to provide age-specific care and effective transitional care.

Content and frequency of LTFU

- Disease follow-up determined by nature of disease itself (not covered further in this chapter; see individual disease chapters).
- In general, LTFU determined by treatment received (taking account of specific treatment or patient-related risk factors, see Specific late adverse effects 📖 pp.298–310), rather than by the disease *per se*
  - use this information to develop specific LTFU plan for each patient, which will:
    - include information about particular LAE risks faced by the patient;
    - provide guidance about important elements of clinical history/ examination/specific investigations required;
  - content of plan may influence when, where, and by whom patient seen, e.g. post-HSCT patients need to be seen in medically supervised hospital clinic;
  - treatment may evolve over time, necessitating different content for LTFU plan even for the same underlying disease;
  - further information about how to construct a LTFU plan is provided in the UKCCSG Late Effects Group Therapy Based Long Term Follow Up Practice Statement.
- Little knowledge about optimal frequency of LTFU, but in general needs to be more frequent (e.g. yearly) for survivors of HSCT, CNS tumours, other intensive treatment.
- Survivors and their families want appropriate information about their treatment, actual present and potential future LAEs, health promotion, and relevant lifestyle issues (insurance, employment, travel, fertility, sexuality etc). Can be delivered in numerous ways, e.g. verbally, written, computer media (including internet), survivor groups.

Further information

UKCCSG. (2005) How to use this practice statement. In: Late effects group therapy based long term follow up practice statement, 2nd edn. Available at: http://www.ukccsg.org.uk/public/ followup/PracticeStatement/index.html. (accessed 2 April 2009).

Specific late adverse effects

The severity of LAEs may vary greatly between individual patients, despite apparently similar risk factor profiles. The timing of onset of LAEs is very variable. Although many will manifest themselves within a year of completing treatment, others such as secondary malignancies or endocrinopathies may only become evident several years afterwards or even later. The management recommendations given below apply to patients perceived to be at risk of the particular LAE (on the basis of treatment received and risk factor profile).

Quality of life

Any survivor of childhood malignancy, regardless of quantity and nature of treatment received, is at risk of potentially disabling late psychosocial adverse effects that may impair quality of life considerably.

Clinical features

There are numerous manifestations, including:
- Difficulty with family, social relationships.
- Emotional problems, including anxiety, depression.
- Concern about physical appearance, future health, functioning.
- School problems, including reduced attendance and poor performance.
- Difficulties in obtaining and maintaining employment.
- Sexual dysfunction.
- Problems with obtaining life insurance, mortgages, related issues.

Risk factors

May occur in any survivor. More likely in intensively treated patients.

Prevention

- Promote healthy lifestyle, including regular exercise and healthy diet.
- Provide advice about the avoidance of risk behaviours.
- Provide written health promotion material where appropriate.

Management

- Allow time for the opportunity for discussion at LTFU clinic.
- When appropriate, consider referral to Psychologist or Social Worker.

Secondary malignancy

Survivors at ↑ risk of wide variety malignancies 2° to previous treatment.

Clinical features
- Solid malignancies, especially thyroid, breast, CNS, bone, soft tissue sarcomas, typically occur 10 years or later after treatment.
- Haematological malignancies, predominantly acute myeloid leukaemia (AML) and myelodysplasia (MDS), typically occur relatively early (4–6 years) after treatment.

Risk factors
- **Radiotherapy:** all tissues in RT field at risk of subsequent solid tumours.
- **Chemotherapy:** especially epipodophyllotoxins (e.g. etoposide, VP-16) and alkylating agents (e.g. cyclophosphamide). Main risk is AML/MDS. May contribute to risk of some solid tumours (e.g. bone).
- **Familial cancer syndromes:** especially heritable retinoblastoma, Li Fraumeni syndrome, neurofibromatosis type I, Fanconi anaemia (Constitutional aplastic anaemia 📖 pp.372–378).

Prevention
Advise avoidance of high risk behaviours, especially smoking and excessive exposure to strong sunlight.

Early detection
- Patient education about risk of 2° malignancy and importance of promptly reporting new symptoms/signs.
- Encourage:
  - regular self-examination e.g. of breast, testes;
  - participation in relevant screening programme (e.g. Department of Health programme of breast screening for high risk adult female survivors of Hodgkin disease, i.e. those treated with mediastinal RT in childhood).
- Increased index of suspicion in higher risk patients, especially those with familial cancer syndromes.
- Consider referral to Clinical Geneticist in patients with history of familial cancer syndrome.

Management
- Careful clinical examination (especially of RT field) in LTFU clinic.
- Early and appropriate investigation of new/worrying symptoms/signs.

Neurological/neuropsychological

May be severe and persistent, sometimes progressive.

Clinical features
- **CNS:**
  - leucoencephalopathy → focal motor signs, spasticity, seizures, ataxia, neuropsychological dysfunction, as described in the next main point;
  - 2° malignancy

- vascular stenosis/occlusion → seizures, TIAs, CVAs, dementia;
- RT necrosis → neurocognitive/neuropsychological dysfunction;
- myelopathy → para/quadriplegia, sphincter dysfunction.
- **Neuropsychological:**
  - functional (gross or fine motor) disabilities;
  - cognitive impairment affecting intelligence, attention, learning skills, memory, verbal, and visual-spatial skills.
- **Peripheral nervous system:** peripheral neuropathy.

Risk factors

- **Leucoencephalopathy and neuropsychological toxicity:**
  - underlying malignancy commoner in CNS tumours;
  - CNS RT;
  - intrathecal chemotherapy;
  - young age at treatment.
- **CNS vasculopathy, necrosis:** CNS RT.
- **Myelopathy:**
  - spinal RT;
  - chemotherapy (i.e. persistence of acute toxicity).
- **Peripheral neuropathy:** chemotherapy, especially cisplatin (mainly sensory) and vincristine (chronic toxicity rare but acute neuropathy may fail to recover fully).

Management

- Physiotherapy and/or Occupational Therapy assessment where appropriate.
- Leucoencephalopathy and neuropsychological toxicity:
  - careful educational assessment with school support, careers guidance;
  - consider neuropyschological assessment.
- **Vasculopathy:** surgery in selected cases.
- **RT necrosis/myelopathy:** long-term medical management difficult, seldom successful. Steroids may alleviate severity of acute onset.
- **Peripheral neuropathy:**
  - consider neurophysiological investigations;
  - drug treatment (e.g. gabapentin) for painful neuropathy.

Visual

Clinical features

- Lacrimal gland dysfunction with impaired tear production may → corneal ulceration and scarring.
- Cataracts (posterior subcapsular).
- Rarely keratitis, uveitis, chorioretinopathy, optic neuritis.

Risk factors

- RT to field including eye → lacrimal gland dysfunction, cataracts.
- Steroids may contribute to cataract formation.
- Chemotherapy agents may (very rarely) contribute to visual toxicity, e.g. fludarabine, vincristine (case reports of blindness, usually acute onset with no/limited recovery).

Management
- Artificial tear replacement for lacrimal gland dysfunction.
- Surgical removal of cataracts (± insertion of lens implant).

Auditory

Clinical features
- Hearing impairment and its consequences:
  - delayed speech development;
  - impaired educational and social functioning.

Risk factors
- Platinum chemotherapy, especially cisplatin:
  - cisplatin dose >400mg/m^2;
  - age at treatment <5 years.
- Prior RT to field including middle ear.
- Other ototoxic treatment (e.g. aminoglycosides).

Management
- **Investigation:** pure tone audiogram (school age children), behavioural audiometry in younger children (otoacoustic emissions or auditory brainstem responses may be helpful).
- Refer Ear, Nose and Throat (ENT), or Audiometry ± Speech Therapy if symptomatic hearing loss.
- Consider 'pre-emptive' referral in infants treated with cisplatin or high-dose carboplatin.
- Liaise with Education and Community Paediatric services in children with significant hearing impairment.

Craniofacial/dental

Clinical features
- Abnormal/hypoplastic craniofacial and orbital skeletal growth → cosmetic deformities, not maximally apparent until after pubertal growth completed.
- **Dental abnormalities:**
  - wide range including dental dwarfism/hypoplasia/agenesis, enamel dysplasia, failure of eruption, impaired calcification or root development;
  - ?increased risk of dental caries (conflicting evidence).

Risk factors
- Cranial/facial RT.
- Chemotherapy.
- Young age at treatment.

Management
- **Craniofacial abnormalities:** regular assessment of craniofacial growth (clinical photographs may help), refer to Maxillofacial surgeon during puberty if facial reconstruction indicated.

- **Dental abnormalities:** regular dental assessment, consider referral to Paediatric Orthodontist. Avoid adrenaline-containing local anaesthetics in recipients of RT (in view of risk of osteoradionecrosis).

Endocrine

Hypothalamic-pituitary axis (HPA)/growth
Clinical features
- Growth hormone (GH) deficiency → growth impairment.
- Early or delayed puberty or attenuated pubertal growth spurt.
- Multiple pituitary hormone deficiency. Hormones lost sequentially – GH (lost first, most commonly affected), LH/FSH, ACTH, TSH.

Risk factors
- RT to field including brain (i.e. involving pituitary) or spine (affecting spinal growth).
- Brain tumours (even without RT).
- HSCT (especially if conditioned with TBI after previous cranial RT).

Management
- 6-monthly monitoring of height/weight, plotted on centile charts. Monitor sitting height in recipients of TBI, craniospinal or abdominal RT (to detect impaired spinal growth).
- 6-monthly pubertal staging (from about 10 years age):
  - testicular volume (TV) in boys (using orchidometer) as a marker of pubertal development;
  - LH, FSH, testosterone (boys), oestradiol (females).
- Consider bone age measurement in recipients of TBI or cranial RT, brain tumour survivors.
- Refer to or see with Paediatric Endocrinologist if:
  - slow height velocity (<25th percentile);
  - height <10th percentile;
  - early puberty (<9 years female, <10 years male);
  - RT dose >30Gy to HPA;
  - TBI;
  - discrepancy between pubertal stage and growth (reduced pubertal growth spurt in GH deficiency).
- Dynamic GH testing and GH treatment in some patients (with endocrinology supervision).

Thyroid

Clinical features
- Hypothyroidism (usually 1°, occasionally 2° to pituitary failure).
- Hyperthyroidism (rare).
- Hyperparathyroidism (rare).
- Thyroid tumour.

Risk factors
- RT to field including thyroid.
- ^{131}I-MIBG (^{131}I-metaiodobenzylguanidine) treatment.

- Busulphan conditioning in HSCT (very occasionally → hypothyroidism).
- Pituitary RT (→ 2° hypothyroidism).

Management
- **Annual thyroid function tests** (T_4, TSH): start thyroxine if:
  - compensated hypothyroidism (↑TSH, ↔T_4) – adjust dose to suppress TSH;
  - overt hypothyroidism (↑TSH, ↓T_4) – adjust dose to suppress TSH and restore T_4 to high normal value.
- **Annual neck palpation:** if abnormal, perform ultrasound, refer to Endocrinologist/surgeon if nodule confirmed.

Pancreatic

Clinical features
- Diabetes mellitus.
- Metabolic syndrome: hyperinsulinaemia, impaired glucose tolerance, hyperlipidaemia ± hypertension ± obesity.

Risk factors
Not clearly identified, may include abdominal RT.

Management
In high risk patients, e.g. survivors of HSCT:
- Monitor urinalysis for glycosuria.
- Fasting blood glucose and lipids.
- HbA_{1c}.
- Glucose tolerance test if ↑ fasting glucose.

Gonadal/reproductive

Severity of gonadal toxicity very variable. Recovery of established gonadal failure is documented but uncommon (especially rare after HSCT).

Male
Clinical features
- Sertoli cell failure: oligo- or azoospermia/subfertility/infertility.
- Leydig cell failure: hypogonadism → low serum testosterone, delayed/arrested puberty (rare), ↑ risk reduced bone mineral density (BMD).
- Erectile dysfunction, ↓ libido.
- ↓ Muscle bulk.
- Fatigue.

Risk factors
- RT to field including testes.
- Chemotherapy:
  - *alkylating agents* – BCNU, busulphan, CCNU, chlorambucil, cyclophosphamide, ifosfamide, melphalan, mustine, nitrogen mustard, thiotepa;
  - cisplatin, cytarabine arabinoside, dacarbazine, procarbazine.

Management

- Consider sperm banking in adolescent males *before* giving potentially gonadotoxic therapy.
- 6-monthly pubertal staging (see Specific late adverse effects, Endocrine, Hypothalamic-pituitary axis (HPA)/growth 🕮 p.303).
- 6-monthly growth monitoring until normal pubertal growth spurt established.
- When/if appropriate:
  - discuss need for contraception (even if considered to have impaired fertility);
  - semen analysis;
  - refer to Endocrinologist if poor growth, delayed puberty, or risk of hypogonadism (high testicular RT dose);
  - refer to specialist in Reproductive Medicine for fertility counselling +/– treatment.

Female

Clinical features

- **Ovarian failure:**
  - hypogonadism (↓ serum oestradiol → vaginal dryness, hot flushes, irritability in post-pubertal females);
  - delayed/arrested puberty;
  - amenorrhoea;
  - subfertility/infertility;
  - ↑ risk early menopause, reduced BMD, cardiovascular morbidity.
- **Uterine damage:** ↑ risk of adverse pregnancy outcome (e.g. premature delivery, low birth weight infant, foetal loss).

Risk factors

- RT to field including ovaries
- Chemotherapy (see list in Secondary malignancies, Gonadal/reproductive, Male 🕮 pp.300, 304).

Management

- 6-monthly pubertal staging (see Secondary malignancies, Endocrine, Hypothalamic-pituitary axis (HPA)/growth 🕮 p.303) and growth monitoring (see Secondary malignancies, Gonadal/reproductive, Male 🕮 pp.300, 304).
- When/if appropriate:
  - discuss need for contraception (even if considered to have impaired fertility);
  - advise about risk of premature menopause;
  - refer to Endocrinologist if poor growth, delayed puberty, risk of hypogonadism;
  - refer to specialist in Reproductive Medicine for fertility counselling (including increased risk of adverse pregnancy outcome) +/– treatment;
  - refer patients with high-risk pregnancies to Obstetrician *early*.

Cardiac

Clinical features
- Cardiomyopathy → cardiac failure.
- Early onset coronary artery disease (CAD).

Risk factors
- Chemotherapy (→ cardiomyopathy):
  - anthracyclines and related drugs – doxorubicin (Adriamycin), daunorubicin, epirubicin, idarubicin, mitozantrone;
  - Amsacrine.
- RT (→ CAD).
- Higher risk patients/situations include:
  - previous acute anthracycline cardiotoxicity;
  - total anthracycline dose >250mg/m^2 (especially >450mg/m^2), but may occur rarely after lower doses;
  - treatment with both anthracycline *and* RT;
  - female sex > male;
  - strenuous exercise (e.g. weight-lifting);
  - pregnancy;
  - patients on treatment with GH and/or sex steroid;
  - co-existing congenital heart disease.

Management
- Take history of cardiac symptoms.
- Advise avoidance of lifestyle risk factors for CAD.
- Measure blood pressure.
- Regular echocardiograms in patients treated with anthracycline. If abnormal, repeat more frequently, discuss with or refer to Cardiologist.
- Refer pregnant patients with risk factor(s) to Obstetrician.

Respiratory

Clinical features
- **Restrictive lung disease:** abnormal pulmonary function tests (PFTs), pulmonary fibrosis.
- **Obstructive lung disease:** most commonly in context of HSCT → chronic GvHD.
- Bronchiectasis (following previous lower respiratory tract infection).

Risk factors
- Chemotherapy: BCNU, CCNU, busulphan.
- RT to field including pulmonary tissue (including spinal).
- Thoracic surgery.
- HSCT.

Management
- Baseline PFTs at end of treatment, and regularly thereafter if symptomatic or if initial PFTs abnormal.
- Advise pneumococcal and annual influenza immunization in patients with established lung disease.

Gastrointestinal

Clinical features
- Strictures, including oesophageal → dysphagia.
- Malabsorption (intestinal, including post-surgical; rarely pancreatic).
- Intestinal obstruction (usually post-surgical).
- Vitamin B_{12} deficiency (after terminal ileum resection).

Risk factors
- RT to field including GIT.
- GIT surgery.

Management
- Imaging as indicated.
- Vitamin B_{12} replacement in appropriate patients.

Hepatic

Clinical features
- Abnormal liver function tests (LFTs).
- Hepatosplenomegaly.
- Chronic liver disease, occasionally with portal hypertension.

Risk factors
- Chemotherapy (usually → acute toxicity, rarely → chronic damage) – actinomycin D, busulphan, methotrexate, thiopurines (especially 6-thioguanine).
- Radiotherapy.
- Hepatic surgery.
- Multiple blood product transfusions, especially before hepatitis C screening was introduced (1991).

Management
- Regular LFTs in at risk patients.
- Abdominal US in patients with hepatosplenomegaly.
- Consider referral to Gastroenterologist/Hepatologist.

Renal

Clinical features
- **Glomerular:**
    - *subclinical* – high urea/creatinine, reduced GFR (common);
    - chronic renal failure (rare);
    - end stage renal failure (very rare).
- **Tubular:**
    - *Proximal* – reduced electrolyte reabsorption →
        - hypophosphataemia → hypophosphataemic rickets (HR) (ifosfamide);
        - hypomagnesaemia (cisplatin), may → convulsions, tetany or arrythmias if severe;

- *Distal* – nephrogenic diabetes insipidus (NDI) (ifosfamide) (rare).
- *Proximal/distal* – renal tubular acidosis (RTA) (ifosfamide) (rare).
- General:
  - hypertension;
  - proteinuria.

Risk factors
- Nephrectomy.
- RT to field including renal tissue (including TBI, spinal).
- **Chemotherapy:**
  - *Nitrosoureas* (BCNU, CCNU).
  - *Platinum drugs* –
  - *cisplatin* – especially if dose rate >40mg/m^2/day;
  - *carboplatin* – renal toxicity similar in nature, but much less frequent and usually much less severe than after cisplatin.
  - *Ifosfamide* –
    - especially if cumulative dose >80g/m^2;
    - ?greater toxicity if <5 years old at treatment.
  - Methotrexate (high-dose IV).
  - Melphalan.
- Other drugs, e.g. aminoglycosides, amphotericin B, cyclosporin A.
- Urinary tract obstruction/pre-existing renal dysfunction due to tumour.

Management
- Measure BP.
- Urinalysis for proteinuria (if ≥++, measure urine protein:creatinine ratio, if >100mg/mmol, discuss with Nephrologist).
- Monitor growth.
- Monitor biochemical profile:
  - *U&Es.*
  - *Tubular function* –
    - *ifosfamide* – measure HCO$_3$, Cl, Ca, PO$_4$, alkaline phosphatase, calculate renal tubular threshold for phosphate (Tm$_p$/GFR)
      Tm$_p$/GFR = Sp - (Up × Scr)/ Ucr
      where S = serum, U = urine concentration, p = phosphate, and cr = creatinine concentration;
    - *cisplatin/carboplatin* – Mg.
- Electrolyte supplementation as clinically indicated.
- Specific treatment as clinically indicated for HR, RTA, NDI.

Lower urinary tract

Clinical features
- Haemorrhagic cystitis (HC).
- Bladder hypoplasia: small volume, urinary frequency.
- Bladder fibrosis: irritability, rarely urinary retention.
- Urethral stricture.
- Bladder malignancy (rare).

Risk factors
- RT.
- Previous history of severe HC caused by:
  - RT;
  - chemotherapy (cyclophosphamide, ifosfamide).
- Bladder surgery.

Management
- Urinalysis, microscopy, culture.
- Regular urine cytology if previous severe HC or if new symptoms.
- Where appropriate, refer to Urologist for cytoscopy or urodynamics.

Skeletal

Clinical features
- Reduced BMD → risk of low impact or vertebral crush fractures.
- Scoliosis.

Risk factors
- Steroids.
- RT (including TBI, cranial, craniospinal, spinal).
- Endocrinopathy: GH deficiency, gonadal failure.
- Chemotherapy: standard ALL treatment protocols, ?methotrexate, ?ifosfamide.
- For scoliosis: spinal or thoracic surgery, young age at treatment.

Management
- Consider BMD measurement (DEXA scan) in survivors of HSCT, ALL, medulloblastoma, or if history of fractures or back pain.
- Where appropriate, refer to specialist (in Bone Disease, Spinal Surgery).

Skin

Clinical features
- Pigmented naevi.
- Skin malignancies: melanoma, basal cell carcinoma, squamous cell carcinoma.
- Drug toxicity (e.g. from steroids, extravasation damage).
- RT changes: atrophy, fibrosis, telangiectasia, altered pigmentation, alopecia (commoner after higher cumulative RT dose to scalp).

Risk factors
- All chemotherapy.
- RT (any site).
- Other drug treatment, including steroids.

Management
- Regular inspection of skin.
- Photograph suspicious skin lesions, where appropriate refer to Dermatologist.
- Provide general advice: avoidance of/protection against excessive sunlight/UV radiation, warning signs of skin lesions.

Immunological/splenectomy or hyposplenism

- Immune function recovers satisfactorily within 6–12 months of stopping treatment in most patients receiving standard chemotherapy.
- Timescale of recovery after RT is uncertain, but probably shorter.
- Recovery usually slower after HSCT (allogeneic > autologous, mismatched or unrelated donor > HLA-matched sibling donor).
- Patients who have undergone splenectomy or high dose splenic RT (>40Gy), and HSCT survivors (especially if conditioned with TBI, which → functional hyposplenism), are at increased risk of encapsulated bacterial infection:
  - immunize with pneumococcal (both conjugate and polysaccharide), *Haemophilus influenzae* type b (Hib) conjugate and meningococcal C conjugate vaccines;
  - *antibiotic prophylaxis* – usually phenoxymethylpenicillin (amoxicillin may be acceptable alternative in children) or erythromycin (if allergic to penicillin);
  - warn about risks of malaria.
- Advise booster immunizations 6 months after completion of standard chemotherapy, and re-immunization when adequate immunological reconstitution has occurred after HSCT, and patient is at least 6 months off immunosuppressive treatment.

Further information

Detailed guidance concerning immunization after treatment is available on the RCPCH website at: http://www.rcpch.ac.uk/publications/recent_publications/Immunocomp.pdf and summarized in Immunization pp.270–275.

Surgical late adverse effects

Significant long-term morbidity may occasionally occur after:

- Neuro-/spinal surgery.
- Ophthalmic/orbital surgery.
- Faciomaxillary/head/neck surgery.
- ENT surgery.
- Dental surgery.
- Thoracic surgery (cardiac, pulmonary).
- Abdominal surgery (gastrointestinal, hepatic).
- Genitourinary/pelvic surgery.
- Orthopaedic surgery (including amputation, endoprosthesis).

Ideally, LTFU should involve both surgical and paediatric oncological teams, and include assessment of:

- Anatomy/structure.
- Physiological function.
- Psychological adaptation.

NB. Ensure patient/family/GP are informed about need for antibiotic prophylaxis for dental (and other bacteraemic) procedures in patients with endoprostheses. Patients at higher risk of LAEs include survivors of:

- **CNS tumours:** late toxicity caused by the tumour itself or by its treatment (surgery, RT, chemotherapy) affecting:
  - *physical health* – dental, auditory, neuro-endocrine function/growth impairment, thyroid function, 2° tumours;
  - *mental health* – cognitive function, behaviour;
  - *social health* – education, employment, daily living activities.
- **HSCT:** affecting any organ, tissue, body system, 2° to additive toxicity (Haemopoietic stem cell transplantation, Late complications and long-term follow-up 🕮 p.199):
  - Previous treatment.
  - Conditioning chemoradiotherapy (often incorporating TBI).
  - Consequences of chronic GvHD (allogeneic HSCT), including:
    - immune-mediated cytopenia;
    - delayed immune reconstitution;
    - *visual* – keratoconjunctivitis sicca;
    - *oral* – xerostomia, lichenoid or atrophic lesions;
    - *respiratory* – obstructive airways disease;
    - *gastrointestinal* – stricture, malabsorption;
    - *hepatic* – cholestatic damage;
    - *renal* – proteinuria, nephrotic syndrome;
    - *peripheral nervous system* – neuropathy, myasthenia gravis, vasculitic syndromes;
    - *musculoskeletal* – polymyositis, sclerodermatous joint contractures;
    - *skin* – lichenoid or sclerodermatous lesions;
    - *serosal* – effusions (pleural, pericardial, peritoneal);
    - adverse effects of immunosuppression;
    - 2° malignancy (skin, oral cavity).

The future

- There is an important need to identify and develop effective models of care for LTFU, delivering most benefit to survivors and their families, with maximum efficiency for health service resource use.
- There is justifiable concern that chronic LAEs may increase with time and interact unfavourably with the normal ageing process, leading to increasing impairment of vital organ systems (e.g. cardiac, pulmonary, renal) in early/mid-adulthood, with increased risk of premature major illness or early death.
- Protective agents may be developed to prevent damage to normal tissues by cytotoxic treatment.
- Genetic risk factors may be identified for development of LAEs in individual patients, explaining why some patients develop severe LAEs and others with similar risk factors do not.
- Newer agents may have as yet unknown LAEs and continued clinical research is vital to document nature of and risk factors for LAEs of new treatments. Therefore, all phase III randomized trials should include investigations of LAE issues.

Benign haematological diseases

Haemoglobinopathies

Introduction

A comprehensive review of haemoglobin (Hb) disorders is beyond the scope of this book. However, some children with malignant disease will happen also to have a haemoglobinopathy. In some units, staff looking after paediatric oncology patients will provide cross-cover for services looking after sickle cell disease and other haemoglobinopathies. An overview of these conditions is therefore included.

Inherited haemoglobin disorders due to globin chain gene abnormalities fall into two categories:

- **Structural variants:** qualitatively abnormal Hb molecules usually due to a single amino acid substitution [e.g. sickle cell Hb (HbS)].
- **Impaired synthesis disorders**, in which the rate of production of qualitatively normal alpha (α) or beta (β) globin chains results in an imbalance of globin chains (the thalassaemia syndromes).

Single copies of abnormal genes are often carried asymptomatically (e.g. sickle cell trait, beta-thalassaemia trait). Homozygosity or double heterozygosity for pathologically interacting abnormalities often results in clinical disease.

Laboratory diagnosis

In addition to the assessment of FBC indices, reticulocyte counts, and film appearances, structural Hb variants are demonstrated by electrophoretic techniques. Most routine hospital laboratories use a combination of high pressure liquid chromatography (HPLC) and iso-electric focusing (IEF). Sickle solubility testing (e.g. Sickledex test) provides a rapid screening test for the presence of HbS, which is useful for out-of-hours emergency testing. It does not distinguish between sickle cell trait and homozygous sickle cell disease, or the doubly heterozygous sickle disorders (see Sickling disorders ☐ pp.318–322). In combination with FBC indices and film appearances however, immediate clinical decisions may be made.

Mass spectrometry may be required to demonstrate some electrophoretically silent unstable haemoglobins, and molecular analysis may be necessary to determine thalassaemia genotypes for genetic counselling. These techniques are generally only available in national reference laboratories.

Sickling disorders

Sickle cell haemoglobin (HbS) is a β-globin chain structural abnormality due to substitution of valine for glutamic acid at position 6. The carrier state – sickle cell trait – may confer a degree of protection against malaria, accounting for the gene distribution in Afro-Caribbean, Middle Eastern, and some Indian and Mediterranean populations. HbS-containing red cells deform when deoxygenated, resulting in vasocclusive 'crises'. Susceptibility depends on the proportion of HbS present.

Sickle cell trait

Heterozygotes with an HbS gene from one parent and a normal HbA β-globin gene from the other parent have the HbAS carrier state, known as sickle cell trait. These individuals have around 40% HbS (lower if coincidental alpha-thalassaemia trait). They have normal blood counts and red cell indices, and are asymptomatic unless oxygen saturation falls <40%, when sickling may occur with severe hypoxia. Screening for sickle cell trait is indicated prior to anaesthesia in individuals of non-Northern European descent. Screening of partners for HbS and potentially interacting β chain abnormalities is appropriate for genetic counselling.

Sickle cell diseases (SCD)

When the proportion of HbS is >55%, clinical sickling may occur. Homozygous sickle cell disease (HbSS) is the commonest genotype, but double heterozygosity for other β-globin disorders may result in clinical sickle cell disease:

- S/beta-thalassaemia.
- SC.
- SD^{Punjab}.
- SO^{Arab}.

Co-inheritance of alpha-thalassaemia trait or genes that promote persistence of HbF production may confer a less severe clinical phenotype in affected patients.

Clinical features

- The effects of this β chain variant tend not to become apparent until about 6 months of age since foetal Hb predominates at birth.
- Patients with sickle cell disease have a chronic haemolytic anaemia with pallor and jaundice. Long-term folic acid supplementation is appropriate.
- May develop pigment gallstones.
- Splenomegaly may be present in infants and young children, but the spleen auto-infarcts due to sickling with increasing age and by adulthood most patients have blood film features of hyposplenism (target cells, Howell-Jolly bodies; raised platelets).
- A predisposition to life-threatening pneumococcal infection is present from infancy, and prophylactic penicillin (lifelong) and pneumococcal vaccination are indicated.
- Also have a predisposition to the development of salmonella osteomyelitis, which should be considered if there is a prolonged episode of localized bone pain.

- Avascular necrosis may develop in the heads of the long bones.
- As in other haemolytic anaemias, aplastic crises due to temporary loss of compensatory reticulocytosis may occur (e.g. parvovirus B19 infection).
- Increased risk of stroke in SCD. Children at higher risk can be identified by transcranial Doppler (TCD) measurement of vascular flow rates. Regular exchange transfusion to maintain HbS levels <30% corrects the increased risk for high risk individuals. Annual TCD screening is recommended for children between the ages of 2 and 10 years.
- Oral hydroxycarbamide [formerly called hydroxyurea (HOH)] increases the proportion of HbF and reduces the frequency of complications in SCD. This therapy may be considered in individuals with serious or frequent SCD complications. Allogeneic haemopoietic stem cell transplantation (HSCT) is potentially curative and may be considered for high risk individuals.

Acute presentations in sickle cell diseases

Intercurrent vaso-occlusive episodes give rise to a variety of acute presentations:

Painful crisis

Localized sickling causing localized vaso-occlusion in bone or soft tissue. Frequently precipitated by intercurrent infection, cold exposure, dehydration, alcohol, or menstruation. Presents with localized severe pain. Many episodes are managed at home with oral analgesia. More severe episodes may require hospital admission for parenteral analgesia and hydration.

Dactylitis

Common presentation in early childhood. Swollen hands and/or feet due to sickling in metacarpal/metatarsal bones.

Splenic sequestration

Rare, but potentially life-threatening. Occurs in early childhood before splenic autoinfarction (Sickling disorders, Clinical features, 📖 pp.318–319). Sudden severe anaemia associated with massive splenic enlargement. May be associated with hypotension/collapse. Transfusion may be lifesaving. Parents should be taught to examine for splenomegaly.

Acute chest syndrome

Pulmonary sickling resulting in chest X-ray (CXR) shadowing and hypoxia with a high mortality. May be precipitated by infection. ITU/PICU support and consideration of exchange transfusion (Sickle cell diseases, Management of acute complications 📖 pp.320–321) may be necessary if pO_2 <70mmHg in air.

Mesenteric syndrome

Intra-abdominal sickling may mimic surgical emergencies (e.g. appendicitis, cholecystitis) Imaging/experienced surgical assessment should be undertaken in addition to supportive care before consideration of emergency surgery.

Stroke

Acute neurological deterioration is an emergency and exchange transfusion (Sickle cell diseases, Management of acute complications 📖 pp.320–321) should be considered.

Priapism

Sustained painful erection is a common complication in older boys and men. A hot bath and encouragement of micturition may be helpful. Ice should not be used. Alpha-adrenergic stimulators may be useful. Anti-androgen treatment may help to prevent recurrent episodes.

Management of acute complications

Appropriate management of the acutely unwell SCD patient consists of:
- Initial assessment, ensuring recognition of the potential clinical issues.
- Immediate supportive care, instituting symptom control.
- Non-specific measures designed to minimize the duration of any sickling episode.
- Consideration of the necessity (or otherwise) of transfusion therapy (top-up or exchange).
- Any additional specific therapy required.

Assessment

In addition to the clinical history and examination, immediate assessment should include measurement and documentation of:
- Temperature.
- Pulse rate, blood pressure.
- Respiratory rate, arterial oxygen saturation (SaO_2).
- Pain score.
- Presence of organomegaly (sequestration syndromes).
- Asymmetrical neurological signs (stroke).
- Priapism (post-pubertal boys).

Investigation should include FBC and reticulocytes, renal and liver function tests, inflammatory markers, transfusion specimen. CXR if respiratory symptoms/signs or hypoxia.

Supportive care
- Analgesia: if pain severe and not controlled by non-opioids (paracetamol and/or ibuprofen) give opioids either:
  - *Oral regimen* – oral morphine stat, followed by every 3h as necessary, then start oral slow release morphine with dose adjustment at 24h if necessary.
  - *Parenteral regimen* – morphine IV/SC/IM, repeated every 20min until pain is controlled, then every 2–4h IV/SC as required. If infusion or patient-controlled analgesia (PCA) system used, there must be protocols for monitoring respiratory rate, hypoxia, and sedation, and appropriately experienced staff.
  - Continue non-opioid analgesia (paracetamol and/or ibuprofen as above). Consider single injection of IM ketorolac (non-steroidal anti-inflammatory drug, NSAID).

- *Laxatives* (e.g. lactulose) – should be prescribed routinely with opiates, other adjuvants as necessary, including antipruritics (e.g. hydroxyzine), anti-emetics (e.g. cyclizine).
- Monitor pain, sedation, respiratory rate, oxygen saturation every 30min until pain controlled and then every 2h. Give rescue doses of analgesia for breakthrough pain (50% of maintenance dose every 30min). Omit opioid if respiratory depression (respiratory rate <10/min) and if severe respiratory depression/sedation occurs, give naloxone IV.
- **Fluid replacement:** oral fluid intake >60mL/kg/24h should be encouraged. If not possible due to, e.g. nausea/vomiting, then IV fluid should be given.
- **Oxygen:** no evidence base for routine use, but if respiratory symptoms or signs, or SaO$_2$ <95% in air, oxygen should be given.
- **Antibiotics:** routine antibiotic administration (other than continuation of prophylactic penicillin) is not required unless there is clinical suspicion of infection (fever >38°C, localizing symptoms/signs), in which case a broad spectrum cephalosporin (+ a macrolide, e.g. erythromycin if there are respiratory signs) is appropriate.
- **Transfusion:** blood transfusion is not routinely required in sickle crises. The Hb often falls temporarily 1–2g/dL below baseline. Any decision to transfuse should be discussed with a haematologist. An extended red cell phenotype should be undertaken and appropriate blood for transfusion selected to minimize the risk of alloimmunization (Blood transfusion 📖 pp.231–243). Transfusion may be undertaken in 2 ways:
  - *Top-up* – simple transfusion aiming to increase oxygen carrying capacity. Consider if Hb has fallen >2g/dL below baseline *and* Hb <5g/dL, *and* patient symptomatic. A low reticulocyte count (aplastic crisis) makes transfusion more appropriate. Target Hb should be 10 g/dL (Blood transfusion 📖 pp.231–243) to avoid viscosity problems with higher haematocrits.
  - *Exchange transfusion* – reducing the proportion of HbS to below 30% is indicated for some serious sickle complications, e.g.
    - acute chest syndrome with persistent hypoxia (SaO$_2$ <60%);
    - acute neurological symptoms (stroke);
    - multi-organ failure.
    May be considered for other unresponsive acute episodes. Exchange is ideally accomplished using an automated cell separator, but partial exchange transfusion may be achieved manually if this is not immediately available.

Other β-globin chain variants

HbC
Apart from the potential interaction with HbS, HbC (gene prevalent in West Africa) is benign. Homozygosity is associated with mild anaemia. Causes prominent target cells on blood film.

HbD
Potential interaction with HbS as above. Otherwise benign. May have microcytic indices.

HbE

Microcytic indices in homozygotes and heterozygotes is usual. Clinically benign.

Unstable haemoglobin variants

Rare variant haemoglobins usually inherited as autosomal dominant. Clinical syndrome of chronic mild compensated haemolysis. Heinz bodies (red cell inclusions due to denatured globin) visible on blood film with supravital staining. Mass spectrometry sometimes required to confirm diagnosis in electrophoretically silent variants. May develop pigment gallstones.

High affinity haemoglobin variants

May cause a physiological polycythaemia (raised Hb/haematocrit) associated with a raised erythropoietin level, e.g. Hb Olympia.

Thalassaemia syndromes

Introduction
Reduced or absent production of qualitatively normal α or β globin chains. Clinical phenotypes include:
- **Silent carriers:** asymptomatic with normal indices.
- **Thalassaemia trait** (thalassaemia minor): microcytic indices with normal or borderline Hb level.
- **Thalassaemia intermedia**: significant anaemia, but not transfusion dependent.
- **Thalassaemia major**: transfusion dependent anaemia.
- **Hydrops fetalis**: fatal *in utero*.

Diagnosis is suggested by microcytic hypochromic red cell indices in the absence of iron deficiency or inflammation. An elevated Hbα_2 distinguishes presumed alpha-thalassaemia trait from beta-thalassaemia trait.

Alpha-thalassaemias
There are normally 4 α chain genes per cell, 2 from each parent (normal genotype designated $\alpha\alpha/\alpha\alpha$).

Silent alpha-thalassaemia ($\alpha-/\alpha\alpha$)
Have a normal Hb, but on average MCV/MCH slightly lower than the normal population, albeit overlapping with the normal range.

Alpha-thalassaemia trait ($\alpha-/\alpha-$ or $\alpha\alpha/--$)
Reduced MCV/MCH, with normal or borderline Hb. Normal HbA$_2$ distinguishes it from beta-thalassaemia trait.

HbH disease ($\alpha-/--$)
Moderate anaemia (Hb around 7–8g/dL). Usually transfusion independent. May develop splenomegaly and pigment gallstones. HbH (tetramer of β chains) bodies in red cells on supravital staining.

Hydrops fetalis ($--/--$)
Incompatible with survival to term.

- The A-/ genotype is sometimes designated α^+ and the — genotype α^0. The α^0 genotype is not found in Africa, but is common in Asian and Far Eastern populations.
- The genotype in alpha-thalassaemia trait can only be determined with certainty by molecular testing. This may be necessary for genetic counselling in couples who both have apparent alpha-thalassaemia trait if one or both are of Asian/Far East origin.
- Haemoglobin Barts (tetramer of γ chains) is present at birth in alpha-thalassaemia syndromes.

Beta-thalassaemias

There are only two β chain genes per cell. Thalassaemic genes may confer reduced (β^+) or absent (β^0) β chain production.

Beta-thalassaemia trait

Normal (or slightly reduced) Hb. Microcytic hypochromic indices in the absence of iron deficiency. Elevated HbA_2. Only clinical significance (apart from genetic implication) is that MCV cannot be used as a surrogate marker of iron status.

Homozygous beta-thalassaemia

- Some β^+ homozygotes may have a thalassaemia intermedia phenotype, but most homozygous beta-thalassaemia patients will be transfusion dependent.
- In the absence of transfusion support severe anaemia and massive organomegaly develop together with growth impairment and bone remodelling due to marrow expansion (ineffective erythropoiesis).
- Regular transfusion in order to maintain the Hb at or >10g/dL prevents these complications. An extended red cell phenotype should be undertaken and appropriate blood for transfusion selected to minimize the risk of alloimmunization (Blood transfusion 📖 pp.231–243).
- Long-term iron chelation therapy with parenteral desferrioxamine (or oral deferasirox or deferiprone) is required to prevent iron overload.
- Allogeneic HSCT (potentially curative) may be considered.

Haemostasis and thrombosis

Models of haemostasis

The simplest way to think about coagulation is a simple 'see-saw', where the factors that promote blood clot formation (the clotting factors, platelets etc) are counter-balanced by the factors that switch the process off (the natural anti-coagulants and fibrinolytic system). In a healthy situation the system is regulated so that blood clots form at the site of vessel injury, but do not extend to block the vessel.

Coagulation cascade

The coagulation cascade is now considered a slightly old-fashioned model, but is still useful as it links into the basic clotting tests:
- Intrinsic pathway (factors XII, XI, VIII and IX – assessed by the APTT [activated partial thromboplastin time]).
- Extrinsic pathway (factor VII – assessed by the PT [prothrombin time]).
- These link together to form the final common pathway (factors X, V, II, I).

Coagulation network

A newer model of coagulation, incorporating:
- Initiation by tissue factor exposure.
- Complexes with factor VII.
- Followed by factor X activation and a small amount of thrombin (IIa) generation.
- Once thrombin is generated, a series of amplification and propagation reactions occur leading to a thrombin burst, which leads to the conversion of fibrinogen to fibrin.

Platelets

Platelets are produced from megakaryocytes in the bone marrow and circulate as small anucleate cells. Their average life span is about 10 days. Platelets are vital for normal haemostasis. If activated by damaged endothelium or thrombin, platelets adhere, undergo a shape change, and subsequently release the content of their granules, which encourages further platelet activation.

Cellular model of haemostasis

This combines the features of several models of coagulation (including platelets, since many of the clotting factors are activated on their surface), and emphasizes the important roles of endothelial cells and von Willebrand factor (VWF).

Laboratory investigation of bleeding problems

Laboratory tests should be guided by the clinical picture. A basic clotting screen usually includes activated partial thromboplastin time (APTT), pro-thrombin time (PT), thrombin time (TT), and fibrinogen. If the clotting times are prolonged, a mixing study is carried out (where normal plasma is added to the tube – correction suggests a factor deficiency and a failure to correct suggests the presence of an inhibitor – most commonly a lupus anticoagulant). Platelets should by assessed by a full blood count and blood film.

- **APTT:** assesses the intrinsic clotting pathway. Prolonged in factor VIII, IX, XI, XII deficiency. Also prolonged in disseminated intravascular coagulation (DIC), by heparin or in presence of a lupus anticoagulant.
- **PT:** assesses the extrinsic clotting pathway. Prolonged in factor VII deficiency. Also prolonged in liver disease, vitamin K deficiency, warfarin (monitored by International Normalized Ratio [INR]) – a standardized PT.
- **TT:** prolonged by heparin, D-dimers or hypo/dysfibrinogenaemia.
- **Reptilase time:** useful to confirm a prolonged APTT is due to heparin (the reptilase time is normal).
- **Specific factor assays:** should be performed if a prolonged APTT or PT corrects on the addition of normal plasma.
- **Platelet count:** performed as part of an automated FBC. Also generates mean platelet volume (MPV), which indicates platelet size. Platelet count be spuriously low due to platelet clumping or in the presence of giant platelets.
- **Blood film:** for platelet size and morphology.
- **Bleeding time:** now rarely performed (particularly in children), and difficult to standardize. Causes scars.
- **Platelet function analyser** (PFA): useful screening test for platelet disorders.
- **Platelet aggregation:** aggregation in response to agonists (adrenaline, collagen, arachadonic acid, ADP, ristocetin most widely used). Aggregation patterns are characteristic for platelet disorders (see Inherited platelet disorders 🕮 p.346).
- **Thrombin generation assays:** new laboratory test to measure individual thrombin generation. Currently has mainly research applications.

Neonatal haemostasis

Normal haemostasis in neonates

Levels of coagulation factors are different in neonates compared with those in adults. Most procoagulant and anticoagulant factors are present at around 50% of adult levels at birth and rise to adult levels within the first 6 months of life. Exceptions to this are: factor VIII and fibrinogen, which are at adult levels at birth, VWF, which is higher than adult levels at birth, and factor V, which is low at birth, but rises to adult levels by day 5 of life. Despite low levels of many of the procoagulant factors, neonates have a shortened bleeding time and are protected from bleeding due to elevated VWF levels factor, particularly the haemostatically-active high molecular weight VWF multimers.

Laboratory assessment

PT, TT, and fibrinogen levels in the neonate do not differ significantly from that seen in adults. However, mostly due to the reduction in levels of the vitamin K-dependent factors, the APTT is prolonged. Different laboratory reference ranges exist for neonates/infants of differing gestational and post-natal ages.

Assessment and management of the bleeding neonate

Most haemostatic problems in the neonate are acquired. However, congenital bleeding disorders can present at this time and a family history of a bleeding tendency may not always be present. A careful history is important in determining the cause of bleeding.

Important points in the history include:
- Nature of the bleeding.
- Underlying conditions, especially sepsis, liver disease, prematurity, severe metabolic disease, all of which can predispose to the development of DIC.
- Family history of a bleeding tendency or a known inherited bleeding disorder.
- Maternal history of immune thrombocytopenia or prior history of neonatal alloimmune thrombocytopenic purpura NAITP.
- Maternal drugs, especially warfarin, anticonvulsants, antituberculous agents.

Differential diagnosis
- DIC.
- Haemorrhagic disease of the newborn (HDN) (Haemolytic disease of the newborn 📖 pp.348–349) or vitamin K deficiency bleeding.
- Congenital bleeding disorder.
- Thrombocytopenia:
  - NAITP;
  - maternal ITP;
  - congenital thrombocytopenia.
- Iatrogenic: surgical, anticoagulant agents.

Laboratory investigation
- PT/APTT/TT/Clauss fibrinogen.
- FBC, especially platelet count.
- D-dimers.
- Blood film, looking for abnormal platelet morphology (congenital platelet disorder) or red cell fragmentation (DIC).
- Coagulation factor assays if PT/APTT prolonged.
- Factor XIII level if indicated (see Factor XIII deficiency 📖 p.344).
- Specific tests of platelet function if indicated (Inherited platelet disorders 📖 p.346).

A few notes on blood sampling
- Take a peripheral venous sample wherever possible.
- If blood is taken from a central line, avoid heparin contamination by discarding the first aliquot of blood.
- Do not overfill or underfill the sample tube.
- Difficult venepuncture or slow sampling can result in activation of the coagulation system, causing shortening of the PT/APTT and thrombocytopenia due to platelet clumping.

Management of DIC in the neonate
- Treat the underlying cause, e.g. antibiotics for sepsis.
- Ensure correction of acidosis and hypothermia, which can exacerbate bleeding.
- If bleeding, correct the coagulopathy:
  - maintain PT/APTT at <1.5 × normal by infusion of 10–15mL/kg virally-inactivated plasma;
  - maintain fibrinogen at >1g/dL by infusion of 10mL/kg cryoprecipitate;
  - maintain platelet count at >50 × 10^9/L by infusion of 10–15mL/kg platelet concentrate;
  - replace vitamin K.
- If thrombosis is the major clinical manifestation, treatment with heparin and replacement of anticoagulant proteins by infusion of virally-inactivated plasma may be appropriate.
- Monitor laboratory parameters frequently, i.e. PT, APTT, Clauss fibrinogen and D-dimers.

Management of a congenital bleeding disorder in the neonate
Bleeding due to a congenital bleeding disorder is best treated by replacement of the missing coagulation factor by the administration of a coagulation factor concentrate, e.g. factor VIII concentrate in haemophilia A. In order to avoid exposure to donor plasma, recombinant products (where available) are preferred. Dosing and frequency of administration is dependant on the severity of the underlying disorder and the severity of the bleeding event. Seek expert advice.

If bleeding is severe and a factor deficiency is expected it may be necessary to give virally-inactivated plasma (10–15mL/kg) pending the results of specific coagulation factor assays.

Investigation of a mild bleeding disorder in the neonate

Due to the low levels of many of the procoagulant factors at birth, diagnosis of mild bleeding disorders can be difficult. Testing should be deferred until the child is at least 6 months of age. Mild bleeding disorders are unlikely to cause problems before then unless major surgery is required. This is true for mild haemophilia A or B, type 1 von Willebrand disease, and mild platelet function disorders. Molecular testing, if appropriate, can help to make the diagnosis.

Important specific bleeding symptoms in the neonate

Bleeding in the neonate can manifest as:
- Post-surgical bleeding (including post-circumcision bleeding).
- Bleeding from venepuncture/heel prick/intramuscular injection.
- Cephalohaematoma.
- Pulmonary haemorrhage.
- Intracranial/intraventricular haemorrhage.
- Bleeding from the umbilical stump.
- Bruising.

Some bleeding symptoms are suggestive of specific underlying congenital bleeding disorders and may require further investigation, even if the basic coagulation screen is normal. Discussion with an expert is required.

Intracranial/intraventricular haemorrhage
- Severe haemophilia A or B.
- Factor XIII deficiency.
- Factor VII deficiency.
- Factor X deficiency.
- Type 3 von Willebrand disease.

Bleeding from the umbilical stump
- Factor XIII deficiency.
- Congenital afibrinogenaemia/dysfibrinogenaemia.

Prevention of bleeding in the neonate

Platelet transfusion

It is common practice to transfuse platelets to maintain a platelet count of $>20 \times 10^9$/L in a well, term neonate, $>30 \times 10^9$/L in a well preterm neonate and $>50 \times 10^9$/L in a sick neonate.

Infusion of virus-inactivated plasma

10–15mL/kg recommended prior to invasive procedures with a risk of bleeding in neonates with PT/APTT $>1.5 \times$ normal.

Haemophilia A

- Factor VIII (FVIII) deficiency.
- X-linked.
- 1 in 30,000 male births.

Family history is absent in 1/3rd of cases (due to new mutations). Classified according to baseline level of FVIII:

- **<1%:** severe (apparently spontaneous bleeding into joints and muscles)
- **1–5%:** moderate (bleeding after minor trauma; spontaneous bleeding unusual).
- **5–30%:** mild (bleeding usually only after significant trauma or surgery).

Genetics

Factor VIII gene is on X chromosome (26 exons). Causative mutations for mild, moderate, and 50% of severe cases are scattered throughout the gene. The other 50% of severe cases are due to the same mutation (the 'flip-tip' inversion in intron 22). Female offspring of affected males are 'obligate carriers'

Clinical features

Previously children with severe haemophilia presented with joint or muscle bleeding when they started weight bearing (age 1–2 years). Now earlier presentation is common due to bruising (often raised or 'chunky' – with a small palpable haematoma in the middle of the bruise). May be confused with non-accidental injury (NAI), so it is important to check clotting screen in all cases of possible NAI.

The natural history of severe haemophilia was previously bleak, with recurrent joint bleeds leading to progressive arthropathy with associated disability. This has been transformed by the use of factor VIII prophylaxis (Management, Severe haemophilia A ☐ p.335).

Moderate and mild haemophilia A may present at any age, either with bruising or bleeding after trauma or surgery.

Investigations

Hallmark of haemophlia is isolated prolongation of APTT. All the other clotting tests are normal. Diagnosis is made by specific factor VIII assay.

Management

Recombinant factor VIII is the treatment of choice. Several types are available, clinically all the same, but do vary in manufacturing process and formulation. This treatment is expensive, so it is not readily available in many parts of the world.

If recombinant factor VIII is unavailable, plasma-derived factor VIII (virus-inactivated to prevent HIV and hepatitis transmission) can be used.

Before factor VIII concentrates were available, crypoprecipitate was used, but this is no longer recommended.

Dose calculation

[Target FVIII level (%) − baseline FVIII level] × body weight (kg)/2
e.g. for major bleeding in a 20kg patient with severe haemophilia = (100 − 0)
× 20/2 = 1000 units.

Factor VIII is available in different vial sizes − round up to nearest vial size.

Minor bleeds may respond to a single dose of factor VIII, but for more significant bleeds, depending on the clinical situation, follow-up doses may be required. For serious bleeding or major surgery, it may be appropriate to use a continuous infusion of factor VIII.

Severe haemophilia A

- Bleeding episodes treated with factor VIII replacement.
- Aim to raise factor VIII level to at least 50% for joint/muscle bleeds or 100% for severe bleeding, such as intracranial.
- Maintain a haemostatic level of factor VIII for a few days (duration according to severity of initial bleed) to prevent re-bleeding.
- Prophylaxis with factor VIII is used in severe haemophilia to prevent bleeding, factor VIII injections are given 1–3 times per week depending on age.
- A port-a-cath may be required for venous access in small children.

Moderate haemophilia A

Usually require factor VIII replacement (calculate dose as for severe haemophilia A).

Mild haemophilia

- May respond to DDAVP. Usually there is a 3–5-fold increase in the baseline factor VIII level, so if the baseline level is >10% DDAVP is usually useful. Give IV (over 30min as infusion) or SC.
- **Dose:** 0.3µg/kg (maximum dose 20µg).
- **Side effects:** flushing, hypotension (occasional severe) and hyponatraemia (fluid restrict for 24h − important to avoid rare hyponatraemic convulsions). Repeated doses of DDAVP may be poorly tolerated or associated with tachyphylaxis.

Laboratory monitoring

Most factor VIII concentrates and DDAVP can be monitored using a standard one stage factor VIII assay.

B-domain deleted recombinant factor VIII (marketed as Refacto in the UK) must be monitored by a 2-stage assay or using a specific laboratory standard, so it is important to inform the laboratory if the patient is receiving this type of factor VIII.

Organization of care for inherited bleeding disorders

It is important to adopt a multidisciplinary approach to the care of patients with haemophilia and other inherited bleeding disorders. In the UK there is a national network of 'Comprehensive Care Centres' (CCC) co-ordinated by the UK Haemophilia Centre Doctors' Organisation (UKHCDO). A CCC should be able to provide all aspects of care.

Management of pregnant haemophilia carrier and during the neonatal period

A woman with a family history of haemophilia should receive genetic counselling and carrier status should be confirmed by genetic testing. For severe haemophilia, pre-implantation genetic diagnosis or antenatal diagnosis are available. Many female carriers decline these options and management of the pregnancy and delivery is according to foetal sex (determined by US). Close communication between the obstetric team and the haemophilia centre is vital. A delivery plan should be clearly agreed. Normal vaginal delivery is preferred – Caesarean section should be performed for obstetric reasons only (it does not protect baby from bleeding). Instrumental delivery (ventouse or traumatic forceps) should be avoided (risk of intracranial or subgaleal bleeding).

Cord blood sample for factor VIII level

- **Severe haemophilia:** easy to diagnose confidently.
- **Mild/moderate haemophilia:** factor VIII may be falsely high at birth, so it is important to repeat when older.

For severe haemophilia, give factor VIII therapy if any concern about neo-natal bleeding – some advocate a single treatment with factor VIII at birth to protect against risk of neonatal intracranial haemorrhage (ICH) (~2%). This is controversial as it may be associated with a risk of inhibitor development when older (Inhibitors in children with haemophilia 📖 pp.336–337).

Inhibitors in children with haemophilia

Inhibitors (allo-antibodies against infused factor VIII) are detected in up to 30% of children – many are transient, but about 5–10% are clinically significant.

Risk factors

- Haemophilia A (more common than in haemophilia B).
- Large deletion in factor VIII gene.
- Younger age of first exposure (controversial).
- No convincing evidence that the risk is greater with any particular FVIII product.

Clinical presentation

May be picked up by routine screening. The risk is greatest around 10th treat-ment exposure. Associated with poor response to treatment (or develop-ment of anaphylaxis in haemophlia B).

Laboratory tests

Inhibitor is quantified using the Bethesda assay (Bethesda units, BU). May be low titre (<5BU) or high titre. Inhibitor levels usually increase if on-going factor VIII treatment.

Clinical management
- **Low titre and transient:** no treatment required as the inhibitors disappear.
- **High titre:** stop FVIII treatment. Treat bleeding with a bypass agent (either recombinant factor VIIa or FEIBA). When inhibitor titre falls to <5BU, start immune tolerance induction (intensive therapy involving high dose factor VIII and sometimes additional immunosuppression; response seen in 70%, but may take many months). Management of inhibitor patients who fail to respond to this treatment is difficult – treat on demand with bypass agents. Prophylaxis with bypass agents is controversial.

Haemophilia B (Christmas disease)

- Factor IX deficiency.
- X-linked.
- Clinical and laboratory features identical to haemophilia A, but specific factor assay reveals low factor IX, rather than factor VIII.

Genetics

Factor IX gene is on X chromosome (9 exons). Mutations are scattered throughout gene. Rare haemophilia B Leyden is androgen responsive – factor IX level improves at puberty.

Management

Recombinant factor IX concentrate is the treatment of choice. Longer half-life than factor VIII, so daily treatment is usually sufficient for bleeding episodes.

Initial dose calculation

[Target factor IX level (%) – baseline factor IX level] × body weight (kg) e.g. for major bleeding in a 20kg patient with severe haemophilia B = (100 – 0) × 20 = 2000units. Monitor factor IX levels to determine frequency of dosing.

If recombinant factor IX is not available, use purified plasma-derived factor IX (virus-inactivated) or prothrombin complex concentrate (also contains other clotting factors, so is associated with a risk of thrombosis ⚠; monitor factor IX levels carefully).

von Willebrand disease

Due to either a quantitative or qualitative defect in VWF.

Clinical features originally described by Dr Eric von Willebrand in a large kindred in the Aland Islands (the index case exsanguinated during menstrual period in adolescence). Clinical severity is highly variable due to large number of different underlying molecular defects.

Functions of VWF

VWF is a large multimeric protein with a pivotal role in haemostasis, which is synthesized in endothelial cells and megakaryocytes and circulates as a large multimeric protein (of varying molecular weights). A cleaving protease (called ADAMTS13) prevents ultra-large multimers from forming (Other non-malignant causes of peripheral blood cytopenias, Haemolytic uraemic syndrome/thrombotic thrombocytopenic purpura pp.386–387).

VWF has several different functions. Forms a bridge between damaged endothelium and platelets as part of platelet plug formation (high molecular weight multimers most important). It is also a carrier protein for factor VIII (reason for diagnostic confusion between some types of VWD and haemophilia A).

Classification of VWD

- **Type 1:** mild quantitative reduction in VWF.
- **Type 2:** qualitative defects in VWF.
  - *Type 2A* – absent high molecular weight multimers;
  - *Type 2B* – increased interaction between VWF and platelets (associated with thrombocytopenia);
  - *Type 2M* – normal multimer pattern;
  - *Type 2N* – reduced binding of factor VIII (N is for Normandy – originally found in a French family).
- **Type 3**: severe quantitative reduction in VWF.

Genetics

VWD genetics is complex. VWF gene is on chromosome 12.

- Type 1 inheritance is usually autosomal dominant. Mutations in VWF gene in approximately 50% of cases. Underlying molecular defect in remaining 50% remains unclear. Non-genetic factors also influence baseline VWF level, e.g. ABO blood group (blood group O have lower levels than A, B, or AB), exercise, pregnancy, menstrual cycle, oral contraceptive pill. Distinguishing between individuals with mild type 1 VWD and those at the bottom of the normal range is difficult.
- Type 2A is usually autosomal dominant. Caused by defects in VWF multimerization or increased proteolysis. Type 2A mutations cluster in the VWF A2 domain.
- Type 2B is caused by a mutation in the VWF gene at the platelet binding site which leads to a gain of function (VWF binds platelets more strongly than normal) and associated thrombocytopenia. Usually autosomal dominant. Mutations cluster in the VWF A1 domain.
- Type 2M is usually autosomal dominant. Mutations in VWF A1 domain.

- Type 2N is autosomal recessive. Affected individuals are homozygous or compound heterozygotes for mutations in the VWF factor VIII binding region.
- Type 3 is autosomal recessive. Molecular defects include large deletions.

Clinical features

Mucocutaneous bleeding is the hallmark – nosebleeds, gastrointestinal (association with angiodysplasia), menorrhagia (may be severe particularly in adolescent girls). May bleed after trauma and surgery. Bleeding into joints is uncommon, but may happen in severe type 3 VWD.

Laboratory tests

The APTT may be prolonged if factor VIII level is low. The correct diagnosis and classification of VWD requires several tests:
- To quantify (VWF antigen).
- To assess function (the VWF ristocetin co-factor is the most widely used functional assay, but VWF collagen binding assay is used in some labs; factor VIII binding assay is required to diagnose 2N subtype).
- Multimer analysis.

The following are typical laboratory abnormalities for each sub-type:
- **1:** reduced VWF antigen and functional tests.
- **2A:** slightly reduced VWF antigen, markedly reduced VWF ristocetin cofactor, absent high molecular weight multimers.
- **2B:** platelet count usually slightly low ($75–100 \times 10^9$/L). VWF antigen is normal or slightly low. VWF ristocetin cofactor is decreased. RIPA (ristocetin-induced platelet agglutination) is increased.
- **2M:** slightly reduced VWF antigen; markedly reduced VWF ristocetin cofactor, normal VWF multimers (distinguishes 2M from 2A).
- **2N:** low factor VIII (must distinguish from haemophilia A), reduced factor VIII binding.
- **3:** absent VWF (VWF antigen <1%). markedly reduced VWF ristocetin cofactor and factor VIII, absent VWF multimers.

Clinical management

The aim of treatment is to elevate VWF level to secure haemostasis or prevent bleeding after surgery. Anti-fibrinolytics are useful for mucosal bleeding:
- **Type 1:** usually responds to DDAVP (see mild haemophilia A). Intranasal DDAVP may be useful to control menorrhagia.
- **Type 2:** may respond to DDAVP; if poor response use VWF plasma concentrate.
- **Type 3:** VWF plasma concentrate.

Acquired VWD

Most commonly associated with Wilms' tumour. Check VWF level prior to biopsy.

Factor XI deficiency

Factor XI deficiency is the one inherited bleeding disorder that does not follow the usual rules. There is a poor correlation between the baseline factor level and the severity of the bleeding tendency. Previously, it was thought to be restricted to certain ethnic groups (e.g. Ashkenazi Jews), but it is now recognized to be widely dispersed in all populations.

Clinical features
- Mucosal bleeding.
- Bleeding after trauma or surgery.
- Joint bleeds rare.

Laboratory features
Usually prolonged APTT. May be very long if factor XI is very low. Some patients with mild factor XI deficiency may have a normal APTT – clinical bleeding may occur in some individuals with a factor XI level as high as 70u/dL.

Clinical management
Bleeding can be treated by raising the factor XI level, either by FFP infusion (preferably virus-inactivated) or by factor XI concentrate (close monitoring of factor XI levels as associated with a risk of thrombotic side effects).

Factor V deficiency

- Very rare.
- Factor V gene is on chromosome 1.
- Platelets contain about 20% of the factor V in the circulation.

Clinical features
- Autosomal recessive. Consanguinity may be present.
- Predominantly mucosal bleeding.
- Joint bleeds may occur after trauma.
- Post-surgical bleeding.

Laboratory features
- Prolonged PT and APTT.
- Confirm by specific factor V assay.

Clinical management
- No factor V concentrate available – use FFP (virus-inactivated).
- Aim for factor V level >15% for normal haemostasis.
- Anti-fibrinolytics may be useful.

Factor VII deficiency

Factor VII is vitamin K-dependent. Factor VII gene is on chromosome 13.
Autosomal recessive.
Incidence of severe factor VII deficiency (<2%) is 1:500,000.

Clinical features
- Poor correlation between factor VII level and bleeding problems.
- Mucosal bleeding is common [epistaxis, menorrhagia (iron deficiency)].
  Joint bleeds unusual.
- Occasional CNS bleeding in neonatal period.

Laboratory features
- Isolated prolongation of PT.
- Specific factor VII assay (N.B. Low levels in neonatal period may make
  diagnosis difficult).

Clinical management
- Treat bleeding episodes with FFP (virus-inactivated) or plasma VII
  concentrate. Frequent infusions may be needed due to short plasma
  half life of factor VII. Level of 10–15% is required for normal
  haemostasis.
- Recombinant factor VIIa can be used for severe factor VII deficiency –
  low dose required e.g. 20µg/kg every 6h.

Factor X deficiency

Factor X is vitamin K-dependent. Factor X gene is on chromosome 13.
Autosomal recessive.
Incidence of severe factor VII deficiency (<2%) is 1:1,000,000.

Clinical features
- **Heterozygotes:** mild bleeding tendency.
- **Compound heterozygotes/homozygotes:** variable factor X level
  (0–5%) with variable clinical bleeding phenotype. Mucosal bleeding
  (epistaxis, menorrhagia – may be severe).

Laboratory features
- Both PT and APTT are prolonged.
- Use specific factor X assay to confirm diagnosis (may be low in
  neonatal period).

Clinical management
- No pure factor X concentrate available.
- Use FFP (virus-inactivated) or prothrombin complex concentrate.
- Aim for factor X level of 15–20% for normal haemostasis.

Factor XIII deficiency

Very rare. Autosomal recessive. Consanguinity may be present.

Clinical features
- Severe deficiency causes bleeding from the umbilical stump in the neonatal period (85%).
- High risk of ICH without regular treatment.

Laboratory features
- Normal clotting screen, so diagnosis may be missed or delayed.
- Specific factor XIII assay required.

Clinical management
- Factor XIII replacement for severe deficiency – start as soon as diagnosis established.
- Long half-life, so treatment only required 4–6 weekly.
- Aim to maintain trough factor XIII >3–5%.

Factor XII deficiency

Causes confusion since it is not associated with bleeding despite prolonged APTT.

There may be a paradoxical association with thrombosis (uncertain in children). The original patient (John Hageman – 'Hageman Factor') died of thrombosis.

Clinical features
- Usually entirely asymptomatic.
- Often picked up when coagulation screen performed for an unrelated reason.

Laboratory features
- Isolated prolongation of APTT.
- **Heterozygotes:** mildly prolonged APTT, slightly reduced factor XII level.
- **Homozygotes:** markedly prolonged APTT, factor XII level <1%.

Clinical management
- No intervention required.
- Not at risk of bleeding after surgery or other invasive procedures.

Rare factor deficiencies

Factor II deficiency

Very rare. Gene on chromosome 11. Consanguinuity may be present. Prolonged PT and APTT. Treat with prothrombin complex concentrate.

Combined factors V and VIII deficiency

Rare. Autosomal recessive. Consanguinuity may be present. Mutations in *ERGIC-53* gene on chromosome 18. Defects in this protein cause abnormal intracellular trafficking of several proteins including factors V and VIII. Usually mild clinical bleeding problems.

Combined deficiency of vitamin K-dependent clotting factors (VKDCF)

Rare. Autosomal recessive. Consanguinuity may be present. Variable clinical severity – most severe may present in neonatal period with ICH. Factors II, VII, IX, and X reduced. Prolonged PT and APTT. May respond to vitamin K administration. If bleeding, use FFP (virus-inactivated).

Inherited platelet disorders

All inherited platelet disorders are rare. Associated with a variable clinical bleeding phenotype, including skin bleeding (petechiae), mucosal, post-traumatic, and post-surgical bleeding. Suspect if clotting screen is normal.

Glanzmann thrombasthenia

Autosomal recessive. Reduced or absent platelet glycoprotein IIb/IIIa. Normal platelet count/size. Reduced/absent platelet aggregation to all agonists except ristocetin. Confirm by flow cytometry/genetic analysis.

Treat mucosal bleeding with anti-fibrinolytics. Recombinant factor VIIa for significant bleeding/surgery. Platelet transfusion reserved for life-threatening bleeds (risk of anti-platelet antibody formation).

Inherited giant platelet disorders

Often confused with ITP. Usually present early in life – consider if the usual ITP picture is absent.

Bernard Soulier syndrome

- Rare. Autosomal recessive. Defective platelet glycoprotein 1b-IX-V complex.
- Thrombocytopenia, giant platelets on blood film, variable bleeding (tends to improve with age).
- Platelet aggregation studies – reduced platelet agglutination with ristocetin (normal response with other agonists).

May-Hegglin anomoly

Mild to moderate thrombocytopenia. Giant platelets on blood film. Inclusions in neutrophils (Dohle bodies). Variable bleeding problems (occasionally severe). Now classified as *MYH9*-related thrombocytopenia syndrome (along with Sebastian, Fechtner, and Epstein syndromes) – mutation disrupts non-muscle myosin, which causes defective megakaryopoiesis.

Grey platelet syndrome

Very rare. Thrombocytopenia, large agranular platelets, variable bleeding. Defect in packing of platelet secretory granules.

Other congenital thrombocytopenias

CAMT (congenital amegakaryocytic thrombocytopenia)

- Mutations in the *MPL* gene. Variable thrombocytopenia – may be severe. Risk of progressive bone marrow failure.
- Often need HSCT.

TAR (thrombocytopenia and absent radii)

Thrombocytopenia often improves with age.

WAS (Wiskott-Aldrich syndrome)

- X-linked. Eczema, immunodeficiency.
- HSCT may be needed.

Inherited platelet function defects

- Dense granule disorders, e.g. Hermansky-Pudlak syndrome, Chediak-Higashi syndrome.
- α-granule disorders, e.g. grey platelet syndrome.

Fibrinogen problems

Fibrinogen is produced in the liver. Normal plasma level is 1.5–4g/L. Made up of 3 different chains (genes all on chromosome 4).

Fibrinogen is cleaved by thrombin to produce fibrin, which is vital for clot formation.

Inherited fibrinogen problems

Afibrinogenaemia

Very rare. Consanguinity often present.
Variable bleeding:
- Joint bleeds.
- CNS bleeding.
- Miscarriages.
- Pregnancy-associated bleeding.
- Poor wound healing.

Marked prolongation of PT, APTT, and TT. Treat with fibrinogen concentrate.

Hypofibrinogenaemia

- Rare.
- Less severe bleeding.
- Prolonged TT.

Dysfibrinogenaemia

- Uncommon.
- Highly variable clinical phenotype:
  - 1/3rd asymptomatic;
  - 1/3rd bleeding tendency (severity variable);
  - 1/3rd prothrombotic (underling mutation causes net gain of function).
- Prolonged TT and reptilase time.
- Molecular defect may give information about likely clinical problems.
Treatment dictated by clinical circumstances – if bleeding, use fibrinogen concentrate or cryoprecipitate.

Acquired fibrinogen problems

Disseminated intravascular coagulation

- Low fibrinogen and associated consumptive coagulopathy.
- Many triggers (sepsis, malignancy, trauma, shock).
- Treat underlying cause.
- Haemostatic support if bleeding (Neonatal haemostasis, Assessment and management of the bleeding neonate, Management of DIC in the neonate 📖 pp.330–331).

Haemorrhagic disease of the newborn

Vitamin K is required for the γ-carboxylation of the vitamin K-dependant coagulation factors (factors II, VII, IX and X). Deficiency and/or antagonism of vitamin K activity can result in a bleeding tendency. When this occurs in the neonate it is referred to as HDN.

Risk factors

Neonates are physiologically at risk due to:
- Lack of gut flora to synthesize vitamin K.
- Reduced capacity of liver to produce coagulation factors.
- Prematurity.
- Cholestatic liver disease or GI tract pathology. Results in reduced vitamin K absorption.
- Maternal drugs, including warfarin, anticonvulsnats, antituberculous agents.
- Breastfeeding (20-fold increased risk compared with formula-fed infants).

Clinical features

Early HDN
- Occurs within first 24h of life.
- Tends to present with ICH or cephalohaematoma.
- Usually associated with maternal drugs (see above).

Classical HDN
- Occurs at 1–7 days of life.
- Tends to present with bruising, umbilical cord bleeding, post-circumcision bleeding, or gastrointestinal bleeding.
- Occurs almost exclusively in breast-fed infants.

Late HDN
- Occurs at 3–8 weeks of life.
- Can present with ICH.
- Often associated with cholestatic liver disease.

Investigation
- The neonate with HDN usually has an isolated raised PT, but APTT may also be raised if severe.
- Levels of vitamin K-dependant factors (see above) are reduced.
- More specialized tests to confirm vitamin K deficiency or antagonism include:
  - measurement of PIVKAs (proteins induced by vitamin K absence – non γ-carboxylated factors II, VII, IX and X), which are raised;
  - serum vitamin K levels, which are low.
- TT, fibrinogen, and platelet count are normal.

Management

Urgent administration of IV vitamin K 1mg (given SC if unable to gain IV access) will correct PT/APTT within 4–6h.

If severe or life-threatening haemorrhage is present, consider administration of FFP (10–15mL/kg) or a prothrombin complex concentrate (PCC) – contains vitamin K-dependant factors).

Prevention

Vitamin K is routinely given to newborn infants in order to prevent HDN. Traditionally, it was administered as a single dose of IM vitamin K 1mg, but there has been concern about an increased risk of childhood malignancy in children given IM vitamin K at birth. This remains controversial. Some centres now instead use repeated oral doses for the first 6–12 weeks of life in breastfed infants and reserve IM vitamin K for high-risk infants.

Idiopathic thrombocytopenic purpura

- Common condition in children.
- May occur at any age. Most patients are 2–5 years old (M=F).
- Often preceded by a virus infection (80%).

Pathophysiology

Auto-antibodies bind to platelets leading to peripheral destruction – removed prematurely from the circulation (mainly in spleen, but also liver).

Clinical features

Most present as acute ITP, with history of recent virus infection followed by sudden onset of bruising and petechiae (may be widespread, often most marked on legs). Blood blisters in mouth. Serious bleeding very unusual. Occasional gastrointestinal bleeding. Intracranial bleeding is rare.

Laboratory features

- Isolated thrombocytopenia (usually platelet count <20 × 10⁹/L). FBC otherwise normal.
- Blood film shows giant platelets.
- ITP is a diagnosis of exclusion.
- Clotting screen is normal.
- Bone marrow examination (if performed – Idiopathic thrombocytopenic purpura Clinical management, FAQs 🕮 p.350) shows normal marrow with plentiful megakaryocytes.
- Platelet-associated antibodies are detectable, but this test is rarely useful in practice.

Clinical management

Spontaneous remission occurs in >80%, usually within 2–4 weeks. No treatment is required unless serious or troublesome bleeding (treat the patient not the platelet count). Repeat FBC after a few days to ensure no new features developing; thereafter, do not repeat FBC if petechiae still present, since it will only confirm platelet count still low.

A small minority of children have serious bleeding. If treatment is required, a short course of prednisolone or intravenous immunoglobulin is used.

FAQs

What is the risk of serious bleeding in a child with ITP?

The risk is very low. Risk of ICH is probably about 1 in 1000. Most children can be looked after safely out of hospital – they can go to school, but should avoid activities with risk of trauma.

Open access is given to ward. Warn parents of symptoms/signs of serious bleeding (headache, vomiting, black stools).

Is a bone marrow examination always required in children with ITP?

No. It is only required if any atypical features are present or if thrombocytopenia does not improve within a few months.

Differential diagnosis

Consider other causes of thrombocytopenia if any atypical clinical or laboratory features.

Rarely the following conditions are confused with ITP:

- WAS (small platelets on blood film; eczema).
- Bernard Soulier (or other congenital thrombopathy).
- Type 2B VWD.
- Congenital amegakaryocytic thrombocytopenia.
- Fanconi anaemia/aplastic anaemia (low platelets often the first sign of bone marrow failure).
- Leukaemia (often the condition parents are most worried about, but isolated thrombocytopenia is an extremely rare presentation of leukaemia).

Micro-angiopathic haemolytic anaemias

Characterized by thrombocytopenia, red cell fragmentation, spherocytes, reticulocytosis and high LDH. There are many underlying causes.

Congenital thrombotic thrombocytopenic purpura (TTP)

- Rare; usually presents early in life.
- Often have thrombotic problems, but may bleed due to thrombocytopenia. Mutation in ADAMTS13 gene (reduced protease required for cleavage of large VWF multimers). Treat with plasma infusions.

Idiopathic TTP

Rare in children; caused by an antibody against ADAMTS13. Plasma exchange required.

Haemolytic-uraemic syndrome (HUS)

Haemolytic anaemia. Thrombocytopenia. Acute renal failure.

Thrombosis in childhood

Introduction
Thrombotic events are rare in childhood. However, they are occurring more frequently over time as a complication of successful treatment of previously fatal conditions (prematurity, malignancy, congenital heart disease).

Incidence
Annual incidence is 0.7–4.9 per 100,000 children.

Epidemiology
Incidence is highest in neonates (due to raised haematocrit, relatively high VWF/FVIII levels, small vessels) and adolescents (due to obesity, thrombophilia, oral contraceptive pill (OCP), connective tissue disorders, e.g. systemic lupus erythematosus (SLE).

Risk factors
Idiopathic thrombosis is rare (<5% of thrombotic events).
The most important risk factor is a central venous access device (CVAD), present in 92% of neonatal thrombosis and 64% of thrombosis in older children. Other frequent risk factors include:
- Malignancy (in 23% of thrombotic episodes).
- Congenital heart disease (15%).
- Trauma (15%).
- TPN.
- Infection.
- Nephrotic syndrome.
- Surgery.
- Inflammatory bowel disease.
- SLE.
- OCP.
- Sickle cell disease.

Venous thrombosis can also occur in the presence of congenital vascular anomalies, e.g. IVC agenesis, thoracic outlet syndrome, May–Thurner syndrome, popliteal vein entrapment, venous malformation.
Cardiac catheterization is a major cause of arterial thrombosis.

Symptoms and signs
- **Deep venous thrombosis** (DVT): pain, swelling, warmth, erythema of limb (may be upper limb if CVAD-related and line is sited in upper venous system), CVAD malfunction.
- **Pulmonary embolism** (PE): dyspnoea, pleuritic chest pain, haemoptysis, hypoxia, tachycardia.
- **Cavernous sinus venous thrombosis** (CSVT): headache, focal weakness/paraesthesia, lethargy, seizures, distension of superficial scalp veins.
- **Arterial thrombosis:** pain, pallor, cool limb, absent, or reduced pulses.

Investigation

- **Doppler ultrasound:** can be used to diagnose lower limb/jugular DVT or arterial thrombosis. Lacks sensitivity for upper limb DVT.
- **Venography:** may be essential in diagnosis of upper limb DVT and neonatal venous thrombosis.
- **VQ scan/CT pulmonary angiography** (CTPA): for diagnosis of PE.
- **CT venogram/MR venogram:**– for diagnosis of CSVT.
- **D-dimers:** a negative D-dimers result may be helpful in ruling out a venous thrombotic event. D-dimers is often raised due to underlying disease rather than thrombosis.

Thrombophilia testing

- Generally not recommended in children.
- Fewer than 10% of children with thrombosis have a thrombophilic abnormality, especially if the thrombotic event was CVAD-related. Testing is expensive and can have long-term implications for the child and family members.
- Testing may be informative in spontaneous thrombosis in an adolescent. A child should ideally only be tested when they are old enough to understand and to give consent.
  First-line thrombophilia testing would include:
- Antithrombin level.
- Protein C and S levels.
- Genetic analysis for Factor V Leiden mutation and prothrombin gene mutation *G20210A*.
- Lupus anticoagulant screen and anticardiolipin antibodies.

Treatment of paediatric thrombosis

Due to the lack of data from RCTs, data is extrapolated from adult studies. Treatment is often individualized and based on the prior experience of the treating physician.

Conservative management

May be appropriate if asymptomatic, CVAD-related thrombosis and alternative venous access exists so that line can be removed. Repeat diagnostic imaging after 24–72h and anticoagulate if clot extends.

Anticoagulant therapy

Duration
- Current practice varies, but generally takes 6 weeks to 3 months.
- Alter duration depending on aetiology (e.g. shorter duration if transient risk factor, longer duration if spontaneous event or known thrombophilia).

Anticoagulant agent
Unfractionated heparin (UFH)
- May be optimal choice if there is a high risk of bleeding or a potential need for urgent reversal.
- Given IV.
- See Table 23.1 for dosing.

Low molecular weight heparin (LMWH)
- Preferred option if low risk of bleeding.
- Can be administered at home by a parent or carer.
- See Table 23.2 for dosing.

Warfarin
Difficult to manage in children due to:
- Variable dose requirements with age.
- Effect of intercurrent illnesses and medications on warfarin metabolism.
- Effect of vitamin K intake in diet (more vitamin K in formula feed than in breast milk causing warfarin resistance).
- Only available in tablet form.
- Needs frequent monitoring with INR leading to time taken off from school.

If warfarin is used, parents usually have a home monitor (e.g. Coagucheck) for capillary INR testing.
See Table 23.3 for dosing.

Thrombolytic therapy

Can be considered in life- or limb-threatening thrombotic event:

- PE with cardiorespiratory compromise.
- Organ-threatening thrombotic event, e.g. bilateral renal vein thrombosis.
- Arterial thrombosis with threatened limb.
- Ischaemic stroke if presenting within 3h.
- Extensive upper or lower limb DVT (may reduce the risk of post-thrombotic syndrome).

Children <1 year of age require infusion of virally-inactivated plasma as a source of plasminogen prior to thrombolysis. Serious bleeding occurs in 5–10% of children treated with a recombinant tissue plasminogen activator, e.g. Alteplase.

FAQs

What if a child is on anticoagulant therapy, but needs an invasive procedure, e.g. intrathecal administration of chemotherapy?

Anticoagulant therapy should be stopped prior to the procedure:

- **UFH:** 4h.
- **LMWH:** 18h for enoxaparin, 24h for tinzaparin.
- **Warfarin:** 4 days.

If high risk of recurrence (thrombotic event was within last 4 weeks or was CSVT), may need UFH 'bridge', while subtherapeutic.

How should I anticoagulate a child who is thrombocytopenic due to chemotherapy?

LMWH in therapeutic doses is safe if platelets >30 × 10^9/L. If platelets <30 × 10^9/L, can either stop LMWH until platelet recovery, or continue LMWH at therapeutic doses with platelet transfusions to maintain platelets >30 × 10^9/L (preferred option if high risk of recurrence, as above).

Prevention

- Thromboprophylaxis is recommended in some clinical settings, using LMWH e.g. tinzaparin SC 50U/kg od.
- Consider in children with malignancy, severe trauma, thrombophilic abnormality or nephrotic syndrome.
- Thromboprophylaxis can be used in children with a previous CVAD-related thrombotic event who require a further line, starting the day after line insertion and continuing until removal.

Neonatal thrombosis

Arterial thrombosis (34%), renal vein thrombosis (22%) and portal vein thrombosis are more frequent in neonates.

Thrombotic events are associated with CVADs, infection, asphyxia, and dehydration.

If the neonate has necrotic skin lesions and/or extensive thrombosis, consider purpura fulminans, which is homozygous deficiency of protein C/protein S. Test protein C/S levels in baby and parents (parents likely both to have heterozygous deficiency). Treat with virally-inactivated plasma (15mL/kg) or protein C concentrate.

Complications of thrombosis in childhood

Venous thrombosis

Short term
- Loss of venous access.
- SVC obstruction.
- Organ dysfunction (renal vein thrombosis/renal failure).
- Mortality (PE, CSVT).

Long term
- Post-thrombotic syndrome (chronic pain, swelling and skin changes of affected limb).
- Organ dysfunction:
  - renal vein thrombosis/renal failure;
  - portal vein thrombosis/portal hypertension, hypersplenism, variceal bleeding;
  - CSVT/neurological deficits, neuropsychometric problems.

Arterial thrombosis

Short term
Vascular compromise.

Long term
Discrepant limb length.

Anticoagulation in children

Dosing and dose adjustment of unfractionated heparin

- **Loading dose:** 75U/kg IV over 10min.
- **Initial maintenance dose:**
  - ≤1 year of age – 28U/kg/h IV;
  - >1 year of age – 20U/kg/h IV.
- **Monitoring:** check APTT (anti-factor Xa preferred if child <1 year of age) 6h after starting treatment, 4h after rate change and at least every 24h.

See Tables 23.1–23.3.

Table 23.1 Heparin infusion adjustment

APTT (s)	Anti-factor Xa (U/mL)	Bolus (U/kg)	Hold (min)	Rate change (%)
<50	<0.10	50	–	↑ 20
50–59	0.10–0.34	–	–	↑ 10
60–85	0.35–0.7	–	–	No change
86–95	0.71–0.89	–	–	↓ 10
96–120	0.90–1.20	–	30	↓ 10
>120	>1.20	–	60	↓ 15

Table 23.2 Dosing and dose adjustment of low molecular weight heparin

	Therapeutic dose	Prophylactic dose
Enoxaparin		
≤2 months of age	1.5mg/kg SC bd	1.5mg/kg SC od
>2 months of age	1mg/kg SC bd	1mg/kg SC od
Tinzaparin	175U/kg SC od	75U/kg SC od

Monitoring
- Check anti-factor Xa 4–6h after dose, aim for anti-factor Xa 0.5–1.0U/mL, adjust by 10–20% until therapeutic level achieved.
- Monitoring of prophylaxis is not required unless concerned about accumulation due to renal failure, in which case check trough level to confirm clearance.

Table 23.3 Dosing and adjustment of warfarin

Day of therapy	INR	Dose of warfarin
Day 1	–	0.2 mg/kg PO od (maximum 5 mg)
Days 2–4	1.1–1.3	Repeat initial loading dose
	1.4–3.0	50% of initial loading dose
	3.1–3.5	25% of initial loading dose
	>3.5	Hold until INR <3.5 then restart at 50% of previous dose

Monitoring

INR every 2–3 days until stable; at least once every 4–6 weeks once stable.

Emergency reversal of anticoagulant therapy

Introduction

Anticoagulant therapy can result in bleeding. This occurs particularly if patient is over-anticoagulated, but can occur when patient is within the therapeutic range.

Reversal of UFH

If the infusion is stopped, anticoagulant effect is reversed within 4h. For severe bleeding give protamine sulphate, 1mg per 100U heparin given in the preceding hour; maximum dose 50mg (see BNF for details). Repeat APTT 15min after protamine sulphate.

Reversal of LMWH

- Half-life is longer than for UFH. The anticoagulant effect of enoxaparin lasts for 18h, and that of tinzaparin for 24h if given at therapeutic doses.
- Protamine sulphate will reverse some of LMWH effect, but is less predictable than for UFH.
- Consult an expert for advice if urgent reversal is required.

Reversal of warfarin

- The effect of warfarin lasts for 3–5 days after the last dose.
- Oral vitamin K reverses warfarin within 24h, IV vitamin K within 4–6h.
- FFP or PCC (prothrombin complex concentrate, containing factors II, VII, IX, and X) reverses warfarin immediately.
- Action taken depends on severity of bleeding and risk of thrombosis when warfarin is reversed.

No bleeding

- If INR >5.0, hold warfarin for 1–2 days, repeat INR before restarting.
- If INR >8.0, risk of bleeding is significant, give vitamin K PO 30µg/kg.

Minor bleeding
- Stop warfarin.
- Give vitamin K 30µg/kg, IV or PO depending on speed of reversal required.

Major bleeding
- Life-, sight- or limb-threatening, e.g. intracranial, gastrointestinal with haemodynamic compromise, compartment syndrome:
- Stop warfarin.
- Give vitamin K, IV, 5mg.
- Give PCC, IV, 30U/kg over 10min. Repeat INR 15min after PCC.
- Virally-inactivated plasma at 15mL/kg is an alternative if PCC is not available.

Bone marrow failure

Aplastic anaemia

Definitions

Aplastic anaemia (AA) is characterized by:
- Pancytopenia:
  - granulocyte count ≤1.5 × 10^9/L (for practical purposes usually regarded as neutrophil count ≤1.5 × 10^9/L);
  - platelet count ≤50 × 10^9/L;
  - haemoglobin ≤10g/dL.
- Hypocellular bone marrow.
- In absence of neoplastic infiltration or fibrosis of bone marrow.

Severe aplastic anaemia (SAA) is defined by:
- Bone marrow cellularity <25% (or 25–50% when <30% residual cells are haemopoietic).

And at least two of:
- Neutrophil count <0.5 × 10^9/L.
- Platelet count <20 × 10^9/L.
- Reticulocyte count <40 ×10^9/L.

Very severe aplastic anaemia (VSAA) is present when the criteria for SAA (as above) are met and neutrophil count <0.2 × 10^9/L.

Non-severe aplastic anaemia (NSAA), also called moderate aplastic anaemia (MAA) or hypoplastic anaemia (HA), is present when the criteria for SAA are not met.

Epidemiology

- Incidence of AA in children (0–15 years age) is 1–3 per million person years in Europe/North America. Higher incidence in Asia, especially the Far East where post-hepatitis AA is much commoner.
- Most (>70%) children with acquired AA have SAA at initial presentation.
- Slight male preponderance.

Aetiology

Acquired
- **Idiopathic:** the commonest group (>70–80% of AA).
- **Post-infectious:** 5–8% of AA in Europe/North America, but accounts for a higher proportion of AA in Asia/Far East.
  - *Viral infections:–*
    - viral hepatitis is commonest infectious cause – usually non-A non-B non-C, but AA has been reported after hepatitis A, B, C, or other viral causes of hepatitis (e.g. adenovirus);
    - herpes family viruses (e.g. EBV, CMV, HHV6, VZV);
    - HIV;
    - parvovirus B19 (rare, more typically causes red cell aplasia);
    - measles;
    - mumps;
    - rubella.
  - *Non-viral infections* – rare, but described in literature, e.g. tuberculosis.

- **Drug-induced:** pancytopenia is a predictable adverse effect of most cytotoxic agents (chemotherapy, radiotherapy to a field including bone marrow), but numerous other drugs may cause bone marrow failure, usually idiosyncratically. Drug-induced AA is considered to be rare in children, but accounts for up to 20% of AA in case series of adults dating from the 1980s. The commonest reported associations are with:
  - *antibacterials* – e.g. chloramphenicol, sulphonamides, methicillin;
  - *antimalarials* – e.g. chloroquine, pyrimethamine;
  - *anticonvulsants* – e.g. phenytoin, carbamazepine;
  - *other central nervous system-acting drugs* – e.g. phenothiazines;
  - *anti-inflammatories* – e.g. phenylbutazone, indomethacin, gold salts, penicillamine;
  - *anti-thyroid drugs* – e.g. carbimazole, propylthiouracil;
  - *oral hypoglycaemic agents* – sulphonylureas.
- **Exposure to chemicals or toxins:** account for <5% AA
  - benzene;
  - other organic chemicals, which may be present in numerous products including paints, glues, insecticides (e.g. DDT).
- Other associations include:
  - *Paroxysmal nocturnal haemoglobinuria* (PNH) – a clonal disorder characterized by intermittent episodes of intravascular haemolysis and haemoglobinuria (classically occurring at night). May be complicated by venous thrombosis, or by bone marrow failure/ myelodysplasia (the commonest presentation in children). The affected clone of haemopoietic cells and their progeny are susceptible to complement lysis. They lack several GPI anchor-associated membrane antigens (e.g. CD55 and CD59). Flow cytometry of white blood cell and pre-transfusion red cells looking for CD55/59 expression forms the basis of a screening test for PNH. Infusions of the monoclonal antibody eculizumab ameliorate haemolysis and the risk of thrombosis. Marrow failure may require immunosuppressive treatment and/or consideration of HSCT as in idiopathic AA, depending on severity.
  - *Autoimmune disease* – e.g. systemic lupus erythematosus (SLE), rheumatoid arthritis.
  - Pregnancy.
  - Starvation.

Constitutional
- Fanconi anaemia (FA).
- Dyskeratosis congenita (DKC).
- AA arising as a consequence of another bone marrow failure disorder:
  - congenital amegakaryocytic thrombocytopenia (CAMT);
  - Schwachman-Diamond syndrome (SDS);
  - Diamond-Blackfan anaemia (DBA).

These conditions are described separately below.

Acquired aplastic anaemia

Pathogenesis

Three main pathophysiological processes have been suggested as possible mechanisms for the development of acquired AA:

- **Cell-mediated autoimmunity directed against haemopoietic stem or progenitor cells:** supportive evidence includes the presence of abnormal T cell populations in patients with AA, and most importantly the success of immunosuppressive treatment (IST) in treatment. The mechanism by which identified agents (such as viruses and toxins) lead to AA may involve their ability to bind with endogenous molecules to induce an autoimmune response against haemopoietic stem cells.
- **Primary haemopoietic stem cell defects:** the ability of haemopoietic stem cell transplant (HSCT) to cure AA supports this mechanism, especially given evidence that bone marrow stroma remains of host origin after successful HSCT for AA.
- **Abnormalities of bone marrow stroma or microenvironment:** may be relevant in a minority of patients with AA.

The evidence is strongest for the role of autoimmunity and the use of IST is based on this premise. However, AA may be due to any of several mechanisms operating individually or collectively, including autoimmunity and direct cytotoxicity (e.g. by viruses).

Telomere shortening is characteristic of DKC and a relatively common finding in patients with FA, SDS and acquired AA.

Clinical presentation

The presenting features of acquired AA are those of bone marrow failure:

- **Anaemia:** pallor, lethargy, dyspnoea on exertion, headaches.
- **Thrombocytopenia:** petechiae, unexplained or excessive bruising or bleeding (especially cutaneous or mucosal, e.g. gingival).
- **Neutropenia:** increased frequency and severity of infections, especially bacterial and fungal.

Typically, the duration of history is a few weeks or months. Longer histories raise the suspicion of a constitutional bone marrow failure syndrome.

A full history should be taken to seek evidence of a possible causative factor, e.g. viral infection within the last few months, drug ingestion (Aplastic anaemia, Aetiology 📖 pp.362–363).

Investigation

Confirmation of diagnosis and exclusion of other diagnoses

- **Haematology:**
  - *FBC*, reticulocyte count, film.
  - *HbF* (blood should be taken <u>before</u> transfusion) – usually ↑ as a manifestation of 'stressed' haematopoiesis.
  - *Coagulation profile* – to exclude other causes of bruising/bleeding.
  - *Blood group/antibody screen* – to guide transfusion.
  - *Haematinics* – iron studies (including ferritin), vitamin B_{12}, folate (Other non-malignant peripheral blood cytopenias 📖 pp.379–394);

- Hb electrophoresis, glucose-6-phosphate dehydrogenase (G6PD) deficiency (in relevant ethnic groups) (Haemoglobinopathies 📖 pp.315–326, Other non-malignant peripheral blood cytopenias 📖 pp.379–394);
- Bone marrow aspirate and trephine biopsy:
  - cellularity;
  - exclusion of leukaemia or other malignant infiltration;
  - iron stain;
  - reticulin stain;
  - cytogenetics (including fluorescent *in situ* hybridization [FISH] for abnormalities of chromosomes 5 and 7) – to evaluate possible Z of myelodysplasia (MDS) (Myelodysplasia 📖 pp.423–430), although clonal abnormalities (especially trisomy 8, but also occasionally monosomy 7) may occur in AA even in the absence of morphological features of MDS.
- **Biochemistry:**
  - Electrolytes, renal function.
  - *Liver function* – ↑ liver enzymes may suggest recent hepatitis.
  - *LDH* – ↑ in haemolytic anaemia.
- **Virology:**
  - *Serology* – herpes family viruses (CMV, HSV, EBV, VZV), hepatitis viruses (A, B, C), parvovirus B19 (including IgM), adenovirus, measles.
  - *PCRs* – may be helpful in specific cases, especially HHV6, parvovirus B19.
  - Consider testing for HIV.
- Consider investigations for other infections as a possible cause (e.g. tuberculosis) or complication (e.g. fungal) of AA if suggested by history or examination findings. May need to include:
  - microbiology;
  - serology;
  - imaging;
  - biopsy/other diagnostic procedures.
- **Immunology:**
  - *immunoglobulins* – ↓ in ~10–15% patients;
  - *autoantibody screen* – usually negative, but presence of autoantibodies may suggest that AA is part of a systemic autoimmune disease.
- **Imaging:** abdominal ultrasound – looking for urinary tract abnormalities suggestive of FA.
- GPI anchor-associated membrane antigens (CD55/59) (blood should be taken *before* transfusion) – reduced levels in erythrocytes and leucocytes in PNH.

- **Diagnosis of constitutional bone marrow failure syndromes:**
  - *Chromosomal fragility test* (Constitutional aplastic anaemia, Fanconi anaemia 📖 pp.372–373) – should be performed in all patients, even in the absence of any signs suggestive of FA, which is characterized by impaired DNA repair. Peripheral blood lymphocytes are cultured with a clastogenic agent [either diepoxybutane (DEB) or mitomycin C (MMC)], with appropriate control experiments, to quantify spontaneous and DEB or MMC-induced chromosomal breakages, which are increased in FA.
  - Consider molecular genetic investigation for other constitutional bone marrow failure syndromes (DKC, CAMT, SDS), but negative test results do not necessarily exclude these clinical diagnoses.
- HLA typing of patient and 1st degree relatives (parents, siblings) – to expedite planning if HSCT is required.

Differential diagnosis
- Constitutional AA.
- Aplastic presentation of acute leukaemia (especially ALL) – sometimes referred to (rather loosely) as 'pre-leukaemia'.
- Hypoplastic myelodysplasia (Myelodysplasia 📖 pp.423–430).
- **Pearson's syndrome:** a rare mitochondrial DNA deletion disorder, which may occur sporadically or be maternally inherited:
  - typically presents with macrocytic anaemia +/– variable severity of thrombocytopenia/neutropenia, and failure to thrive, in infancy/early childhood;
  - anaemia then usually improves during first 4 years of life;
  - bone marrow aspirate reveals characteristic vacuolation of granulocyte and eryrthroid precursors, with ring sideroblasts (Δ MDS);
  - diagnosis confirmed by mitochondrial DNA testing;
  - numerous and potentially life-threatening sequelae include Kearns-Sayre syndrome (opthalmoplegia, ataxia, cardiac conduction defects), metabolic (lactic acidosis), exocrine pancreatic dysfunction, and cardiomyopathy.

Management
Supportive care
Meticulous supportive care is a fundamental component of management of bone marrow failure.
- **Blood product transfusion support:**
  - *Try to minimize the number of transfusions* – early HSCT experience in AA demonstrated an increased risk of graft rejection in multiply transfused recipients, assumed to be related to increased allosensitization to HLA antigens –
    - Red cell transfusions are given to reduce symptoms due to anaemia. Decision to transfuse is guided by presence of symptoms rather than primarily by Hb concentration threshold – may be able to delay transfusion until Hb is below ~7g/dL. As well as reducing allosensitization, reduction in intensity of blood transfusion support may also reduce the likelihood of iron overload.

- Platelet transfusions should be given to treat active bleeding or when platelet count <5 × 10⁹/L (or <10 × 10⁹/L if patient is bleeding, unwell or febrile).
- All blood products used in UK are now leucodepleted (to prevent transmission of variant Creutzfeldt-Jakob disease) – this has the added benefit of reducing allosensitization.
- Despite leucodepletion (which greatly reduces risk of CMV transmission), many units still use CMV-negative blood products for CMV-seronegative patients (or sometimes for all patients).
- **Other measures to reduce risk or severity of bleeding:**
  - norethisterone controls or prevents menstrual bleeding;
  - topical tranexamic acid may control mucosal bleeding (e.g. oral).
- Prevention and treatment of infection is of paramount importance, especially given the usually long-term nature of AA and its treatment.
  - *General measures to reduce likelihood of infection* –
    - promote sensible personal hygiene;
    - oral/dental care;
    - avoidance of fungal exposure, e.g. from hay, building work.
  - *Prophylaxis* –
    - *antibacterial* – although use of prophylactic oral broad spectrum antibiotics (e.g. ciprofloxacin) may reduce the incidence of Gram –ve bacterial infection, routine use is not usually recommended due to concerns about the emergence of antibiotic resistance;
    - *antifungal* – very important since long-term severe neutropenia is a major risk factor for potentially lethal invasive fungal infection; a triazole antifungal (e.g. itraconazole) is the most practical (oral) and effective means of preventing serious fungal infection;
    - *cotrimoxazole prophylaxis* against *Pneumocystis jirovecii* is vital in patients undergoing HSCT, but generally regarded as unnecessary in untreated AA or during IST, and is usually avoided in view of the theoretical risk of impairing bone marrow recovery;
  - *Treatment* of suspected or documented infection should be prompt and aggressive in view of the potentially serious implications (including severe morbidity or death) of uncontrolled infection:
    - immediate institution of empirical broad spectrum IV antibiotics in any neutropenic AA patient with fever (Infection 📖 pp.207–230);
    - early addition of empirical antifungal treatment (timing and nature varies according to local policies) in patients with febrile neutropenia who do not respond to initial IV broad spectrum antibiotic treatment;
    - use of haemopoietic growth factors (usually G-CSF) is seldom indicated or effective, but short-term use may be appropriate in the presence of severe bacterial or fungal infection in a severely neutropenic patient.

- **Venous access:**
  - Essential in patients undergoing IST or HSCT.
  - May be valuable in patients (especially young children) requiring frequent venous cannulation for transfusions, antibiotics, etc.
  - A tunnelled CVAD (e.g. Hickman line) is vital in the context of HSCT, but it is feasible and often desirable to use a vascular port device (e.g. Port-a-cath) in patients undergoing IST due to lower complication (e.g. infection) rates.

Observation

Initial observation (with ongoing appropriate supportive care) is usually undertaken for 2–6 weeks (and sometimes longer in stable patients):

- Whilst awaiting the results of initial investigations, especially chromosomal fragility testing (for FA), which will influence choice of treatment strategy.
- To confirm the diagnosis of AA (by excluding alternative diagnoses, e.g. MDS) and exclude reversible bone marrow suppression (e.g. after viral infection).
- To establish the severity of AA, specifically NSAA (when further observation may be indicated) as opposed to SAA or VSAA (which require definitive treatment as soon as possible).

Choice of definitive treatment strategy

IST is indicated as initial definitive treatment when a patient with acquired SAA or VSAA does not have a HLA-identical sibling donor.
   HSCT is appropriate:

- As initial definitive treatment when a HLA-identical sibling donor is available in a patient with SAA or VSAA.
- After failure of 1 or (traditionally) 2 courses of IST in a patient with SAA or VSAA who has an acceptably matched alternative donor.
- In patients with constitutional AA (e.g. FA) who are transfusion-dependent and who have a HLA-identical donor (related or unrelated).

Immunosuppressive treatment (IST)

Although several different protocols exist with different preparations, doses and durations, contemporary IST protocols for AA usually incorporate a combination of a polyclonal anti-lymphocyte antibody preparation, a corticosteroid and ciclosporin A. Response is slow over at least 3–4 months, and is traditionally not assessed formally until 6 months. Failure to respond by 6 months prompts reassessment to either give a 2nd course of IST (classically with an alternative anti-lymphocyte antibody preparation) or consider HSCT.

Anti-lymphocyte antibodies

Given by prolonged intravenous infusion, typically daily for 4–5 days (dose and scheduling depends upon preparation and protocol used).
   The activity of polyclonal antibodies against T cells [e.g. anti-lymphocyte globulin (ALG) and anti-thymocyte globulin (ATG)] was first reported in 1970 in the context of failed bone marrow transplantation (some patients with AA due to acute radiation poisoning who had been conditioned for transplant with ALG showed autologous marrow reconstitution).

Further studies in the late 1970s and 1980s confirmed that IST, based on ALG or ATG, was an effective treatment for AA, even when not followed by HSCT. Several preparations remain available with no good evidence of differences in efficacy. Traditionally, most IST protocols (especially in the UK) have used equine ATG, but rabbit ATG has been used for 2nd courses when no response has been observed to a 1st course of equine ATG. However, equine ATG has recently been withdrawn in the UK.

Corticosteroids

Typically IV methylprednisolone or prednisolone 1–2mg/kg/day is given from days 1–5 (as prophylaxis against reactions to the anti-lymphocyte antibody), and then gradually tapered (and converted to oral preparations) to stop by about day 21–28.

High dose steroids (most commonly methylprednisolone) were used as single agent treatment of AA for many years before the introduction of ALG. Therefore, most early IST protocols incorporated additional corticosteroids, with the intention of providing further immunosuppression, as well as prophylaxis against infusional reactions and serum sickness due to the antibody preparation.

However, there is no evidence that high-dose steroids improve the response rate above that seen with anti-lymphocyte antibodies alone, whilst their use is associated with considerable short- and long-term toxicity. Therefore, contemporary IST protocols use lower doses primarily to prevent reactions to ALG/ATG.

Ciclosporin A

Oral ciclosporin A to maintain trough levels of 100–150µg/mL.

- Although some protocols start ciclosporin on day 1, others delay its introduction until steroids have stopped to avoid excessive toxicity (especially hypertension).
- Typical starting dose is 5mg/kg/day, divided into 2 doses, but start with a lower dose if patient is on a triazole (which will increase serum levels of ciclosporin).

Trials in the 1990s demonstrated further improvements in survival when ciclosporin was added to anti-lymphocyte antibodies and steroids.

Other agents

The addition of androgen treatment (usually with oxymetholone) to IST with anti-lymphocyte antibodies and steroids may improve the initial response rate, but a survival benefit has not been demonstrated.

The combination of growth factors (usually G-CSF) and contemporary IST protocols (as above) has also been investigated in recent years. Neutrophil recovery may be enhanced, whilst the patient is still on G-CSF, but sustained benefit or improvements in infection rates, overall haematological responses or survival have not been shown.

Haemopoietic stem cell transplant (HSCT)

Until recent years, the majority of HSCTs performed in AA were HLA-identical sibling donor bone marrow transplants (BMTs).

Conditioning and GvHD prophylaxis protocols for conventional HLA-identical sibling donor BMTs have usually comprised:

- IV cyclophosphamide 50mg/kg/day days –5 to –2 (total dose 200mg/kg).
- IV ALG: preparation, dose and schedule varies with protocol, but often given days –5 to –3.
- IV ciclosporin A from day –1.
- Short course IV methotrexate (Preparation for haemopoietic stem cell transplantation, Graft versus host disease prophylaxis 📖 p.176).

During the last decade, the success rate and, therefore, the use of alternative donor HSCTs (especially unrelated donor transplants) has increased, due to:

- **Improved donor selection:** ideally fully matched (with high resolution HLA-typing) donors should be used whenever possible to reduce the risk of graft failure and GvHD, which are the commonest causes of adverse HSCT outcome in AA.
- Increased use of fludarabine in conditioning protocols (to reduce graft rejection).
- Improved use of serotherapy and other GvHD prophylaxis strategies.
- Improved supportive care which has reduced severe morbidity and mortality due to post-HSCT infection.

Complications

Complications of bone marrow failure itself

The most feared and potentially lethal complications of AA itself are:

- Bleeding.
- Infections:
  - Bacterial;
  - fungal – comprise about a third of infections in AA, high mortality rate.

Complications of treatment

Supportive care

- Blood product transfusions (Blood transfusion 📖 pp.231–244)
  - transfusion reactions;
  - blood-borne infection;
  - iron overload.
- Drug toxicity, e.g.
  - *nephrotoxicity* – aminoglycosides, amphotericin;
  - *hepatotoxicity* – triazoles.

IST

- Reactions to anti-lymphocyte antibodies:
  - *Infusion toxicity* – fever, rigors, rash, hypotension, or hypertension, bronchospasm, diarrhoea, vomiting, and anaphylaxis; managed by paracetamol, chlorphenamine ± hydrocortisone, promethazine, pethidine, salbutamol, adrenaline as indicated by nature of reaction.

• *Serum sickness* - typically presents between days 7 and 14, with fever, rash, arthralgia, myalgia, pleuritic chest pain, platelet consumption; managed by giving IV hydrocortisone or increasing dose or duration of prednisolone.

▶ When infusion toxicity or serum sickness present with fever, it is still important to start empirical IV broad spectrum antibiotics in case the fever is due to genuine concurrent infection.

• Increased immunosuppression with increased risk of a wide range of infections, including viral.
• Specific drug toxicity:
  • *Corticosteroids* – especially weight gain, hypertension, hyperglycaemia, behaviour/mood disturbances. Avascular necrosis is a rare, but serious late adverse effect of prolonged high dose steroids, which are therefore usually avoided;
  • *Ciclosporin A* – nephrotoxicity (monitor U&Es, Mg), hypertension, neurotoxicity (Preparation for haemopoietic stem cell transplantation, Graft versus host disease prophylaxis 🕮 p.176), hirsutism.

HSCT

(Haemopoietic stem cell transplantation, Complications 🕮 pp.180–197).

Prognosis

Spontaneous recovery of established bone marrow failure is rare (<10%). Untreated AA has a very high mortality from infection or haemorrhage (historically 70–90% at 5 years). Although aggressive supportive care may increase the duration of survival, only a small minority of patients survive without definitive treatment (IST or HSCT).

Contemporary treatment has transformed the prognosis of AA, especially in children:

IST

• 80% have a 5-year survival rate.
• Relapse of AA may occur in up to 30% patients at 5 years, requiring further treatment in 10–20%.
• Survival curve does not plateau due to risk of development of clonal disease (PNH or MDS/AML) in a small proportion of patients (commoner in adults).
• Long-term complications are rare.

HSCT

• 80–95% have a 5-year survival rate.
• There is a much lower relapse risk, although late graft rejection is well documented. However, may be followed by autologous marrow recovery.
• Short- and long-term complications commoner → small, but significant transplant-related mortality (<5% in HLA-identical sibling BMTs).

Constitutional aplastic anaemia

Several rare inherited bone marrow failure syndromes (IBMFSs) are described, many of which may lead to AA. They may constitute up to 25% of cases of AA in children.

The clinical features of IBMFSs vary in terms of:

- Age and speed of onset.
- Haematological features:
  - Some IBMFSs lead to pancytopenia (e.g. FA, DKC);
  - Others predominantly present with monocytopenias –
    - *neutropenia* – e.g. Kostmann disease (severe congenital neutropenia);
    - *anaemia* – e.g. Diamond-Blackfan anaemia (DBA);
    - *thrombocytopenia* – e.g. thrombocytopenia absent radii (TAR) syndrome.
- Associated clinical features.
- Mode of inheritance.

Only those IBMFSs that usually present with AA are described in detail in this chapter.

Fanconi anaemia

The prototype and commonest IBMFS, with numerous characteristic clinical associations. Progressive onset of marrow failure occurs in ≥90% of patients, nearly always within 1st two decades of life.

Epidemiology and genetics

- Rare, but well described (>1000 cases reported in literature).
- Occurs in all racial and ethnic groups.
- Autosomal recessive. Heterozygote frequency ~1 in 200.
- At least 13 'FA genes' have been identified. These gene mutations mediate their effects by impairment of DNA repair mechanisms.

Clinical presentation

Very variable. May present with:

- Classic phenotype with several characteristic physical abnormalities (see below) with bone marrow failure at initial presentation or developing at a later stage.
- Bone marrow failure without any physical abnormalities (about 30% of FA patients have no identified somatic abnormalities).

Characteristic physical abnormalities include:

- Short ± slender stature.
- **Limb anomalies:** absent or hypoplastic thumb ± radii, hand (clinodactyly, hypoplastic thenar eminences), legs (including congenital dislocation of hip), feet (club foot, abnormal toes).
- **Other skeletal abnormalities:** head/facial (microcephaly, hydrocephalus), neck, spinal (vertebral, ribs), numerous others.
- Developmental delay.
- **Eyes:** morphological ± visual abnormalities.
- **Ears:** morphological abnormalities, conductive deafness.
- **Cardiac:** congenital heart disease, e.g. persistent ductus arteriosus, ventricular, or atrial septal defect.

- **Urinary tract abnormalities:** ectopic, hypoplastic, dysplstic, or absent kidneys.
- **Gonadal:** morphological abnormalities, most (but not all) males are azoospermic.
- **Gastrointestinal:** atresia of oesophagus, duodenum or jejunum, tracheo-oesophageal fistula (TOF), anal abnormalities.
- **Skin:** café *au lait* patches, generalized hyperpigmentation.

Timing of onset of initial haematological manifestations is very variable, ranging from birth to >30 years age, but is usually in 1st or 2nd decade of life (median 7 years).
- First manifestation is usually thrombocytopenia, but MCV often already elevated at this time (reflecting stressed erythropoiesis).
- Followed by gradual evolution of anaemia and neutropenia progressing to pancytopenia over a period of many months or years.

FA is a cancer predisposition syndrome:
- **Increased risk of myeloid malignancies:** myelodysplasia (MDS) occurs in 30% and may progress to acute myeloid leukaemia (AML), which develops in 10% of FA patients. A high degree of suspicion may be required to diagnose MDS expeditiously in a patient with evolving bone marrow failure. Surprisingly rapid changes in FBC should prompt consideration of bone marrow aspirate/biopsy with cytogenetic analysis (looking for, e.g. monosomy 7). Onset of MDS warrants reconsideration of HSCT options, whilst HSCT is usually performed as soon as possible in FA patients with AML, in view of their poor tolerance of most chemotherapy strategies.
- **Solid tumours:** especially head/neck/oral and gynaecological/anorectal squamous cell carcinomas. Treatment of these malignancies is difficult in view of the limitations placed on chemotherapy and radiotherapy by the DNA repair sensitivity, and prognosis is poor.

Diagnosis
FA should be suspected in any patient presenting with bone marrow failure, especially if the history is unusually long (more than a few months) and/or in presence of suggestive phenotypic features (as above).

Chromosomal fragility test (MMC or DEB) should be performed (Acquired aplastic anaemia, Investigation 📖 pp.364–365).

Management
The only curative treatment available at present is HSCT, but it is possible that gene therapy may be feasible in the future.
- Although autologous haemopoetic stem cell (usually bone marrow) harvest before bone marrow failure supervenes may provide back-up stem cells for possible use if graft failure complicates future HSCT or as a substrate for possible gene therapy in the future, this procedure is not performed routinely since harvest yields are usually very poor.
- Initial management usually comprises careful observation during earlier stages of bone marrow failure. Supportive care aims to prevent or treat complications of bone marrow failure (Acquired aplastic anaemia, Supportive care 📖 pp.366–368). Blood product transfusions should be avoided if at all possible, and further treatment should be instituted once they are becoming necessary (or ideally shortly before this timepoint).

- **Androgens:** generally regarded as a 'holding' or 'delaying' measure in patients without a HLA-identical sibling donor, but very long-term and apparently sustainable haematological responses (several years) are sometimes observed, especially when low doses are used. Oxymetholone may be commenced at a low dose (e.g. 0.5–1mg/kg/day), increasing up to about 2mg/kg/day if required to achieve a response, then subsequently reduced to the lowest possible dose that maintains an acceptable blood count and prevents transfusion needs. This may involve giving oxymetholone every 2nd–5th day and accepting low Hb, e.g. 8–9g/dL, and platelet counts, e.g. $20–30 \times 10^9/L$, as long as symptoms and complications are avoided:
  - this may allow stabilization of counts and clinical condition for months or years;
  - pretreatment and ongoing investigations.
- **Growth factors:** short-term experience of use of G-CSF to improve neutrophil count is encouraging, but long-term use limited by concern that it may increase risk of AML/MDS.
- HSCT is appropriate:
  - In patients with a HLA-identical sibling (or other related) donor (in whom FA has been excluded by chromosomal fragility testing), when bone marrow failure has progressed sufficiently to predictably necessitate blood product transfusion support, or (more rarely) cause other significant complications (e.g. infections). A trial of androgens is usually avoided in such patients in view of previous evidence that their use may adversely affect HSCT outcome, although this may no longer be the case with modern conditioning regimens.
  - In patients without a HLA-identical related donor, alternative donors may include mismatched related donors or unrelated (matched or mismatched) donors. Historically, the outcome has been much poorer in alternative donor HSCTs, due to the high incidence of graft failure, GvHD and/or infection. Therefore, most such patients have received a trial of androgens, with HSCT being delayed until loss of androgen response or the development of significant side effects. More recent experience suggests that use of well matched donors (chosen with high-resolution HLA typing), improved supportive care, contemporary conditioning and GvHD prophylaxis protocols have reduced these risks, although information about long-term outcome is awaited.
  - In patients developing MDS or AML.
- FA patients are extremely sensitive to agents causing DNA damage, especially alkylating agents and radiotherapy, necessitating the use of low dose conditioning regimens:
  - Cyclophosphamide usually given at a total dose of 20–40mg/kg (compared with 120–200mg/kg for non-FA patients), given over 4 days.
  - Radiotherapy [total body irradiation (TBI) or total lymphoid irradiation (TLI)] usually given at 4–6Gy (compared with ~12–14.4Gy for non-FA patients), usually given over 1–3 fractions.

Radiotherapy has been removed from more recent protocols in the hope of reducing the risk of 2° malignancy, although this remains controversial.

- Fludarabine can be given safely at full dose (total dose 125–150mg/m² over 5 days).
- GvHD prophylaxis usually includes ciclosporin A, short-course methotrexate, and serotherapy (e.g. ATG or CAMPATH).

- Post-HSCT relapse of MDs or AML is very difficult to manage. Rarely, donor lymphocyte infusion (DLI) may be considered, but this treatment may be complicated by severe GvHD, which is poorly tolerated by FA patients.

Complications

- **Androgens:**
  - There are several important side effects, including:
    - virilization (especially important in girls);
    - premature closure of epiphyses;
    - abnormal LFTs – ↑ enzymes, cholestasis;
    - structural liver changes – peliosis hepatis (development of multiple vascular cavities in liver) 9 hepatocellular carcinoma.
  - Pretreatment tests include LFTs and liver ultrasound, which should be repeated regularly during treatment (LFTs every 1–2 months, ultrasound every 6–12 months).
- **HSCT:** FA patients are at risk of all the usual complications of HSCT (Haemopoietic stem cell transplantation 📖 pp.163–200), but particularly vulnerable to:
  - *2° malignancy* – the already increased risk of solid tumours, especially squamous cell carcinomas, in FA patients is even higher in HSCT recipients. Occurrence of GvHD is a major risk factor, and use of radiotherapy in conditioning may be. However, the increased risk of myeloid malignancy (AML, MDS) in FA patients is removed by *successful* HSCT.
  - *Endocrine complications* – including short stature ± GH deficiency, hypothyroidism, abnormal glucose/insulin metabolism, metabolic syndrome, and dyslipidaemia. These are inherent to FA, even in non-transplanted patients, but it is likely they will be commoner still in survivors of HSCT (although little long-term data is available yet).
- Long-term follow-up is very important in all FA patients, whether or not they have been transplanted, and should include careful regular surveillance for the many documented complications (as above).

Prognosis

Without HSCT, the prognosis of FA is poor with nearly all patients dying of bone marrow failure or malignancy by the 3rd or 4th decade of life.

Until recently, results of HSCT have been far better with HLA-identical sibling donor (~70% 5-year survival) than with unrelated donor (URD) transplants (~20–30%), but newer conditioning and GvHD prophylaxis protocols have been reported to improve the survival after URD HSCT to ~50%.

Dyskeratosis congenita

Rare form of ectodermal dysplasia, complicated by bone marrow failure and cancer predisposition.

Epidemiology and genetics

- Very rare – about 200 cases reported across all racial and ethnic groups.
- Most cases are males, usually with X-linked recessive inheritance (mutation located in *DKC1* gene on Xq28), but autosomal recessive (AR) and autosomal dominant (AD) inheritance also described.
- DKC is now known to be characterized by marked telomere shortening, and the AD form is associated with mutation of *TERC* gene (RNA component of telomerase), located on 3q.

Clinical presentation

Reported cases and the international DKC registry have documented the clinical features and complications.

- Characeristic mucocutaneous features during the 1st decade of life:
  - abnormal skin pigmentation;
  - nail dystrophy;
  - oral leukoplakia.
- Progressive bone marrow failure occurs, usually during 2nd decade of life, in 50–70% of patients with X-linked and AR DKC, but only ~20% of those with AD form.

Other manifestations of DKC may include:

- **Ophthalmological:** excessive tearing (2° to obstructed nasolacrimal duct), conjunctivitis, loss of eyelashes.
- **Dental:** increased rate of decay and tooth loss.
- **Gastrointestinal:** oesophageal strictures, hepatomegaly.
- **Skeletal:** osteoporosis, scoliosis, avascular necrosis (especially if treated with steroids).
- **Urinary tract:** phimosis, hypospadias, urethral stenosis, horseshoe kidney.
- Immunodeficiency.
- Interstitial pulmonary disease.

Cancer occurs in 10–15% of patients, usually in 3rd and 4th decades of life. Similar range of malignancies to that seen in FA, but solid tumours are commoner than AML/MDS in DKC.

Diagnosis

Chromosomal fragility testing is normal. Therefore, a diagnosis of DKC is made clinically based on the characteristic features. Mutation analysis of *DKC1* and *TERC* genes is now feasible allowing molecular genetic diagnosis in X-linked and AD, but not AR, forms.

Management and complications

- Similar to FA, including supportive care.
- Androgens may delay progression of bone marrow failure, but sustained response is unlikely.
- Neutropenia may be ameliorated by G-CSF or GM-CSF, but longevity of response and safety of long-term use is unknown.

- Experience with HSCT is more limited than in FA, but demonstrates considerable early and late morbidity and mortality due to infection, GvHD and organ toxicity (especially pulmonary). Hence, conditioning treatment protocols without TBI and/or busulfan are recommended.
- Gene therapy may be feasible in future.

Prognosis
HSCT is the only curative treatment, with a 3-year survival rate of ~50–60% post-HSCT from published case reports. Without HSCT, the mean age of death (usually due to bone marrow failure or malignancy) in X-linked and AR disease is approximately 30 years, although mortality appears to be much lower in AD DKC.

Other syndromes that may present with pancytopenia

- **Congenital amegakaryocytic thrombocytopenia:** very rare (only ~50 cases reported in literature). X-linked and AR forms described.
  - usually, but not always, associated with mutations in *c-mpl* gene (which encodes the thrombopoietin receptor) on chromosome 1; presents at birth or during early childhood with isolated thrombocytopenia, which evolves to AA within months or years;
  - increased risk of AML/MDS;
  - isolated thrombocytopenia can be managed by supportive care including platelet transfusions, but HSCT is only definitive treatment for established AA.
- **Schwachman-Diamond syndrome:** rare (~300 published cases reported). Inheritance appears to be AR. Associated with mutations in *SBDS* gene on chromosome 7.
  - Characterized by haematological and non-haematological features:
    - *haematological* – neutropenia develops in most patients by early childhood l pneumonia and other infections, and may be followed by anaemia and thrombocytopenia in ~25%. AML or MDS occurs in ~5–10% of patients;
    - *non-haematological* – exocrine pancreatic insufficiency (→ steatorrhoea and failure to thrive), short stature, skeletal, and other congenital abnormalities.
  - HSCT is potentially curative for haematological aspects of SDS, but has high morbidity and mortality with frequent organ toxicity (especially cardiac).
- **Diamond-Blackfan anaemia:** classically presents with isolated anaemia from birth or very early infancy, but additional neutropenia and thrombocytopenia may become evident during childhood, and occasionally progress to AA. Most cases occur sporadically, with a minority (~20%) of familial cases. Physical abnormalities (e.g. short stature, facial dysmorphisms) may be seen in up to 40% of patients. *RPS19* mutations on chromosome 19 have been described in 25% of patients. Although usually treated with blood transfusions and/or corticosteroids, HLA-identical sibling HSCT is a potentially curative therapy for uncomplicated DBA, whilst an alternative donor transplant may be appropriate in severe AA associated with DBA.

- Even rarer IBMFSs that may cause pancytopenia include:
  - *Seckel syndrome* – autosomal recessive; severe intrauterine and post-natal growth retardation, microcephaly, developmental and cognitive impairment, typical facies;
  - *Dubowitz syndrome* – probably autosomal recessive, intrauterine and post-natal growth retardation, microcephaly, developmental and cognitive impairment, hyperactivity, eczema, facial abnormalities.

Other non-malignant causes of peripheral blood cytopenias

Cytopenias due to shortened peripheral blood cell survival caused by immune, mechanical, or constitutional damage to blood cells are considered in this chapter, as well as some causes of reduced production due to inflammation or haematinic deficiency.

Cytopenias in children with malignant disease are due to replacement of healthy bone marrow by the underlying malignant disease and/or reduced marrow production of haemopoietic cells as a result of the suppressive effects of chemotherapy and/or radiotherapy. Primary bone marrow failure syndromes and hypoplastic/aplastic anaemia are rarer and are considered elsewhere (Bone marrow failure ☐ pp.361–378).

Immune thrombocytopenia (ITP)

Childhood ITP is typically an acute self-limiting illness in an otherwise well child. There is an abrupt onset of a petechial rash associated with an isolated numerical thrombocytopenia, with otherwise normal blood counts and film appearances. There is frequently a history of recent intercurrent infection. The commonest outcome is spontaneous recovery within a few weeks. A minority of cases run a more chronic course.

Principles of good management

- Avoidance of invasive investigation (e.g. marrow examination, over-frequent blood count monitoring) in typical cases where the working diagnosis is robust.
- Avoidance of unnecessary therapeutic intervention when spontaneous recovery is the likely outcome ['most parents and patients can live quite comfortably with petechiae and low platelets awaiting spontaneous recovery provided their physician can' (Dickerhoff, 1994)].
- Recognition of atypical features either at presentation or later, when alternative diagnoses need to be considered. ITP is always a 'working diagnosis'.
- Appropriate intervention with specific therapy when circumstances require it. Treatment decisions should always be made on the basis of symptoms, and not the numerical level of the platelet count.

Incidence

Rare in infancy, but may occur at any other age, typically in childhood between the ages of 2–10 years. Incidence is similar to that of childhood acute lymphoblastic leukaemia (ALL; approximately 50 per million person years). Most childhood cases have an abrupt onset and will remit spontaneously within a few weeks. About 10–20% will continue to produce autoantibody and remain thrombocytopenic for over 6 months (chronic ITP). The overwhelming majority of these children will eventually make a spontaneous recovery after a variable time course sometimes lasting several years.

Typical clinical features

- Easy and spontaneous bruising, petechial rash, mucosal bleeding (e.g. gingival, epistaxis, menorrhagia), usually of abrupt onset. 10–20% cases will have a more insidious onset, and a higher proportion of these may go on to a more chronic course.
- Otherwise well child.
- Commonly, there will be a history of a recent intercurrent infection or immunization.
- Serious or life-threatening spontaneous bleeding is exceedingly rare.
- The level of symptoms (bleeding) is less than might be expected for an equivalent numerical thrombocytopenia due to marrow failure. This is because the platelets which are present are fresh, and function normally (the autoantibody causes the platelets to be removed from the circulation by macrophages in the spleen and reticulo-endothelial system, but does not compromise their function before they are removed).

Typical laboratory features

- Thrombocytopenia: platelets that are present are often large (younger platelets are bigger).
- Otherwise normal blood counts and film appearances.
- Normal plasma coagulation screen.
- Normal marrow appearances, plentiful megakaryocytes (if a bone marrow aspirate is performed, see Management, Acute presentation, troublesome haemostatic symptoms, p.382).

Some laboratory pitfalls

- The commonest cause of apparent thrombocytopenia is artefact (clot or clumping in the specimen). Repeat if not commensurate with clinical symptoms.
- Platelet antibody studies have no place in the assessment of individual patients with ITP in routine clinical practice.

Atypical clinical features: differential diagnosis

Ill child

Consider:

- Sepsis (e.g. meningococcal)/disseminated intravascular coagulation (DIC):
  - signs of infection;
  - deranged coagulation (low fibrinogen, elevated D-dimers).
- Haemolytic uraemic syndrome (HUS)/thrombotic thrombocytopenic purpura (TTP) (see ⬚ pp.386–387). Microangiopathic blood film, anaemia, jaundice, renal impairment.
- Malignancy, e.g. ALL, acute myeloid leukaemia (AML), myelodysplasia (MDS), non-haematological malignancy involving bone marrow. Marked adenopathy, bulky splenomegaly (a minority of children with ITP may have a just palpable spleen), other cytopenias (e.g. anaemia, neutropenia), leucoerythroblastic picture or primitive cells on blood film.
- Haemophagocytic syndrome: primary or post-viral infection, both which are rare (Haemophagocytic lymphohistiocytosis ⬚ p⬚
- Viral infection: remember HIV (risk factors), EBV.

- Associated autoimmune disease, e.g. connective tissue disease (especially in older girls), autoimmune haemolytic anaemia (AIHA) (anaemia, jaundice, positive direct antiglobulin test (DAT)):

  ITP + AIHA = Evan's Syndrome

Unusually young child (<1 year) (or positive family history)
Consider constitutional or inherited causes of thrombocytopenia:
- Thrombocytopenia with absent radii (TAR), congenital amegakaryocytic thrombocytopenia (CAMT).
- Wiskott-Aldrich syndrome (WAS):
  - small dust-like platelets on blood film, reduced MPV on automated count;
  - associated eczematous rash and immunodeficiency.
- Bernard-Soulier syndrome: giant platelets, platelet function impairment
- May-Hegglin anomaly: Dohle body inclusions in neutrophils on blood film examination. Often have minor/moderate thrombocytopenia.
- Type IIB Von-Willebrand disease (VWD): Family history, plasma coagulation studies.

Neonate
Consider:
- **Neonatal alloimmune thrombocytopenia** (NAITP): usually due to maternal anti-HPA-1a antibodies from HPA-1b mother crossing placenta to an HPA-1a child (HPA = human platelet antigen). Confirm by serological testing, support with appropriate antigen negative platelets.
- **Maternal ITP:** check maternal platelet count and medical history (N.B. when previous splenectomy for ITP, mother's platelet count may be normal even though antibody is still present).

Management
Acute presentation, typical features, minor haemostatic symptoms
- No active treatment required.
- Observation, patient, and parent education, and anticipation of spontaneous recovery is appropriate.

Acute presentation, troublesome haemostatic symptoms
For example, difficult epistaxes.
- Treatment with intravenous immunoglobulin (IVIg) (e.g. 0.8g/kg) or oral prednisolone (4mg/kg/day for 7 days, followed by tapered reduction) may be considered.
- Bone marrow examination (to rule out any possibility of occult ALL) should be considered before steroid treatment.
- Intravenous anti-D immunoglobulin (50µg/kg) is a potential alternative, but only works for RhD-positive patients. Efficacy is equivalent to IVIg and infusion time is shorter. Red cell haemolysis may occur.
- Platelet transfusion is not generally indicated. Transfused platelets are rapidly destroyed by the anti-platelet antibody. They are only indicated in major or life-threatening haemorrhage in the context of ITP.

Chronic ITP

- Therapy is only required for troublesome haemostatic symptoms. IVIg or anti-D immunoglobulin may be repeated in responders, but each infusion may only have an effect for a few weeks. Repeated or prolonged use of steroid is not appropriate in children. The immunomodulatory agents azathioprine and danazol may be useful. Vincristine and cyclophosphamide have been effective, although there is a lack of randomized trial-based evidence. The monoclonal anti-CD20 antibody rituximab 100mg IV weekly (NB adult dose – consider appropriate dose reduction in children) for 4 weeks has demonstrated useful sustained responses in ~65% patients, but there is again no robust evidence base.
- **Splenectomy:** removal of the spleen will achieve a haemostatic platelet count in about 70% of children with chronic ITP, but the potential benefit must be balanced against the possibilities of:
  - spontaneous resolution occurring eventually anyway without surgery;
  - response is not guaranteed;
  - increased risk of post-splenectomy infection.

A radioactive indium-labelled platelet scan demonstrating splenic sequestration may help to predict responders. Vaccination against pneumococcus, HIb, and meningococcus at least 14 days prior to surgery is mandatory.

Life-threatening haemorrhage in ITP

Spontaneous life-threatening haemorrhage (e.g. intracranial haemorrhage, uncontrolled gastrointestinal haemorrhage) in ITP is exceedingly rare. If it does occur, intensive platelet transfusion support, together with both IVIg and high dose IV methylprednisolone, should be administered and consideration given to emergency splenectomy.

Further information

Dickerhoff (1995) Immune thrombocytopenic purpura in childhood – how much diagnosis and therapy is reasonable? *Klin Pediatr 207*, 98–102.

Auto-immune neutropenia of infancy (primary immune neutropenia)

Unusually for autoimmune disease this typically occurs within the first year of life. Children present with an isolated neutropenia with otherwise normal blood counts and film appearances. In contrast to children with anaemia due to marrow failure, infection is rare despite numerically severe neutropenia. Spontaneous recovery usually occurs after a variable number of months.

Diagnosis

Unlike in ITP, antibody studies are clinically very useful. Specific anti-neutrophil antibodies are usually demonstrable and false positive test results are rare. In the UK, neutrophil antibody studies are undertaken in a single national reference laboratory. Marrow examination is often undertaken in order to exclude other pathology. The marrow appearances are either normal or show a moderate 'left shift' in otherwise active granulopoiesis.

Management

Febrile illness during the neutropenic period requires prompt clinical assessment and appropriate antibiotic therapy even though opportunistic infection is rare. There is usually a prompt neutrophil response to granulo-cyte colony stimulating factor (G-CSF) administration. This may be considered in the unwell child with fever and neutropenia, but is not indicated prophylactically in this condition.

Acquired haemolytic anaemias

Haemolysis (shortened red cell survival) is characterized by anaemia, with increased reticulocytosis and unconjugated hyperbilirubinaemia. LDH is raised and if haemolysis is intravascular, there may be haemoglobinuria. Serum haptoglobin is reduced or absent, and there may be haemosiderinuria. Clinically, patients present with pallor and jaundice, and increased splenic red cell destruction may lead to splenomegaly.

Auto-immune haemolytic anaemia

AIHA is rare in childhood, with a whole population annual incidence of 1 in 80,000, i.e. rarer than ITP, but more common than aplastic anaemia. Immune haemolysis is characterized by the presence of antibody on the red cell surface, detected by the direct antiglobulin (Coombs) test (DAT). Spherocytes and tear-drop poikilocytes are often prominent on blood film examination. The thermal characteristics and specificity of the red cell antibody further identify the underlying conditions.

Warm antibody haemolytic anaemia

The commonest form of AIHA in children. It is caused by IgG antibody reacting with antigen on the red cell surface at 37°C. The DAT is positive with IgG detected. Sometimes the antibody is specific for a particular red cell antigen, or it may react with several antigens in a non-specific way. Haemolysis is extravascular (spleen, liver) and haemoglobinuria is unusual. Most frequently idiopathic, but occasionally associated with underlying connective tissue disease (more common in older girls.).

Cold antibody haemolytic anaemia [cold haemaglutinin disease (CHAD)]

Rare, but most frequently seen after mycoplasma infection. Caused by IgM antibody preferentially reacting at 4°C. Agglutination of red cells is seen on blood film examination (at room temperature).

Paroxysmal cold haemoglobinuria (PCH)

Very rare. Precipitated by preceding viral infection. Due to cold reacting IgG antibody with anti-P specificity, which then fixes complement at 37°C (Donath-Landsteiner antibody). Intravascular haemolysis may be brisk and produce life-threatening anaemia with haemoglobinuria.

Management

Depends on severity of anaemia. If cold reacting antibodies are suspected, keeping the patient (and any blood product for transfusion) warm is important.

- Red cell transfusion may be necessary for severe anaemia (e.g. <5g/dL or if there is cardiovascular compromise.) Red cells negative for any antigen for which specific reactivity of the antibody has been demonstrated should be selected. P-negative blood may be available for PCH cases, but may take time to source. It is usually only required for cases requiring repeated transfusion. Transfusions should be given through approved blood warming apparatus if a cold reacting antibody is found.
- **Corticosteroids:** methlyprednisolone IV or prednisolone orally, 1–2mg/kg initially, later tapering according to response. Effective and usually required in warm antibody AIHA, sometimes required in cold reacting antibody cases.
- IVIg is less effective in children with AIHA, and is seldom used.
- Splenectomy may be considered for refractory or persistent cases.
- Rituximab 100mg IV weekly (NB adult dose – consider appropriate dose reduction in children) for 4 doses has been effective, and may be considered in order to try and avoid the need for splenectomy.

Haemolytic uraemic syndrome/ thrombotic thrombocytopenic purpura

This disease spectrum is caused by vascular endothelial damage and is characterized by:

• Thrombocytopenia.
• A microangiopathic picture (red cell fragments with schistoctyes and helmet cells on blood film examination).
• Haemolysis (anaemia, reticulocytosis, unconjugated hyperbilirubinaemia, raised LDH, negative DAT).

In HUS the pathology is principally confined to the renal vascular bed, and presents with renal failure together with the above haematological abnormalities. In thrombotic thrombocytopenic purpura (TTP), the pathology is more widespread. Renal failure may be mild or not evident, but neurological symptoms (headache, confusion, intracranial haemorrhage), unexplained fever and systemic illness with collapse due to myocardial involvement may occur.

Large Von Willebrand factor (VWF) multimers are found in the blood in HUS/TTP. A deficiency in a VWF cleaving protease ADAMTS13 may predispose to familial cases of TTP, and antibodies against ADAMTS13 are sometimes demonstrable in cases of HUS and TTP.

Haemolytic uraemic syndrome

Typical

Verocytotoxin-associated (E. coli 0157)

Typically presents in childhood following an episode of diarrhoeal illness due to *E. coli* 0157, with renal failure, thrombocytopenia and a microangiopathic blood picture. Most cases will resolve spontaneously and require appropriate renal support (managed fluid balance, dialysis if indicated). Platelet tranfusion should be avoided unless there is life-threatening haemorrhage. Plasma exchange may be required for severe or refractory cases. Plasma (FFP) administration may be used alone if exchange facilities are not initially available. Cryoprecipitate-poor FFP has a lower concentration of VWF multimers and may be used in cases refractory to FFP for exchange.

Atypical

• Post-pneumococcal, familial.
• These cases often run a more severe, protracted, or relapsing course, and are more likely to require plasma exchange.

Thrombotic thrombocytopenic purpura

This condition is extremely rare in childhood, but potentially life-threatening. It may be a manifestation of collagen vascular disease. It should be suspected if a systemically unwell child presents with fever, unexplained neurological symptoms, thrombocytopenia, and a microangio-pathic picture. Urgent plasma exchange (or FFP administration prior to organization of plasma exchange) should be considered.

Post-transplant TTP

TTP occuring in the context of allogeneic marrow transplantation may in part be drug related (ciclosporin A, tacrolimus) but is probably multifacto-rial. It is often less responsive to plasma exchange. There are reports of effective responses to rituximab.

Haemophagocytic lymphohistiocytosis (HLH)

A rare, but potentially life-threatening spectrum of disorders character-ized by a proliferation of macrophages phagocytosing red cells, and some-times other nucleated cells and platelets, in the marrow, liver, spleen, and reticulo-endothelial system.

Different categories are sometimes described, but there may be a common genetic predisposition.
- **Post-viral:** virus-associated haemophagocytic syndrome.
- **Primary:** familial, presenting in infancy.
- **Secondary:** associated with underlying autoimmune disease or immunosuppression.

Presentation
- Unwell with fever, weight loss, adenopathy, hepatosplenomegaly, ± CNS symptoms. A maculopapular rash is common.
- Typical investigation findings include blood cytopenias, deranged LFTs, coagulopathy with ↓ fibrinogen, ↑ ferritin, ↑ triglycerides
- Confirmatory tests include demonstration of haemophagocytosis in tissue (bone marrow, lymph node biopsy).

Treatment
Aggressive treatment with a regimen including high dose steroid, ciclosporin A, and etoposide may be life-saving. Haemopoietic stem cell transplantation is sometimes required. Protocol details may be obtained from the Histiocyte Society of America.

Further information
Histiocyte Society of America. Available at: www.histio.org (accessed 6 April 2009).

Inherited causes of haemolysis

Red cell survival may be shortened by inherited abnormalities of haemo-globin (Haemoglobinopathies 📖 pp.313–325), inherited red cell membrane disorders, and inherited red cell enzyme deficiencies.

Inherited red cell membrane disorders

Hereditary spherocytosis

The most common inherited red cell membrane disorder. Prevalence is 1 in 5000 individuals. Different molecular abnormalities exist, causing deficiencies of spectrin, ankryn, protein 4.2 or band 3 in the membrane cytoskeleton. Hereditary spherocytosis (HS) is sometimes autosomal dominant and sometimes recessive. 25% of cases have no family history (i.e. new mutations).

Clinical features

- Haemolysis, manifest with a compensatory reticulocytosis and an unconjugated hyperbilirubinaemia. Anaemia is frequent, depending on severity of haemolysis.
- Splenomegaly.
- Pigment gallstones may develop.
- May present with an 'aplastic crisis' caused by temporary reticulocytopenia due to infection (especially parvovirus B19). Rapid onset of severe anaemia is caused by loss of compensatory reticulocytosis. May require transfusion to tide over the period of reticulocytopenia.
- May present with hyperbilirubinaemia and anaemia in the neonatal period (spherocytosis and negative DAT).

Diagnosis

- Blood film shows polychromasia, spherocytes (NB indistinguishable appearances from AIHA, but DAT negative).
- Eosin-5-maleamide (EMA) test (a flow cytometry test which correlates with the amount of spectrin in red cell membrane) gives a characteristic ratio in HS.
- Osmotic fragility and auto-haemolysis testing are less commonly used since EMA testing has been introduced.
- Family studies (FBC, reticulocytes, film, EMA).

Management

- Folic acid supplementation may be appropriate (increased demand).
- Supportive care (including transfusion) for episodes of severe anaemia due to reticulocytopenia (e.g. neonatal period, post-parvovirus B19 infection).
- Consideration of splenectomy in cases with more severe haemolysis and pigment stone formation (simultaneous cholecystectomy in gallstone cases.). The spleen is the principal site of removal of spherocytes from the circulation. Splenectomy is usually effectively curative of the anaemia, and prevents further pigment gallstone formation, but is not required in mild cases. Ideally should be performed after 5 years of age because of the increased risk of

encapsulated bacterial infection in younger children. Preoperative pneumococcal, meningococcal and *Haemophilus influenzae B* (Hib) immunization is mandatory at least 2 weeks pre-operatively. Indefinite penicillin prophylaxis (erythromycin if allergic) should be given post-operatively.

Hereditary elliptocytosis and hereditary pyropoikilocytosis

The most common presentation of hereditary elliptocytosis (HE) and hereditary pyropoikilocytosis (HPP) in Northern Europe is an incidental condition with autosomal dominant inheritance, causing a preponderance of elliptical cells on blood film examination, but without causing significant haemolysis. Double heterozygosity or homozygosity may be associated with haemolysis, and with more bizarre film appearances and significant HPP.

Inherited red cell enzyme deficiencies

Peripheral blood red cells have no nuclei and cannot synthesize the enzymes required to keep their membrane pumps running. Deficiency in the amount or function (qualitative abnormalities) may shorten red cell survival causing haemolysis (congenital non-spherocytic haemolytic anaemia [CNSHA]). The commonest deficiencies are of glucose-6-phosphate dehydrogenase (G6PD) and pyruvate kinase (PK) and most laboratories will have access to screening tests for these. Other enzymes may be implicated (rare) and referral to reference laboratories may be required. These conditions may manifest as neonatal jaundice, or as a chronic CNSHA.

Glucose-6-phosphate dehydrogenase deficiency

This is common in ethnic populations from endemic malarial areas. X-linked inheritance. Most affected individuals have completely normal health. Episodes of haemolysis may follow exposure to oxidizing agents, and the following drugs and other exposures should be avoided:

- **Antimalarials:** maloprim, primaquin, pentaquine, pamaquine.
- **Other antimicrobials:** dapsone, nalidixic acid, nitrofurantoin, sulphonamides (including cotrimoxazole).
- Contact with mothballs (napthalene).
- **Eating:** Fava (broad) beans, Chinese herbal medicines.

Pyruvate kinase deficiency

Inherited in autosomal recessive manner. More severely affected individuals may be transfusion dependent. Splenectomy (preferably after the age of 5 years) may abolish transfusion dependence. Iron accumulation may occur long-term even in the absence of a transfusion requirement.

Other non-malignant causes of anaemia

Anaemia of chronic disease

Perhaps better termed 'anaemia of inflammation'. Any infective, inflammatory or neoplastic underlying cause of an 'acute phase reaction' ($\uparrow$ ESR, $\uparrow$ CRP, $\downarrow$ albumin, polyclonal $\uparrow$ immunoglobulins) may be associated with a hypochromic (or sometimes normochromic) anaemia. This is due to an inflammatory iron utilization defect. Serum iron is usually low, due to reduced transferrin (or iron binding capacity [IBC]). Transferrin/IBC is increased in iron deficiency (Other non-malignant causes of anaemia, Haematinic deficiencies Iron deficiency 📖 p.391). Serum ferritin is normal or high (ferritin is an acute phase protein).

Haematinic deficiencies

Vitamin B$_{12}$ and folic acid

Deficiencies of either vitamin cause indistinguishable haematological effects: macrocytic anaemia, often associated with leucopenia ± thrombocytopenia, as well as marked anisopoikilocytosis, hypersegmented neutrophils. May be circulating megaloblasts in peripheral blood. Marrow shows megaloblastic changes (characteristic morphological changes in nucleated red cell precursors). Serum LDH raised due to ineffective erythropoiesis. Serum vitamin B$_{12}$ level is low in B$_{12}$ deficiency. Red cell folate level also low in folate deficiency.

Vitamin B$_{12}$ deficiency

Found in foods of animal origin (meat, fish, eggs, dairy products). Requires gastric intrinsic factor for absorption in terminal ileum.

Causes of deficiency

- **Dietary deficiency may occur in strict vegans:** in infants maternal deficiency may contribute.
- **Pernicious anaemia** (PA): commonest cause of B$_{12}$ deficiency in adults. Caused by autoantibodies against intrinsic factor, found in serum in >50% cases. Rare in children. Family history of PA or autoimmune disease is frequent.
- Terminal ileal disease (e.g. inflammatory bowel disease, blind loop syndrome).
- Congenital intrinsic factor deficiency (very rare).
- Inherited transcobalamin II (carrier protein) deficiency (very rare).

Treatment

Administration of parenteral (IM) hydroxocobalamin.

Folic acid deficiency

Found in fruit and vegetables. Destroyed by prolonged cooking. Absorbed in small bowel.

Causes of deficiency
- Dietary (relatively common).
- **Malabsorbtion:** e.g. coeliac disease – look for anti-tissue transglutaminase antibodies (or anti-endomyseal antibodies). Laboratory test should include a screen for selective IgA deficiency.
- Increased demand (e.g. chronic haemolytic anaemia).
- Drugs interfering with folate absorption or metabolism (e.g. phenytoin, sodium valproate, carbamazepine, methotrexate, trimethoprim).

Treatment
Oral folic acid supplementation.

Iron deficiency
Deficiency causes microcytic anaemia. The platelet count may be moderately raised.

Diagnosis
- Blood film shows hypochromia with target cells and rod poikilocytes.
- The red cell distribution width (RDW) is characteristically raised.
- Serum ferritin (reflecting body iron stores) is reduced (NB ferritin is an acute phase protein, and a low normal level may not exclude iron deficiency in the presence of an acute phase reaction).
- ↓ serum iron, ↑ transferrin (or IBC).
- ↑ zinc protoporphyrin (ZPP) level (NB also seen in lead poisoning).

Causes of deficiency
- Dietary.
- Malabsorbtion (e.g. coeliac disease, see above under folate deficiency).
- **Chronic blood loss:**
  - The common adult causes (GI malignancy, peptic ulceration) are rare in childhood.
  - Consider:
    - *Helicobacter pylori* gastritis (serology, breath test);
    - Meckel's diverticulum (radioisotope scan);
    - menorrhagia (consider coagulation disorder).

Treatment
Oral iron supplementation:
- Ferrous sulphate tablets are the best absorbed preparation in older children and adults.
- Ferrous edetate suspension is sugar free, and generally well tolerated by infants and younger children.
- Administer 2–3 times daily, with food to minimize gastric side effects. Continue for at least 2–3 months after correction of haematological indices in order to replenish body iron stores. In cases of genuine intolerance of oral preparations parenteral replacement may be appropriate (IV iron Dextran – may be associated with allergic reaction, and needs to be given in hospital with appropriate supervision. Intramuscular preparations are available, but very uncomfortable and not generally suitable for children).

Malignant haematological diseases

Acute lymphoblastic leukaemia

Acute lymphoblastic leukaemia (ALL) in children is a paradigm for the development of paediatric haematology and oncology over the last 40 years. As it has evolved from being an incurable disease in the 1960s to an overall event-free survival at 5 years now approaching 80%, it has become one of the success stories of modern multi-agent chemotherapy. The history of treatment for childhood ALL highlights the importance of randomized clinical trials, since these formed the basis for the continuous improvement of ALL chemotherapy. In addition, substantial insight into the biology of childhood ALL has been gained that in the future will hopefully translate into improved and more specific treatments with fewer side effects. However, despite the excellent cure rates, ALL treatment still puts a significant burden onto affected children and their families.

Incidence

ALL is the most common malignancy of childhood with an incidence in Europe for children aged 0–14 years of 35 per million person years. This amounts to approximately 370 patients per year in the UK. Boys are slightly more often affected than girls and in Europe the overall incidence appears to be continuing to rise slowly (by 0.8% per year from 1978 to 1997).

Aetiology and prenatal origin

The vast majority of childhood ALL does not appear to be part of any known cancer predisposition syndromes suggesting that, in most cases, it arises from spontaneously occurring genetic alterations. Rearrangement of the immunoglobulin and T cell receptor genes in lymphoid precursor cells may explain their slightly higher genetic instability and likelihood of acquiring chromosomal translocations compared with other cell lineages in the body. Interestingly, the first hit often occurs before birth, as has been shown for ALL with the chromosomal translocation t(12;21). The *TEL/AML1* fusion product formed by this translocation can be detected retrospectively at birth on Guthrie cards or in cord blood samples. However, only a small fraction of children that are *TEL/AML1* positive at birth will go on to develop leukaemia later in life. At least one second event appears necessary, often deletion of the second, non-rearranged *TEL* allele.

Presenting symptoms

The clinical features at presentation mainly reflect *bone marrow failure* and *expansion of the leukaemic clone*:

- Weakness, lethargy, pallor (particularly of lips, mucous membranes, and conjunctivae) due to anaemia.
- Petechiae, nose, and gum bleeding due to thrombocytopenia.
- Febrile infections, sometimes with an unusual or prolonged course due to neutropenia.
- Lymphadenopathy (particularly cervical), hepatosplenomegaly due to leukaemic expansion.
- **Bone pain** due to osseous and periosteal infiltration.
- Non-painful testicular enlargement due to leukaemic infiltration.
- Cranial nerve palsies/facial numbness, headache, meningism due to CNS leukaemia.
- **Superior vena cava syndrome** with distension of the external jugular veins, facial and neck swelling, shortness of breath, cough due to anterior superior mediastinal mass/thymic enlargement/lymphadenopathy (⚠ Do not sedate or anaesthetize these patients; Superior vena cava syndrome 📖 pp.102–103).
- Abdominal pain due to hepatosplenomegaly or abdominal lymph node enlargement (causing intussusception/ileus).
- Rare symptoms and signs, including hypoxia, confusion due to leucostasis (very high white cell count [WCC] >>100 × 10^9/L); visual disturbances due to retinal infiltration or haemorrhage.

Differential diagnosis

- Other types of leukaemia (acute myeloid leukaemia, chronic myeloid leukaemia).
- Other causes of bone marrow failure (aplastic anaemia, myelodysplastic syndromes, inherited bone marrow failure syndromes).
- Other malignancies with widespread bone marrow infiltration [non-Hodgkin lymphoma (NHL), neuroblastoma].
- Other causes of bone pain (rheumatoid arthritis, osteomyelitis).
- Idiopathic thrombocytopenic purpura.

Investigations

If a leukaemia is suspected, the following diagnostic tests are recommended to support the diagnosis and exclude leukaemia-related complications (tumour lysis syndrome, mediastinal mass):

- FBC and blood film.
- Serum electrolytes (including Ca, K, PO$_4$).
- LDH, LFTs, PT, APTT, fibrinogen.
- Creatinine, uric acid.
- CXR.

If FBC or blood film confirm or suggest the diagnosis of leukaemia the nearest Paediatric Haematology referral centre should be contacted to discuss further investigations and management.

Leukaemia-specific diagnostics (Fig. 26.1)

Include:

- Bone marrow aspirate/biopsy (cytology and histology).
- Lumbar puncture to exclude CNS involvement.
- Flow cytometric immunophenotyping of leukaemic blasts to determine cellular lineage and maturation (e.g. B cell precursor ALL, T lineage ALL).
- Cytogenetic and molecular genetic analyses to identify high risk patients (e.g. children with Philadelphia chromosome-positive ALL) who may need to be stratified for more intensive chemotherapy.
- Molecular determination of clonotypic immunoglobulin and T cell receptor rearrangements or flow cytometric determination of leukaemia-associated immunophenotypes (LAIPs) for future assessment of treatment response by minimal residual disease (MRD) monitoring.
- Research protocols may also include whole transcriptome and genome profiling to identify novel risk groups, or leukaemia-specific signalling pathways that can be targeted with novel drugs.

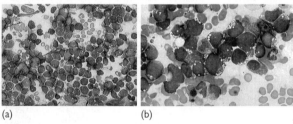

(a) (b)

Fig. 26.1 (a) Bone marrow c ALL (L1). (b) Bone marrow Burkitts morphology (L3) ALL.

Primary management at presentation (including clinical emergencies)

- **Avoid tumour lysis syndrome** (Tumour lysis syndrome 🕮 pp.94–95): Start potassium-free hydration ($3L/m^2/24h$, maximum $4L/24h$) and allopurinol or rasburicase. Monitor WCC, serum electrolytes, creatinine, and uric acid.

- **Consider broad spectrum antibiotics** if child is febrile or has other symptoms and signs indicative of infection.

- Carefully transfuse patients depending on platelet count and haemoglobin (⚠ Avoid hyperviscosity syndrome in patients with high cell counts) after collecting blood samples for blood-borne viral infections (baseline screen). If clinically justifiable, avoid blood or platelet transfusions before transfer to the nearest paediatric haematology referral centre.

- One of the few true **emergency** situations in paediatric haematology/ oncology is the patient with T-ALL/NHL with a **large anterior mediastinal mass** causing superior vena cave syndrome and/or tracheal obstruction (Superior vena cava syndrome 🕮 pp.102–103). Do not sedate or anaesthetize these patients! Most are old enough for a needle aspiration of a malignant pleural or pericardial effusion (common in these patients) to confirm the diagnosis. Always consult with a paediatric haematologist immediately (even at night or at weekends!). In some patients, steroid treatment may need to be started without histological or cytological confirmation.

- Be aware that the **presumed diagnosis** of leukaemia is very **stressful** for the child/young person and his/her parents. Be honest, but reassure the parents that most forms of childhood leukaemia can be treated with at least a good chance of cure.

- Transfer patient to the nearest paediatric haematology referral centre for completion of leukaemia-specific investigations.

Treatment

Treatment of childhood ALL is mainly based on *multi-drug chemotherapy* that includes steroids, methotrexate, vincristine, asparaginase, cytarabine, cyclophosphamide, daunorubicin and 6-mercaptopurine. Treatment usually consists of a 6–12-month phase of more intensive, although mainly outpatient-based, chemotherapy blocks (remission induction, consolidation, and delayed intensification) followed by low-intensity maintenance therapy for a total treatment duration of 2–3 years. In most countries, children will be treated within standardized national treatment protocols.

Infantile ALL is rare (~4% of childhood ALL), but has characteristic clinical and biological features, including:
- High WCC.
- Increased frequency of CNS disease at presentation.
- Immature precursor B lineage (CD10 negative) immunophenotype.
- MLL gene (11q23) rearrangements.

Infants with ALL should be treated on separate protocols that combine both ALL and AML treatment elements as this improves outcome for this distinct subgroup.

CNS-directed therapy An essential element of any treatment protocol for childhood ALL as the blood–brain barrier prevents effective penetration of many chemotherapeutic drugs to the cerebrospinal fluid. Treatment of ALL without CNS-directed therapy in the 1960s was associated with a high rate of CNS relapse. Except for children with CNS leukaemia at diagnosis, most treatment protocols no longer include routine cranial irradiation for CNS-directed therapy because of its long-term consequences. Several studies have shown that intrathecal methotrexate (in some protocols in combination with high-dose IV methotrexate) achieves similar results to irradiation in preventing CNS relapse.

Modern treatment for childhood ALL is *risk-adapted*, i.e. children with a good prognosis receive less treatment than children with a high risk of relapse. Traditionally, the following risk factors have often been used:
- Age <1 year at diagnosis (infantile ALL).
- Age >10 years at diagnosis.
- High WCC (e.g. >50 × 10^9/L).
- T lineage ALL.

Other prognostic markers more directly reflecting the underlying biology include the following cytogenetic aberrations:
- **Favourable prognosis:** high hyperdiploidy (51–65 chromosomes), t(12;21) translocation.
- **Poor prognosis:** t(9;22) translocation (the Philadelphia chromosome), t(4;11) translocation, intrachromosomal amplification of chromosome 21 (iAMP21).

The most important prognostic parameter, however, is response to treatment. Response to treatment is usually quantified by light microscopic assessment of the reduction of blasts in the peripheral blood or bone marrow on day 8, and again in the bone marrow on day 28 of chemotherapy. More recently, clearance of the leukaemia has been additionally assessed by molecular quantification of minimal residual disease (MRD) at weeks 5 (D28) and 11 of treatment. Based on the results of the German BFM group showing >90% survival rate in children with a good response on MRD testing, several trials worldwide are currently investigating whether it is safe to reduce treatment in this favourable ALL subgroup.

Haematopoietic stem cell transplantation (HSCT) is not recommended for most patients with childhood ALL in first remission because of its excellent prognosis with chemotherapy alone. There is controversy on the role of HSCT in certain high risk patients and future studies are needed to prove its benefit. Indications will vary in different countries depending on the treatment protocol used. There is consensus that children and young people with Philadelphia chromosome-positive ALL may benefit from HSCT. The role of imatinib (a small molecule *BCR/ABL* kinase inhibitor) in these patients is currently being evaluated within clinical trials.

Some lessons learnt from recent randomized phase III trials include:

- Response to treatment as measured by blast cell reduction in the peripheral blood after a 1-week course of steroids, and the level of MRD at weeks 5 and 11 of treatment is the strongest predictor of relapse-free survival (German ALL-BFM studies).
- Dexamethasone (6.5mg/m^2/day) as compared with prednisolone (40mg/m^2/day) appears to have a higher anti-leukaemic activity (UK MRC-ALL trials), but may also be associated with a higher incidence of steroid-related complications.
- While 6-thioguanine and 6-mercaptopurine appear to have comparable anti-leukaemic efficacy, 6-thioguanine appears to be associated with a high incidence of veno-occlusive disease (UK MRC-ALL trials).

NB These results need to be interpreted with caution and are dependent on the context of the different treatment protocols.

Treatment-related complications

- Febrile neutropenia.
- Bacterial and fungal infections (including sepsis) due to the treatment-induced immunosuppression.
- *Pneumocystis jiroveci* pneumonia (formerly called PCP).
- Severe varicella zoster infections.
- Nausea and vomiting.
- Hair loss (intermittent).
- Mood and behavioural changes (emotional instability, aggressiveness, depression), often steroid-induced, can be severe, and very stressful for the families.
- Cushing syndrome (steroid-induced), obesity.
- Avascular necrosis of bone (steroid-related).
- Diabetes mellitus (steroid-induced).
- Neuropathy (neuropathic pain, jaw pain, loss of deep tendon reflexes, 'foot drop', constipation; vincristine-induced).
- Allergic reactions to asparaginase, more common after IV as compared with IM administration.
- Coagulopathy (asparaginase-related).
- Sinus venous thrombosis and other thromboembolic complications of asparginase therapy.
- Pancreatitis (asparaginase-related).
- Seizures (following intrathecal methotrexate).
- Transfusion reactions.
- Late adverse effects of treatment (low risk of anthracycline-induced cardiomyopathy, secondary malignancies, infertility).

Prognosis

Outcome of childhood ALL is excellent with an overall 5-year event-free survival rate of 70–80% in published clinical trials in Europe and the US. Certain subgroups, such as patients with t(12;21) translocation or high hyperdiploidy, and in particular patients with rapid leukaemia clearance as assessed by MRD monitoring, may do even better. On the other hand, infantile ALL with t(4;11) translocation, Philadelphia chromosome, or iAMP21-positive ALL, or patients with a poor response to treatment are associated with a high risk of relapse and a 5-year event-free survival rate of <50%. However, as high-risk patients only constitute a small subgroup of all patients, the majority of relapses still occur in standard risk patients.

It is currently been recognized that teenagers and young people (probably up to the age of 30 years) do better on paediatric style protocols. This provides a strong rationale for treating teenagers and young adults on interdisciplinary paediatric/adult teenage cancer wards with common protocols.

Management of relapse

The initial investigation and management of patients with suspected ALL relapse is identical to that of patients at primary diagnosis.

Treatment of ALL relapse is similar to initial treatment, and includes steroids, methotrexate, vincristine, asparaginase, cytarabine, cyclophosphamide, daunorubicin (or other anthracyclines), and 6-mercaptopurine followed by allogeneic bone marrow or peripheral blood stem cell transplantation of high-risk patients.

Overall outcome of first relapse of ALL is 30–50% event-free survival at 5 years, indicating that many children with ALL relapse have a second chance of cure. However, there are big differences in survival depending on whether relapse occurs very early (within 18 months after initial diagnosis), early (i.e. later than 18 months after initial diagnosis, but within 6 months after completing maintenance therapy), or late (later than 6 months after completing therapy). Early and, in particular, very early relapse is associated with a poor prognosis, while some late relapses may even be cured by chemotherapy alone. In ALL with the t(12;21) translocation, late relapse may represent a second leukaemia arising from a common pre-leukaemic clone, rather than a drug-resistant sub-clone that was selected during initial chemotherapy. The site of relapse (isolated bone marrow, extramedullary or combined) is also of prognostic importance and used for therapy stratification, with isolated extramedullary relapse usually having a better outlook. With continuing improvement of first line treatment, the incidence and prognosis of relapsed ALL is changing with fewer overall numbers of patients relapsing but a higher proportion of these having drug-resistant disease.

Acute myeloid leukaemia

Acute myeloid leukaemia (AML) comprises a group of clonal disorders caused by maturation arrest leading to proliferation of abnormal myeloid precursor cells. However, this definition incorporates a wide and heterogenous group of leukaemias (see Classification). The prognosis of paediatric AML was very poor until the introduction of intensive chemotherapy protocols in the 1980s, but has now improved greatly although survival rates still lag behind those for ALL.

Epidemiology

- Incidence of AML for children aged 0–14 years is 6 per million person years, amounting to approximately 70 new cases per year in UK. Stable during childhood except for peak in neonatal period and gradual increase during adolescence.
- Accounts for ~15–20% of all paediatric leukaemia in industrialized countries.
- There is no difference between sexes.
- There is no evidence for changes in incidence over last 20 years.
- There is some evidence of racial differences, with slightly higher incidence reported in Asian and Hispanic children, especially for acute promyelocytic leukaemia (Treatment, Acute promyelocytic leukaemia, 🕮 p.416).

Aetiology

- Cause of AML unknown in most children.
- Environmental factors associated with the development of AML (across all age groups) include ionizing radiation and organic pesticides. Prenatal exposure to maternal tobacco or marijuana use may increase AML risk, but evidence not conclusive.
- Previous chemotherapy (alkylating agents, epipodophyllotoxins, other topoisomerase II inhibitors) may cause 'secondary' AML – typically occurring within 4–7 years of treatment and characterized by an *MLL* gene arrangement. High maternal intake of foods rich in topoisomerase II inhibitors may also be associated with higher risk of *MLL* gene rearranged AML in exposed offspring.
- Increased risk in siblings of patients developing AML in early childhood (up to ~6 years age) – very high concordance (approaching 100% in identical twins) where proband presents in infancy.
- Paediatric AML is relatively unusual in that numerous predisposing conditions are known, although collectively they only account for a small proportion of cases.
  - *Hereditary –*
    - *Down syndrome* (Treatment, Down syndrome–acute myeloid leukaemia 📖 p.416);
    - *bone marrow failure syndromes* – Fanconi anaemia (FA), Schwachman-Diamond syndrome, dyskeratosis congenita, congenital amegakaryocytic thrombocytopenia (Constitutional aplastic anaemia 📖 p.372–378);
    - *other DNA repair disorders* – ataxia telangiectasia, Bloom syndrome (although ALL/NHL commoner than AML in these patients);
    - Kostman n syndrome (severe congenital neutropenia);
    - Neurofibromatosis type I, Noonan syndrome;
    - Diamond-Blackfan anaemia;
    - Klinefelter syndrome.
  - Familial AML is rare, but may be associated with constitutional chromosomal abnormalities (e.g. involving chromosome 7).
  - *Acquired –*
    - myelodysplasia (Myelodysplasia 📖 pp.423–430);
    - aplastic anaemia (Acquired aplastic anaemia 📖 pp.364–371);
    - paroxysmal nocturnal haemoglobinuria (PNH) (Other non-malignant causes of peripheral blood cytopenias 📖 pp.379–394).

Clinical presentation

- **Symptoms/signs of bone marrow failure:**
  - *anaemia* – lethargy, pallor, headaches, occasionally cardiac failure;
  - *neutropenia* – infections;
  - *thrombocytopenia* – increased bruising (often spontaneous), purpura, bleeding (usually mucosal, e.g. oral, epistaxis; occasionally serious internal, e.g. intracranial, or pulmonary, especially in presence of leucostasis).
- **Raised total white cell count** (WCC) (myeloblasts):
  symptoms/signs of leucostasis may occur when WCC >200 × 10^9/l (Hyperleucocytosis 📖 pp.120–121).
- **Infiltration of:**
  - liver +/– spleen → mild/moderate hepatosplenomegaly (15–50%);
  - lymph nodes → lymphadenopathy (10–20%), especially in M4/5 morphology (see Classification (27) 📖 pp.410–412);
  - bone → pain, limp, backache (10–20%).
- **Coagulopathy:** especially in M3 (APL) and M5.
- **Other sites of extramedullary disease** (commoner in M4/5):
  - *skin* (→ nodules – leukaemia cutis; overall occurring in ~1% children, but commoner in infants, extreme cases may present as 'blueberry muffin' baby), gums (hypertrophy) (~10%), CNS (2-4%), testicular (very rare);
  - *granulocytic sarcoma* (chloroma) – extramedullary deposits of immature myeloid cells, commonest sites in children are orbital (→ proptosis), epidural (→ spinal cord compression), lymph nodes, skin, gastrointestinal tract; often associated with t(8;21), and may occur without, or as a prelude to, bone marrow involvement.
- **Fever:** may be related to disease, rather than infection.

Investigations

- FBC.
- Coagulation profile.
- Biochemical profile (including urate).
- Bone marrow aspirate and biopsy:
  - Morphology (see Classification (27), Morphology 📖 p.410).
  - Immunophenotyping (+/– immunocytochemistry) may help in differentiating AML from ALL where morphology is difficult, and in distinguishing certain FAB subtypes (see Classification (27) 📖 pp.410–412). Useful immunophenotypic markers include –
    - CD13, CD33, CD117 (M0 – M7);
    - CD14, CD64 (more suggestive of M4, M5);
    - Glycophorin A (M6);
    - CD41, CD42, CD61 (M7);
    - HLA-DR is negative in M3, but usually positive in other FAB subtypes;
    - CD7 (a T lymphoid marker) is often aberrantly expressed in AML.
  - Useful immunocytochemical stains include –
    - *myeloperoxidase* (MPO) – in granules and/or Auer rods in myeloid and monocytic progenitor cells (M2, M3, M5);
    - *Sudan black* – in granules in myeloid and monocytic precursors;
    - *non-specific esterase* (NSE) – monocytic precursors (M4, M5);
    - *periodic acid-Schiff* (PAS) and terminal deoxynucleotide transferase (TdT) usually negative (although PAS positive in M6).
  - Cytogenetics, and where relevant, molecular genetics (see Classification (27), Cytogenetics and molecular genetics 📖 p.411).
- Lumbar puncture and CSF examination (cell count and morphology).
- In appropriate clinical context, imaging and ?biopsy of possible granulocytic sarcomas or extramedullary disease.

Diagnosis

Morphology is the mainstay of diagnosis, but may be supported by immunophenotyping, immunocytochemistry and/or cytogenetics/molecular genetics.

Classification

Morphology (French-American-British [FAB] criteria) (Fig 27.1)

- M0 – undifferentiated.
- M1 – myeloblastic with no differentiation.
- M2 – myeloblastic with differentiation.
- M3 – promyelocytic (APL).
  - M3v – microgranular variant.
- M4 – myelomonocytic.
  - M4Eo – with eosinophilia.
- M5 – monocytic.
- M6 – erythroleukaemia.
- M7 – megakaryoblastic (AMKL).

With the exception of the association between M2, M3 and M4Eo with good risk cytogenetic abnormalities (Classification (27), Cytogenetics and molecular genetics 📖 p.411). there is no consistent evidence that FAB type has important prognostic significance since intensive chemotherapy has improved the overall survival rates for paediatric AML.

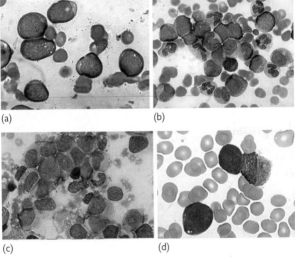

(a)　　　　　　　　　(b)

(c)　　　　　　　　　(d)

Fig. 27.1 (a) Bone marrow of M1 AML showing maturation and an Auer rod. (b) Bone marrow of M2 AML. (c) Bone marrow of acute promyelocytic leukaemia (M3) showing a collection of Auer rods. (d) Bone marrow showing M5 AML blasts.

Cytogenetics and molecular genetics

Good risk cytogenetic abnormalities are shown in Table 27.1.

Table 27.1 Good risk cytogenetic abnormalities

Cytogenetics	Corresponding molecular genetics	Morphology
t(8;21)(q22;q22)	*AML1-ETO*	Usually M2
t(15;17)(q22;q21)*	*PML-RARα*	M3
inv(16)(p13q22)	*CBFβ-MYHII*	Classically M4Eo also M1, M2

* Several other cytogenetic/molecular genetic abnormalities are described in APL, e.g. t(11;17)(q23;q21) associated with PZLF-RARα – these patients are poor responders to ATRA, and t(5:17)(q35;q12-21) associated with NPM-RARα. However, collectively these only account for <5% of patients.

Poor risk cytogenetic abnormalities are less common in children than in adults, but their significance is similar:

- −7 (monosomy 7).
- −5 (monosomy 5).
- del(5q).
- abn(3q).
- t(9;22) (Philadelphia chromosome).
- complex (≥5 abnormalities).

11q23 (*MLL*) rearrangements, with several different partner chromosomes occur in 8–20%, especially:

- Infants (commonly associated with M4/5) – prognostic significance (if any) is unclear.
- Secondary AML – poor prognosis.
- t(9;11)(p22;q23) appears to be associated with good prognosis.

FLT-3 (fms-like tyrosine kinase 3) mutations (internal tandem duplications or point mutations) promote myeloblast proliferation by ligand-independent receptor activation and are associated with poorer outcome, but relevance for treatment in children is not yet clear.

WHO classification

A refined classification of myeloid haematological malignancies has been developed recently by the World Health Organization (WHO), based on morphology, immunophenotyping, and cytogenetics. Although it was not developed specifically with children in mind, a paediatric modification has been published, but not yet applied universally. This approach distinguishes AML from MDS and myelodysplastic/myeloproliferative disorders.

- **AML:**
  - *AML with recurrent genetic abnormalities* – t(8;21); inv(16); t(15;17) and variants; 11q23 rearrangements;
  - *AML not otherwise categorized* (morphologically akin to M0-M7, plus granulocytic sarcoma).

- Myelodysplastic/myeloproliferative diseases
  - myelodysplastic/myeloproliferative disease e.g. juvenile myelomonocytic leukaemia (JMML) (Myelodysplasia, Clinical presentation, Juvenile myelomonocytic leukaemia 📖 pp.423–430);
  - Down syndrome disease –
    - transient abnormal myeloproliferation (Treatment, Down syndrome–acute myeloid leukaemia 📖 pp.416–417);
    - DS-AML.
- MDS (Myelodysplasia 📖 pp.423–430).

Risk stratification

Since 1995, the UK Medical Research Council (MRC) AML 12 and 15 clinical trials have stratified patients (both children and adults) into three risk groups based on cytogenetics (and/or corresponding molecular genetics) and response to the first course of chemotherapy:

- **Good risk:** 30% of children. Good risk genetic abnormalities (as above) — even if other cytogenetic abnormalities present, or if >15% blasts in bone marrow after 1st course of chemotherapy.
- **Standard risk:** 58% of children. Patients in neither good nor poor risk groups.
- **Poor risk:** 12% of children. >15% blasts in bone marrow after 1st course, or with poor risk genetic abnormalities (as above) and without good risk genetic abnormalities.

Treatment

Chemotherapy

Intensification of treatment has improved remission rates, reduced relapse rates, and increased disease-free and overall survival rates.

- Most contemporary AML treatment protocols schedule 4 or 5 courses of intensive chemotherapy delivered as rapidly as possible
  - Typically 1–2 courses of induction chemotherapy – usually based predominantly on anthracyclines and cytosine arabinoside, +/– etoposide +/– 6-thioguanine.
  - Followed by 2–3 courses of consolidation treatment (and/or HSCT) – incorporating above chemotherapy +/– others (e.g. asparaginase, amsacrine, azacytidine).
  - Prior to advent of intensive chemotherapy, many protocols used low-dose maintenance chemotherapy. Contemporary BFM AML protocols still use this approach (6-thioguanine and cytosine arabinoside), but most other national/collaborative AML trial groups have dropped maintenance treatment in the absence of evidence that it improves survival.
- CNS-directed treatment is given with intrathecal chemotherapy (typically 2–6 doses of methotrexate or cytosine arabinoside or triple treatment , i.e. including methotrexate, cytosine and hydrocortisone), and cranial radiotherapy is now usually reserved only for patients with CNS disease at presentation.
- The addition of Mylotarg (an anti-CD33 monoclonal antibody) to intensive chemotherapy is under investigation in Phase III clinical trials. Other monoclonal antibodies directed against specific molecular targets (e.g. FLT-3 activated tyrosine kinase) are undergoing preclinical and early clinical trials in adults.
- The role of HSCT as the last course of consolidation treatment in CR1 has diminished steadily as frontline chemotherapy has improved survival over the last two decades:
  - *autologous HSCT* is no longer included in paediatric AML treatment protocols in CR1 in most countries;
  - *allogeneic HSCT* is performed less frequently – now reserved for poor risk patients only in most paediatric protocols.
- Granulocytic sarcomas respond well to intensive systemic chemotherapy. Local radiotherapy is now used only rarely, usually to provide rapid relief of compressive symptoms (e.g. in spinal cord compression due to epidural masses).

Treatment of relapse

Despite greatly improved frontline chemotherapy, 30–50% of children will still relapse, although a significant proportion of these can still be cured by further intensive chemotherapy usually followed by allogeneic HSCT. Autologous HSCT is sometimes performed, especially in late relapses (e.g. CR1 duration >2 years) and/or when no suitably matched allogeneic donor is available.

- Historically, relapse chemotherapy has usually been similar to frontline chemotherapy (i.e. based on anthracyclines and cytosine), since this still achieves CR2 in many patients.
- However, further anthracycline use associated with a significant risk of serious cardiotoxicity due to high cumulative doses:
  - recent protocols have included fludarabine in an effort to limit the use of further anthracyclines;
  - other investigational strategies to reduce cardiotoxicity risk have included use of liposomal daunorubicin (aiming to reduce cardiac exposure to toxic metabolites) or dezrazoxane (cardioprotectant), but efficacy of these approaches is unproven.
- Likelihood of achieving CR2 is lower in early relapses (~50% if CR1 duration <12 months, compared with ~75% if CR1 duration ≥12 months).
- 5-year overall survival also lower in early relapses (~25% if CR1 <12 months, compared with ~40% if CR1 ≥12 months)
- HSCT usually performed with high-dose conditioning chemoradiotherapy [e.g. busulfan + cyclophosphamide +/– melphalan (BuCy +/– Mel) or cyclophosphamide + total body irradiation (CyTBI)]. HSCT also offers potential of a graft-versus-leukaemia (GvL) effect (Haemopoietic stem cell transplantation 📖 pp.163–200).

Haemopoietic stem cell transplant

In the 1980s and 1990s most paediatric AML trials incorporated HSCT as consolidation treatment in CR1, but this strategy is now usually reserved for higher risk patients only.

Allogeneic HSCT

- Historically offered whenever HLA-identical sibling donor available, but progressively removed from treatment protocols for good and standard risk patients as non-HSCT approaches have improved survival rates to >50%.
- Currently reserved for poor risk patients only. Some trial groups no longer recommend HSCT except in refractory AML (i.e. failure to remit after 2 induction courses) or relapsed AML.
- When HSCT is considered essential, there is increasing experience with, and use of, alternative donors, especially matched unrelated donors.
- Despite widespread use as above, it has been difficult to confirm survival advantage of HSCT, especially as comparative chemotherapy results have improved. Most trials have shown reduced significantly reduced relapse risk, but higher treatment-related mortality rate after HSCT, with no significant difference in overall survival.

Autologous HSCT

Now rarely used by most trial groups (but see Treatment, Treatment of relapse 📖 pp.414–415). Some groups have investigated autologous HSCT in CR1 using peripheral blood stem cells (PBSC) or manipulated bone marrow (purged by in vitro immunological or chemotherapy techniques).

Acute promyelocytic leukaemia

Classically associated with t(15;17) translocation and more recently *PML-RARα* rearrangement (see Classification 🕮 pp.410–411).

Although APL was feared historically due to the high frequency of haemorrhagic complications (sometimes fatal) at initial presentation or during induction chemotherapy, it is now recognized as a good risk subtype especially in children.

- Coagulopathy presents with prominent bruising and may result in severe mucosal (e.g. gastrointestinal) or internal haemorrhage (e.g. intracranial):
  - due to release of anticoagulant factors from intracytoplasmic granules in malignant promyelocytes;
  - coagulation profile typically shows markedly prolonged PT, PTT, and TT with evidence of DIC (↓ fibrinogen, ↑ D-dimers);
  - early introduction of *all*-trans retinoic acid (ATRA) promotes maturation and eventually apoptosis of malignant promyelocytes and reduces the frequency of severe haemorrhagic complications.
- Until recently treated by conventional AML chemotherapy protocols with addition of ATRA during induction (+/– consolidation):
  - some trial groups (especially in adults) have also added intermittent ATRA to conventional maintenance chemotherapy;
  - increasing interest (especially in adults) in efficacy of anthracycline-only protocols (e.g. Spanish approach);
  - increasing use of specific paediatric APL treatment protocols incorporating ATRA, followed by post-treatment molecular monitoring for *PML-RARα* to detect and treat incipient relapse (in expectation of reducing frequency and severity of haemorrhagic complications).
- HSCT no longer recommended in CR1.
- Relapsed APL is usually treated with further chemotherapy (± ATRA), usually followed by allogeneic HSCT. Arsenic trioxide, which (like ATRA) promotes differentiation and apoptosis of promyelocytes, is used increasingly in relapsed APL, since it is able to reinduce remission in patients who have become resistant to ATRA.

Down syndrome–acute myeloid leukaemia

AML is very common in younger children (<5 years age) with Down syndrome (DS), with a 150-fold increased risk (occurs in 1% of children with DS). Most of these children have AMKL. Although other AML subtypes occur occasionally in older DS children, the biological basis and clinical features of DS-associated AMKL are characteristic:

- AMKL occurs during 1st 4 years of life.
- Associated with acquired mutations in *GATA-1* gene, which encodes a transcription factor essential for normal erythroid and megakaryocyte differentiation.
- May be preceded by a phase of MDS which evolves into AML or demands treatment in its own right.
- Up to 10% of neonates with DS may have transient abnormal myeloproliferation (TAM):

- bruising, skin infiltrates, effusions (pleural, pericardial, ascites), hepatomegaly, respiratory distress;
- some infants present with severe hydrops, which may also → stillbirth;
- FBC usually → leucocytosis and circulating blast cells, but normal Hb and neutrophil count; either thrombocytopenia or thrombocytosis;
- usually resolves spontaneously within 1st 3 months of life;
- occasionally necessitates careful low dose chemotherapy (e.g. low-dose cytosine) due to progressive organ infiltration (e.g. liver);
- rarely, may lead to fatal hepatic failure due to liver fibrosis;
- 20–30% of DS patients with TAM develop MDS or AML by 4 years of age.
- DS-AMKL is very responsive to treatment:
  - relapse rare if intensive AML treatment is given;
  - most deaths are due to toxicity, especially infection, rather than leukaemia;
  - cytosine appears to be the most important component of successful chemotherapy;
  - concerns about anthracycline treatment in DS patients, many of whom have history of congenital cardiac disease;
  - therefore, most trial groups are reducing treatment, especially cumulative anthracycline dose, in attempt to reduce treatment-related mortality and severe cardiotoxicity.

Complications of treatment

Acute toxicity of treatment for paediatric AML is frequent and may be fatal:
- Consequences of severe myelosuppression (may be life-threatening):
  - *infection* – especially bacterial and fungal (commonest cause of treatment-related death);
  - haemorrhage.
- *Mucositis* – severe oral pain/ulceration, abdominal pain, diarrhoea, severe nutritional compromise.
- Tumour lysis syndrome (Tumour lysis syndrome 📖 pp.94–95).

The commonest potentially severe late adverse effect of treatment for AML in children is cardiotoxicity. Mild/moderate left ventricular impairment is common, but severe cardiotoxicity leading to cardiac failure is fortunately uncommon.

Other potential late toxicities may include (Long-term follow-up 📖 pp.293–314):
- Late effects of HSCT.
- Late effects of chemotherapy.
- Late effects of cranial radiotherapy (although this is seldom required in absence of HSCT).

Prognosis

The disease-free and overall survival of paediatric AML has improved greatly, especially in good and standard risk patients. Complete remission rates are now consistently >95%, but relapse rates are still >35% and treatment-related mortality (TRM) remains considerable at about 5%, predominantly due to infection.

Although results from UK MRC AML 15 remain immature, initial 5 year survival rates in children have improved compared with AML 10 (Table 27.2).

Table 27.2 5-year survival rates for childhood AML treated in AML 10 and AML 15 trials

	AML 15 (1995–2002)	AML 10 (1988–1995)
Overall survival	66%	58%
Disease free survival	61%	53%
Event free survival	56%	49%

The future

It is likely that we are approaching the limit of success that is feasible with contemporary intensive chemotherapy approaches, and that consolidation with HSCT will only improve long-term survival if HSCT-related TRM is reduced. Therefore, further progress in paediatric AML may rely on the success of targeted treatments with monoclonal antibodies and/or the development of more effective (and hopefully less toxic) cytotoxic drugs.

Acute leukaemia of ambiguous lineage

Several terms have been used previously to describe this heterogenous group of rare acute leukaemias, including:

- Biphenotypic acute leukaemia.
- Bilineal acute leukaemia.
- Mixed lineage (or phenotype) acute leukaemia.
- Hybrid acute leukaemia.
- Acute leukaemia of indeterminate origin (or lineage).

Definitions

The WHO classification of acute leukaemias defines acute leukaemias of ambiguous lineage (ALAL) as:

- Forms of acute leukaemia in which the morphological, cytochemical, and immunophenotypic features of the proliferating blasts lack sufficient evidence to classify as myeloid or lymphoid origin (acute undifferentiated leukaemia) or
- Which have morphological and/or immunophenotypic characteristics of both myeloid and lymphoid cells or both B and T cell lineages (acute bilineal leukaemia and acute biphenotypic leukaemia).

Biphenotypic acute leukaemia

This term is generally used to describe a single population of blasts with uniform expression of a mixture of myeloid and lymphoid (B or T-cell) antigens.

Bilineal acute leukaemia

This term is generally used to describe the presence of two morphologically and immunophenotypically distinct myeloid and lymphoid blast cell populations.

Aberrant antigen expression

In contrast, this is defined as the presence of 'aberrant' myeloid antigen expression by lymphoblasts, or of 'aberrant' lymphoid antigen expression by myeloblasts. It is a common finding in childhood acute leukaemia, and does not have significant therapeutic or prognostic implications. Cases with co-expression of myeloid, B and T-cell antigens, or of B and T-cell markers, are exceedingly rare. Aberrant antigen expression alone does not equate to a diagnosis of ALAL.

ALAL in children

ALAL is rare, representing 3–5% of acute leukaemia (all ages). It is believed to account for an even smaller proportion of childhood leukaemia, although paediatric epidemiological data are lacking.

The clinical features are not clearly distinguishable from those of other acute leukaemias (i.e. symptoms/signs due to bone marrow failure and leukaemic infiltration), although infants may present with multiple skin lesions due to leukaemic deposits.

About 30–40% of cases are Philadelphia chromosome (*BCR-ABL*) positive.

Diagnosis

Diagnosis of ALAL is facilitated by the use of a scoring system, such as that developed by the European Group on Immunological Classification of Leukemias (EGIL). This is based on the number and degree of myeloid/lymphoid specificity of antigens expressed by the leukaemic cells.

Treatment

There is no clinical trial or defined protocol for the treatment of children with ALAL, so treatment varies considerably. Some children receive standard ALL or standard AML chemotherapy, whilst many receive hybrid chemotherapy combinations according to the predominant clinical characteristics and the response to treatment. It is advisable to reassess response regularly with bone marrow aspirates, particularly during the early stages of treatment. Historically, many children with matched donors have undergone haemopoietic stem cell transplantation in first complete remission in view of adverse risk features (e.g. Philadelphia-positive disease, poor initial response) or concerns about the perceived poor prognosis of ALAL, although it is not known whether or not this leads to an improved outcome.

Prognosis

The prognosis of ALAL has been considered to be very poor, although recent evidence suggests that it is better in children than in adults. A small single-institution study reported 2-year survival in children of 75%, which was not significantly different to that of children with ALL or AML. Poor risk features were:
- Age at presentation >15 years.
- Presence of Philadelphia chromosome/*BCR-ABL*.
- Secondary (as opposed to *de novo*) leukaemia.

Myelodysplasia

Definition

The myelodysplastic syndromes (MDS, collectively termed myelodysplasia) incorporate a group of clonal haematopoietic stem cell disorders involving one or more cell lineage(s), characterized by:
- Ineffective haematopoiesis 2° to increased apoptosis → one or more cytopenia(s).
- Disordered differentiation → dysplasia in one or more cell lineage(s).
- Tendency to evolve to AML (reflecting myeloid clonality).

In contrast to acute leukaemia, the blast cell proportion in bone marrow in MDS remains low due to the retention of some differentiation capacity, as well as the increased degree of apoptosis.

Most published information about MDS derives from adult literature. However:
- MDS is much rarer in children than in adults, in whom it is predominantly a disease of the elderly.
- Childhood MDS differs considerably from adult MDS, particularly in:
  - the presence of associated conditions and abnormalities (Acute myeloid leukaemia 📖 pp.405–418, Bone marrow failure 📖 pp.361–378);
  - haematological and morphological features;
  - cytogenetic abnormalities;
  - natural history;
  - response to treatment;
  - prognosis.

Classification

Traditionally, MDS in both adults and children has been classified using the French-American-British (FAB) system, based on the proportion of blasts in the bone marrow:
- Refractory anaemia (RfA).
- Refractory anaemia with ringed sideroblasts (RfARS).
- Refractory anaemia with excess blasts (RfAEB).
- RfAEB in transformation (RfAEB-t).
- Chronic myelomonocytic leukaemia (CMML).

In 2000, WHO revised the FAB classification by:
- Redefining RfAEB-t as AML (by lowering the threshold for diagnosing AML to 20% blasts in bone marrow).
- Subdividing RfAEB according to the marrow blast count (5–9% or 10–19%).
- Reclassifying CMML as a myeloproliferative/myelodysplastic disorder.

However, aspects relevant to paediatric MDS were not addressed adequately, particularly issues related to its association with congenital conditions (especially Down syndrome) and to the diagnosis of CMML. Therefore, a new classification of paediatric MDS has been proposed:

- Myeloproliferative/myelodysplastic disease:
  - juvenile myelomonocytic leukaemia (JMML);
  - chronic myelomonocytic leukaemia (CMML).
- Down syndrome disease (Acute myeloid leukaemia, Treatment, Down syndrome–acute myeloid leukaemia 📖 pp.416–417):
  - transient abnormal myelopoiesis (TAM);
  - DS-AML.
- Myelodysplastic syndrome:
  - refractory cytopenia (<5% bone marrow blasts);
  - RfAEB (5–19% bone marrow blasts);
  - RfAEB-t (20–29% bone marrow blasts; retained as a distinct sub-category in children, in contrast to the new WHO MDS classification, in view of the lack of evidence to indicate whether a threshold of 20% or 30% blasts is better at distinguishing MDS from *de novo* AML).

Some children with AML present with a relatively low bone marrow blast count initially, but progress rapidly to typical and overt AML. They are usually classified as AML, rather than MDS.

Cytogenetics

Clonal cytogenetic abnormalities are present in >60-70% of children with MDS. In contrast to leukaemia, most abnormalities are chromosomal deletions or duplications, whilst translocations are rare.

The commonest abnormalities found in paediatric MDS are:

- Monosomy 7.
- Trisomy 8.
- Trisomy 21 (because it is present constitutionally in children with Down syndrome).

Clinical presentation

Most children with MDS present with symptoms or signs of bone marrow failure (Bone marrow failure 📖 pp.361–378), although the diagnosis may be made incidentally when a blood count performed for other reasons reveals cytopenia, leading to more detailed haematological investigation. Occasionally, children with symptoms and signs (e.g. hepatosplenomegaly) suggestive of acute leukaemia (Acute myeloid leukaemia 📖 pp.405–418) may be found to have RfAEB or RfAEB-t.

History ± examination may reveal an associated inherited or acquired condition, or previous treatment (e.g. chemotherapy) predisposing to MDS.

Rarely, there may be a family history of AML or MDS.

Investigation

- Full blood count:
  - *cytopenia* – mono-, bi- or trilineage cytopenia may be seen;
  - *dysplasia* – wide range of dysplastic features may occur, commonly including abnormal red cell (e.g. poikilocytosis, dysplastic nucleated red cells) and white cell (e.g. hypogranular) morphology, bizarre small or giant platelets;
  - macrocytosis (↑ MCV) common, but not invariable.
- HbF may be slightly elevated (when corrected for age).
- Bone marrow aspirate/biopsy:
  - to exclude acute leukaemia;
  - *cellularity variable* – hypocellular in up to 40%, but may be normo- or hypercellular;
  - *dysplasia* – variable extent and nature;
  - cytogenetics;
  - immunophenotyping is seldom helpful;
  - may be wise to confirm diagnosis with a repeat bone marrow after a few weeks.
- Other investigations (e.g. viral serology or detection) may be indicated in cases where the diagnosis is uncertain.

Minimal diagnostic criteria for paediatric myelodysplasia

At least 2 of:
- At least bilineage dysplasia.
- Clonal cytogenetic abnormality in haemopoietic cells.
- Persistent cytopenia in at least one lineage.
- >5% blasts in bone marrow.

Refractory cytopenia

The term refractory cytopenia (RC) represents a better description than refractory anaemia in paediatric MDS in view of the occurrence of isolated neutropenia or thrombocytopenia, or of cytopenia affecting two or three cell lineages (bi- or tri-lineage MDS).

Prolonged follow-up may be necessary to distinguish RC from other causes of chronic cytopenias (e.g. evolving aplastic anaemia).

Natural history is variable with some patients remaining haematologically and clinically stable over many years of follow-up whilst others may develop advanced bone marrow failure, or more often progress to RfAEB or AML.

Refractory anaemia with ringed sideroblasts

Extremely rare in children.

May be a feature of mitochondrial disease (e.g. Pearson's syndrome, see Bone marrow failure, Acquired aplastic anaemia, Investigation, Differential diagnosis).

Refractory anaemia with excess blasts

Although often relatively indolent, RfAEB usually progresses to AML, albeit with a very variable speed of evolution.

RfAEB in transformation

In terms of classification, the separation between RfAEB-t and AML is clearly arbitrary (as evidenced by the recent changes in classification), whilst the clinical distinction may also be relatively unhelpful. The recognition of a preceding MDS phase may lead to a description of MDS-related AML, rather than de novo AML, but the treatment given is likely to be similar (intensive 'AML type' chemotherapy) and there is no clear prognostic implication.

Juvenile myelomonocytic leukaemia

JMML is extremely rare. It presents in early childhood (range 0–6 years, median 2), with a male predominance (2.5:1).

Suggestive clinical features include various combinations of:
- Marked hepatosplenomegaly.
- Lymphadenopathy.
- Pallor.
- Fever.
- Rash (often facial but non-specific).

Other symptoms include failure to thrive, anorexia, respiratory symptoms (cough, tachypnoea) and frequent infections.

Published diagnostic criteria for JMML are:
- Suggestive clinical features (as above).
- Laboratory criteria (all 3 must be present):
  - persistent peripheral blood monocytosis ($>1 \times 10^9$/l);
  - absence of Philadelphia chromosome or BCR/ABL fusion gene;
  - bone marrow blasts <20%.
- Further criteria (at least 2 required):
  - ↑ HbF (corrected for age);
  - immature myeloid precursors on peripheral blood film;
  - peripheral blood white cell count $>10 \times 10^9$/l;
  - clonal cytogenetic abnormality (including monosomy 7);
  - in vitro hypersensitivity of myeloid precursors to GM-CSF.

Progression of JMML is usually characterized by increasing bone marrow failure, whilst blast crisis is rare (in contrast to CML).

Chronic myelomonocytic leukaemia

CMML is a disease of older adults (again more commonly males), presenting with symptoms of bone marrow failure and/or signs or organ infiltration (hepatosplenomegaly). It may occur very rarely in childhood. WHO diagnostic criteria include monocytosis, absence of Philadelphia chromosome or BCR/ABL, <20% blasts in peripheral blood or marrow, and dysplasia in at least myeloid cell line.

Hypoplastic myelodysplasia

Hypoplastic MDS is extremely rare and does not fit easily into existing classification systems for MDS. Patients (children or adults) present with aplastic anaemia (and are sometimes treated for this with immunosuppressive treatment), but subsequently develop dysplastic and cytogenetic abnormalities in bone marrow, often progressing to AML.

Treatment

Supportive care

Similar to that for patients with aplastic anaemia (Bone marrow failure pp.361–378, Acquired aplastic anaemia pp.364–371, Management pp.366–370).

- Blood product transfusion support.
- Other measures to reduce the risk or severity of bleeding.
- Prevention and treatment of infections.

Observation

May be appropriate in some children with stable RC who are not suffering from complications of bone marrow failure.

Chemotherapy

Intensive chemotherapy (usually following an AML protocol) may be indicated in RfAEB, although these children may still require haemopoietic stem cell transplantation (HSCT) subsequently, depending on their clinical response to treatment and cytogenetic status.

Chemotherapy (e.g. with AML protocols, or cytosine arabinoside + etoposide) has been used in JMML to reduce disease burden (leucocytosis and organomegaly), but response is often poor.

Other drugs

13-cis-retinoic acid

13-cis-retinoic acid may induce maturation and inhibit proliferation of JMML cells in vitro, but evidence for sustained clinical benefit is lacking.

There is very little experience in children of the use of other drugs and no published evidence of long-term benefit. Other treatment strategies sometimes employed in adult MDS include growth factors [e.g. erythropoietin (EPO) ± granulocyte colony stimulating factor (G-CSF)], immunosuppressive agents (e.g. ciclosporin A), immunomodulatory agents (e.g. thalidomide) and non-intensive chemotherapy (e.g. 5-azacytidine).

Haemopoietic stem cell transplant

HSCT may be indicated for:

- RC with blood product transfusion dependence and/or persistent clonal cytogenetic abnormality.
- RfAEB (after initial chemotherapy), especially if poor clinical response to chemotherapy or in presence of poor risk cytogenetics (e.g. monosomy 7).
- HSCT is the only potentially curative treatment for JMML, but relapse is common. Donor lymphocyte infusion (DLI) may control post-HSCT relapse in some patients, suggesting that a graft-versus-leukaemia (GvL) effect is important in this disease.
- Secondary MDS (i.e. 2° to previous chemotherapy) – sustained response to further chemotherapy is unlikely, and HSCT is usually recommended.

Splenectomy

Occasionally used in JMML:

- To treat significant hypersplenism when disease otherwise indolent.
- Reduction of disease burden before HSCT.

Down syndrome disease

- Acute myeloid leukaemia, Treatment, Down syndrome–acute myeloid leukaemia 🕮 pp.416–417.

Prognosis

- Variable.
- RC may be indolent, as may occasional cases of JMML in infants without significant thrombocytopenia or splenomegaly. Occasional cases of RC with monosomy 7 may regress spontaneously.
- In contrast, advanced JMML is often a relentless disease.
- A paediatric MDS prognostic score based on HbF, platelet count, and cytogenetic profile appears to identify children with RC, RfAEB, or JMML who have a better prognosis.

Myeloproliferative diseases

Definition

Myeloproliferative diseases (MPDs) are clonal multipotential haemopoietic stem cell diseases, broadly characterized by:
- Proliferative behaviour, usually associated with:
  - hypercellular bone marrow;
  - increased numbers of one or more cell types in peripheral blood.
- Insidious onset.
- Chronic natural history, but tendency to:
  - progress to bone marrow failure; or
  - transform to acute leukaemia.

MPDs are predominantly adult diseases. Chronic myeloid leukaemia is rare and other MPDs exceedingly rare, in children.

Chronic myeloid leukaemia

Epidemiology
- Although CML appears to be the same disease in molecular terms in patients of all ages (Myeloproliferative diseases, Chronic myeloid leukaemia, Aetiology 📖 p.432), it is much rarer in children than in adults, only accounting for 2-3% of childhood leukaemia.
- Incidence in children 0.6–1.2 per million person years.
- Slight male preponderance (1.2:1).
- Median age at presentation in paediatric age range is 12 years.

Aetiology
- Ionizing radiation is the only definitive causative agent.
- No definite genetic predisposition, although isolated cases have been reported in Down syndrome.

Pathogenesis
The molecular basis for CML is the *BCR/ABL* fusion gene, which codes for an abnormal tyrosine kinase (TK) protein product. In most patients this is visible cytogenetically, represented by the classical Philadelphia chromosome, with a t(9;22)(q34;q11) reciprocal translocation.
- 90–95% of children with CML have the Philadelphia chromosome (Ph^+).
- The *BCR/ABL* fusion gene is present in ~50% of the remainder (2–5% overall) despite no visible Philadelphia chromosome.
- A very small number of paediatric CML patients are both Philadelphia and *BCR/ABL* negative.

Clinical presentation

Chronic phase

Most children (and adults) present in chronic phase (CP), which is characterized by massive proliferation of morphologically normal and differentiated blood cells, including both mature granulocytes and to a lesser extent myeloid precursor cells, involving bone marrow, peripheral blood, spleen, and (less frequently) liver. Symptoms and signs are due to:

- Organ infiltration.
- Metabolic consequences of excessive myeloproliferation.
- ± features of hyperleucocytosis (Hyperleucocytosis 🕮 pp.120–121)

History

Most symptoms are explicable on the above basis, but nevertheless non-specific. Therefore, CML is sometimes diagnosed coincidentally (especially in adults) when a blood count is checked for other reasons, e.g. as a pre-operative check.

- **Organ infiltration:** bone pain, left upper abdominal fullness/discomfort.
- **Metabolic consequences**: systemic symptoms including fever, night sweats, lethargy, weight loss.
- ± Symptoms of hyperleucocytosis (e.g. neurological, visual, respiratory).

Examination

- Pallor.
- Fever.
- Bruising.
- Hepatosplenomegaly.
- ± Signs of hyperleucocytosis (e.g. focal neurological signs, papilloedema, retinal haemorrhages, tachypnoea).

The development of accelerated phase (AP) or blast crisis (BC) is usually accompanied by a progressive increase in systemic symptoms, whilst BC presents with additional symptoms and signs characteristic of acute leukaemia.

Disease phase

- CML is usually diagnosed in CP (for haematological features – see Myeloproliferative diseases, Chronic myeloid leukaemia, Investigation, Diagnosis 🕮 p.434), and may remain in this phase (with or without treatment) for many years.
- AP is characterized by the presence of any one of a number of clinical, haematological or cytogenetic features:
  - *Clinical –*
    - increasing splenomegaly;
    - development of a chloroma;
    - presence of a previous BC.
  - *Haematological –:*
    - WCC rapidly rising (doubling in 5 days) or difficult to control;
    - Hb <10g/dL or platelets $<100 \times 10^9$/L, unresponsive to treatment;
    - platelets $>1000 \times 10^9$/L;
    - blasts >10% but <30% in peripheral blood or bone marrow;

- blasts plus promyelocytes >20% in peripheral blood or bonemarrow;
- basophils plus eosinophils = 20% in peripheral blood.
- Cytogenetic abnormality in addition to Philadelphia chromosome.
- BC may occur in the context of either CP or more commonly AP, and is defined by >30% blasts in peripheral blood and/or bone marrow.

Investigation

Diagnosis

In CP CML:
- FBC:
  - Marked leucocytosis with left shift.
    - total WCC may reach 800 × 10^9/L;
    - median WCC in childhood CML is ~250 × 10^9/L – higher than that seen in adults;
    - severe hyperleucocytosis commoner in children than adults.
  - Platelet count may be normal or show mild/moderate thrombocytosis (median 500 × 10^9/L).
  - Mild normochromic, normocytic anaemia is common, but not invariable.
- Peripheral blood film shows the full range of differentiation of myeloid cells, including neutrophils, myelocytes, metamyelocytes, basophils, eosinophils:
  - absolute basophilia is invariable, and absolute eosinophilia common (80% of patients);
  - blasts may be seen, but usually <1–2%.
- ↑ Serum urate and LDH.
- ↓ Leucocyte alkaline phosphatase (LAP) (in contrast to ↑ LAP seen in leucocytosis 2° to infection), but now rarely used in clinical practice.
- Bone marrow aspirate/biopsy confirm marked hypercellularity:
  - mostly granulocytic ± megakaryocytic;
  - despite hypercellularity, myeloid maturation unremarkable in appearance;
  - blasts present but <10%.
- Cytogenetic analysis: usually performed on marrow, but feasible to analyse peripheral blood samples in some cases:
  - *standard karyotyping* – t(9;22) i.e. Philadelphia chromosome, or variant, in >95%;
  - fluorescent *in situ* hybridization (FISH) or polymerase chain reaction (PCR) analysis nearly always demonstrates a *BCR/ABL* fusion gene.
- Other investigations performed at diagnosis should include:
  - biochemical profile, including serum urate;
  - coagulation profile;
  - blood group;
  - HbF;
  - virology screen;
  - HLA typing of patient and 1st degree relatives (parents, siblings).

Disease phase

Designation of disease phase (CP, AP, or BC) relies on a combination of clinical, haematological (blood and marrow) and cytogenetic features (Myeloproliferative diseases, Chronic myeloid leukaemia, Disease phase 📖 p.433).

Differential diagnosis

Diagnostic difficulties are rare due to the characteristic cytogenetic findings. Possible differential diagnoses (which will all be Philadelphia or *BCR/ABL* negative, except for Ph⁺ acute leukaemia) include:

Chronic phase CML

- **Leukaemoid reaction:** splenomegaly usually absent or mild, infective/inflammatory source usually evident, LAP usually ↑.
- **Juvenile myelomonocytic leukaemia (JMML):** blood film usually shows a greater degree of monocytosis in JMML than in CML, whilst HbF is ↑ and skin involvement/lymphadenopathy common, in JMML but not CML.
- **Other MPDs:** granulocyte series is involved to a relatively much greater extent in CML than in other MPDs.

Blast crisis CML

- **de novo acute leukaemia:** can usually distinguished cytogenetically (no Philadelphia chromosome) and by lack of prior history of CP CML. BC CML is also typified by prominent splenomegaly and peripheral blood basophilia.
- **de novo Ph⁺ acute leukaemia (Ph⁺ AL):** can be much harder to distinguish, but nearly all children with Ph⁺ AL have atypical *BCR/ABL* rearrangements that produce a 190 kd TK protein, in contrast to the typical *BCR/ABL* rearrangements and 210 kd TK protein seen in CML.

Management

General management at initial presentation

- Treat bleeding or infection if present.
- Ensure good hydration and start allopurinol to prevent tumour lysis syndrome. This may not be necessary in the rare patient with a low presenting white cell count (e.g. <20 × 10⁹/L).
- Management of tumour lysis if present (rare) (Tumour lysis syndrome 📖 pp.94–95).
- Leucopheresis may be indicated:
  - in hyperleucocytosis (especially in presence of symptoms or if WCC >300 × 10⁹/L) (Hyperleucocytosis 📖 pp.120–121);
  - to harvest autologous back-up stem cells for storage and possibly future use in the event of graft failure following HSCT (autologous marrow harvest may be performed at a later stage if leucopheresis is not performed at presentation).

Initial treatment

Hydroxycarbamide

Hydroxycarbamide (formerly called hydroxyurea [HOH]) is a short-acting S phase specific cytotoxic agent which normalizes blood count and reduces splenomegaly, but does not normalize cytogenetic abnormalities, nor modify the natural history of CML. Prior to the introduction of imatinib (Myeloproliferative diseases, Chronic myeloid leukaemia, Management, Initial treatment, Imatinib ☐ p.436), hydroxycarbamide was usually started at 15–30mg/kg orally once daily and the dose titrated to reduce WCC without excessive myelosuppression. Other side effects include skin rashes, but are uncommon.

Imatinib

Imatinib (IM) is a small molecule signal transduction inhibitor that acts by targeting specifically the *BCR/ABL* gene protein or other similar TKs. It is now the preferred initial treatment in most patients with CML, and it is anticipated that it will constitute effective long-term treatment for many.

- Usually started in newly diagnosed patients, or after withdrawal of hydroxycarbamide, at 260–340mg/m^2 orally once daily with water (gastric irritant).
- Myelosuppression is common, managed by stopping IM if neutrophils $<1 \times 10^9$/l or platelets $<50 \times 10^9$/L, but since success of treatment appears to be reduced if low doses of IM are given, it appears preferable to support blood count (e.g. by transfusions or G-CSF) rather than stop IM or reduce dose repeatedly.
- Other side effects are common, including gastrointestinal symptoms (nausea, vomiting, diarrhoea), fluid retention ± oedema, cramps, bone pain, skin rashes, abnormal LFTs. In general, these should be managed symptomatically and dose reductions of IM avoided.
- Avoid concurrent use of paracetamol.
- Beware of potential interactions with drugs metabolized by CYP450 2D6 (e.g. codeine) or 3A4 (e.g. carbamazepine).

Long-term treatment

Imatinib

- Long-term IM has been used in adults for about 10 years, and is now being employed in an increasing number of children and adolescents, especially if a suitable well-matched allogeneic HSCT donor is not available.
  - a small percentage of patients (<10%) achieve prolonged molecular remission but most relapse when IM is discontinued;
  - however, no evidence yet that IM is curative.
- Response to treatment should be monitored very carefully using peripheral blood and bone marrow haematological and cytogenetic criteria (Chronic myeloid leukaemia, Response criteria ☐ p.438).

- If a complete molecular response is achieved (i.e. no detectable *BCR/ABL* transcripts using very sensitive methods) and maintained, medium-term evidence from adult studies and shorter-term experience in children suggests that long-term response is likely to be maintained and that it is appropriate to continue IM. However, almost all patients relapse when IM is discontinued.
- However, since IM was only introduced into clinical trials in adults in the late 1990s, information about long-term durability of response remains preliminary. Therefore, continued response monitoring is important, and HSCT should be considered if there is any loss of complete molecular response, or if molecular analysis demonstrates the presence of a *BCR/ABL* mutation associated with a higher risk of IM resistance.

HSCT

- Historically, HSCT has been the mainstay of curative treatment strategies for children and adolescents with CML, and it remains the only treatment with a proven record of very long-term (i.e. >10 years) survival and apparent cure.
- Outcome of transplant is better (in particular, relapse rate is reduced) if HSCT performed in CP rather than more advanced disease (i.e. patients with previous AP or BC).
- Evidence from the pre-IM era shows that the outcome of HSCT is better if transplant is performed within 1 year of initial diagnosis. It is not yet known if this remains true for patients treated with IM.
- Most HSCT protocols employ either cyclophosphamide/total body irradiation (CyTBI) or busulfan/cyclophosphamide (BuCy) conditioning, with additional GvHD prophylaxis in unrelated donor transplants (Haemopoietic stem cell transplantation, Graft-versus-host disease prophylaxis 📖 p.176). CyTBI is usually preferred to BuCy for more advanced disease and for unrelated donor HSCT. There is little experience yet with the use of reduced-intensity conditioning for CML in children.

Others

- Interferon-α (IFN-α) may be indicated in patients intolerant of IM and without a suitable HSCT donor. Most protocols give 3 MIU subcutaneously once daily with concurrent paracetamol to reduce 'flu-like' side effects. Compared to hydroxycarbamide, IFN-α increases the complete cytogenetic response rate and prolongs survival, and occasionally leads to complete molecular response and long-term survival. However, toxicity may prevent long-term treatment. The addition of cytosine arabinoside to IFN-α has not been shown to improve survival.
- Busulfan is no longer used in CML, even in adult practice.
- Newer TK inhibitors are being developed and introduced into clinical practice. Dasatinib may lead to improved response in some patients who are resistant to IM, but the durability of response is often poor. If feasible, such patients should undergo HSCT as soon as possible.

Imatinib or HSCT in chronic phase CML?
- Until the last few years, most children with CML and suitable HSCT donors (either related or unrelated) have been transplanted. Therefore, there is very little experience of even medium-term survival in children treated with IM.
- However, adult data from CP CML treated with IM is very encouraging, and most adults now receive IM as initial treatment, proceeding to HSCT only if intolerant of IM or if response to IM is suboptimal or not maintained.
- Therefore, many collaborative groups now recommend that children with CML should start initial treatment with IM, and either continue with this long-term (with current knowledge, this implies life-long) as long as a complete molecular response is maintained, or undergo HSCT ideally within the first 2 years after diagnosis.
- When fully informed of the potential benefits and risks of each treatment approach, individual patients and families may appropriately elect to follow either an IM (and monitor response) or a HSCT strategy.

Response criteria
Detailed response (and failure) criteria have been developed, primarily for adult patients but still applicable to children.

Different versions are available as experience (especially with IM) has evolved, but all are based on:
- Haematological response – normal blood count and film, resolution of splenomegaly.
- Cytogenetic response – based on karyotypic analysis of marrow; varies from none (>95% Ph+ cells) to complete (0% Ph+).
- Molecular response – based on PCR measurement of *BCR/ABL/ABL* ratio in peripheral blood.

Complications
Complications of treatment
Drug treatment
Drug-related toxicity due to hydroxycarbamide or IM is usually manageable without stopping treatment, but IFN-α toxicity may be severe and necessitate discontinuation.

HSCT
HSCT is associated with a risk of transplant-related mortality (~10–20% in HLA-identical sibling donor and ~30% in unrelated donor HSCT). (Haemopoietic stem cell transplantation, Complications 📖 pp.180–197).

Relapse
- Although successful HSCT reduces the risk of progression to AP or transformation to BC considerably, relapse may occur in up to 25% of patients (over follow-up of up to 20 years). However, early (cytogenetic or ideally molecular) relapse may be treated very satisfactorily by donor lymphocyte infusions (DLI), albeit with a small risk of GvHD and marrow aplasia (Post-haemopoietic stem cell transplantation relapse 📖 p.198).

- Post-HSCT relapse may be:
  - *molecular* – detected by PCR (performed >4 months post-transplant; analysis before this time may reveal a measurable but still falling *BCR/ABL/ABL* ratio);
  - *cytogenetic* – detected by FISH or karyotype analysis;
  - *haematological* – diagnosed by abnormal blood count or marrow appearance consistent with CML.

Transformation

Estimates based on historical adult data suggest transformation rates to BC of 20–35% per year in patients treated with hydroxycarbamide or busulfan, and 10–20% per year during IFN-α treatment. Progression to AP or BC occurs in 1–3% of patients per year during the first 4 years of IM treatment.

Prognosis

- **Interferon-α:** 10 year overall survival in adult studies is ~25–50%, but almost all of these patients have molecularly detectable disease.
- **Imatinib:** adult data show 4–5-year overall survival of 90% and a transformation rate of 1–3% per year.
- **HSCT:** paediatric data show 3-year overall survival rates of 75–90% in HLA-identical sibling donor and 65% in unrelated donor HSCT. A mixed (but predominantly) adult study has shown a 20-year overall survival rate of 40% for HLA-identical sibling donor HSCT.

Other chronic MPDs of childhood

As a rule, chronic MPDs (other than CML) are diseases of older adults and exceptionally rare in children. Except for essential thrombocythaemia (ET), where recent paediatric literature is available, most information about their classification, presentation, treatment, and prognosis is derived from adult-based literature.

Recent investigations have revealed the presence of a mutation in the *JAK2* TK gene (*V617F*) in 80–90% of adults with polycythaemia vera (PV) and 30–50% with ET or chronic idiopathic myelofibrosis (CIMF).

Essential thrombocythaemia

- Incidence 1 in 10 million children/year (60 times lower than in adults)
- Persistent isolated thrombocytosis (>600 × 10^9/L) without other cause (e.g. CML, PV, inflammatory response, hyposplenism).
- Platelet function abnormal.
- Splenomegaly.
- Thrombotic episodes, especially if platelet count >1500 × 10^9/L.
- Transformation, usually to AML or more rarely myelodysplasia (MDS) or myelofibrosis, may occur in ~1% of patients. It may be commoner in patients treated with chemotherapy.
- Management strategies modified from adult experience:
  - observation only may be appropriate if platelet count <1000 × 10^9/L;
  - consider low dose aspirin if platelet count <1500 × 10^9/L (care regarding risk of Reye's syndrome, but this appears to be lower with low dose aspirin, and is probably outweighed by risk of thrombosis due to thrombocytosis; written parent information about Reye's syndrome is available for parents);
  - in patients with higher platelet counts, initial treatment with hydroxycarbamide will reduce thrombocytosis (which may then allow treatment with aspirin alone), followed by either –
    - IFN-α, or if not tolerated;
    - anagrelide (but long-term safety is unproven);
  - consider HSCT only if refractory disease;
  - spontaneous resolution of childhood ET has been reported.

Polycythaemia vera

- Increased red cell mass (haematocrit above age-related reference range), without a reason for 2° polycythaemia (e.g. chronic hypoxaemia, high affinity haemoglobin, raised erythropoietin).
- Plethoric complexion, headaches, dizziness, night sweats, pruritis.
- Low erythropoietin (differentiates PV from 2° polycythaemia).
- Hepatosplenomegaly.
- ± Thrombocytosis ± neutrophilia.
- *JAK-2 V617F* (or rarely other *JAK-2* exon 12) mutations present.
- May be complicated by thrombosis or CNS ischaemia.
- Transformation to AML, MDS or myelofibrosis may occur.
- Management may involve:
  - venesection to lower haematocrit (e.g. to <0.45);
  - consider low dose aspirin;
  - add IFN- α if not responding to above or if progressive disease.
- HSCT very rarely considered. Only if transformed to AML or if previous history of major thrombotic complications.

Chronic idiopathic myelofibrosis

- May be asymptomatic or present with systemic symptoms due to increased metabolic rate (night sweats, weight loss).
- Hepatosplenomegaly, may be massive.
- FBC variable, but typically → anaemia, thrombocytosis, leucocytosis.
- BM → variable cellularity (decreased in advanced disease), progressive fibrosis, often with prominent or bizarre megakarocyte proliferation.
- Diagnosis requires exclusion of other causes of marrow myeloproliferation and/or fibrosis, including CML, ET, PV, M7 AML, hypoplastic MDS and auto-immune disease.
- Transformation to AML in up to 30% of patients.
- Consider trial of steroids to exclude auto-immune disease.
- Advanced disease may merit HSCT.

Lymphoma

Classification

Leukaemia and lymphoma account for 30 and 15%, respectively, of childhood malignancies.

What is the difference between acute lymphocytic leukaemia and lymphoma? Historically, the distinction arose based on the clinical presentation with either bone marrow failure (leukaemia) or lymphadenopathy (lymphoma). This led to treatment developing along separate pathways until it began to be appreciated in the 1980s that it was the stage of differentiation arrest of the malignant lymphocyte precursor, rather than the distribution of disease, that was crucial, and that some lymphomas responded better to leukaemia-type treatment and *vice versa*.

Subsequent relaxed use of terminology in leukaemia has contributed to the confusion experienced by those trying to understand lymphoma classification (Fig. 31.1).

- In the USA, acute leukaemia is described as 'non-lymphocytic' or 'lymphocytic', whereas in the UK the terms 'myeloid' and 'lymphoblastic' are used. The first three of these terms describe lineage, the fourth refers to a morphologically recognisable and phenotypically characterizable T or B lymphocyte precursor [responsible for the majority of cases of acute lymphocytic leukaemia (ALL)]. This is of paramount importance in understanding lymphoma classification.
- By definition, all lymphomas are 'lymphocytic' and, whilst the malignant precursor might well be arrested at the lymphoblastic stage, it may be more primitive (anaplastic) or more mature (Burkitts, diffuse large cell) and therefore 'non-lymphoblastic'.
- A child presenting with common ALL will have the normal bone marrow population replaced by lymphoblasts. Many cases will also have pathological lymphadenopathy, which is eclipsed by the leukaemia diagnosis. However, if a node was sent for histopathological examination it would be reported as showing lymphoblastic lymphoma.
- A child presenting with extensive abdominal Burkitt's (i.e. non-lymphoblastic) lymphoma may be found to have a significant number of malignant cells in the staging bone marrow aspirate. These would be reported by the haematologist as showing ALL, subtype (L3), mature surface immunoglobulin positive - Burkitt's type.
- Thus, lymphoblastic lymphoma/leukaemia and Burkitt's lymphoma/L3 ALL can present as pure leukaemias, pure lymphomas or anywhere inbetween. In contrast it is unusual for the other common childhood lymphomas to infiltrate bone marrow to a significant level.

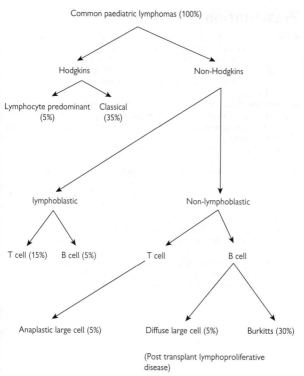

Fig. 31.1 Subtypes of common paediatric lymphomas.

Presentation

- Generally present with lymphadenopathy or consequences of enlarged lymph nodes. Visible lymph nodes usually present as painless node enlargement, whereas internal lymphadenopathy may result in problems related to obstruction of vital organs (gastrointestinal obstruction, renal dysfunction or breathlessness in mediastinal lymphadenopathy).
- Lymphadenopathy in Hodgkin disease (HD) tends to have a more chronic history than that in non-Hodgkin lymphoma (NHL). The presence of B symptoms of fevers, night sweats, and weight loss should be documented.
- Generalized pruritis is a not uncommon feature at diagnosis in HD, but it is not a B symptom.
- Any suggestion of superior vena cava (SVC) obstruction, respiratory disease or especially orthopnoea means that the child will almost certainly have T cell lymphoblastic lymphoma (LL) and a significant risk of acute respiratory decompensation from the effect of a mediastinal mass and possibly pleural effusions.
- Burkitt's lymphoma (BL) can present with the clinical picture of intussusception, or given its short doubling time of 48h, rapidly increasing superficial lymphadenopathy.
- All lymph node areas and the abdomen should be carefully examined for lymphadenopathy and hepatosplenomegaly, and abnormal findings clearly documented for future reference.

Investigations

Initial tests should include:
- **FBC, ESR and film:** microcytic anaemia in HD, leukaemia.
- **U&Es, LFTs, clotting:** renal, hepatic involvement/dysfunction.
- **LDH and urate:** reflect tumour turnover.
- **Viral serology/PCR:** Lymphadenopathy 📖 pp.75–78.
- **CXR:** nodes +/– effusions.
- **CT** (pre-anaesthetic if CXR suspicious): exclude airway obstruction.
- **Node biopsy:** fine needle aspirate (FNA) not sufficient.
- **BM aspirates + biopsy × 2 sites:** NHLs (only if stage IV) or B symptoms in HD.
- **Chromosomes:** anaplastic large cell lymphoma (ALCL) – t(2;5); BL – t(8;14), t(2;8) or t(8;22).
- **LP:** NHL only.
- The timing and order of the investigations is dictated by the age and clinical condition of the patient.
- Most patients will require at least two anaesthetics, one primarily for node biopsy and a second one to insert an appropriate central venous access device. This means that BM and diagnostic/therapeutic LP can be performed at either opportunity depending on other results.
- Prior to anaesthetic, it is mandatory to do a CXR to exclude the potential of airway problems from tracheal deviation or compression.

Mediastinal disease

- Whilst patients with mediastinal disease are able to maintain their airway when awake, the trachea may collapse during anaesthetic induction and they may then not respond to simple endotracheal intubation, precipitating emergency thoracotomy.
- In general, children with mediastinal HD rarely experience this problem and the most concerning group are T cell lymphoblastic NHL. These children commonly have significant pleural effusions from which a small diagnostic specimen can be obtained under local anaesthetic with appropriate care. Once treatment is started effusions rapidly resolve and it is rarely necessary to perform emergency drainage. If, however, it becomes necessary, the aim should be to drain the effusions slowly (especially if the child is anaesthetized) and symmetrically to prevent potentially fatal acute mediastinal shift.
- If the child is too unwell to tolerate any procedures they should be admitted to a high dependency area and started on steroids. The dose intensity should reflect the balance between overall clinical condition and renal function in the face of incipient tumour lysis syndrome. Appropriate diagnostic tests should be performed as soon as the child can safely tolerate them.

Staging and treatment

The treatment modalities are dictated by the type of lymphoma. The intensity and duration of therapy is decided by the stage of disease. Whilst lymphomas can be staged according to the standard system, the implication of stage in deciding treatment is different in each of the main subtypes.

Classical Hodgkin disease

HD is staged according to the distribution of lymph node groups affected:
- **Stage I:** single lymph node group.
- **Stage II:** two or more lymph node groups on same side of diaphragm.
- **Stage III**: lymph node groups on both sides of diaphragm.
- **Stage IV:** remote extranodal disease.

Local invasion of tissues from a clearly involved nodal group is staged by the addition of an 'E'. Additionally, an 'A' or 'B' is assigned depending on the absence or presence (respectively) of B symptoms.

HD is very sensitive to both radio and chemotherapy and it is now uncommon for children to die from this condition. Consequently, there are many treatment options that all have the common goal of cure with minimum long-term side effects. The current UK protocol uses stage to decide between 2, 4, or 6 cycles of monthly chemotherapy (OEPA – Vincristine , etoposide, prednisolone and adriamycin, previously ABVD –adriamycin,bleomycin, vinblastine and dacarbazine or ChlVPP – chlorambucil, vinblastine, procarbazine and prednisolone). This is followed by radiotherapy to all originally involved areas in children who have active disease demonstrable on CT/positron emission tomography (PET) scan after the first two cycles.

In relapsed HD there is a clear role for aggressive 2nd line treatment with reinduction chemotherapy followed by high dose therapy with autologous stem cell rescue and any appropriate local radiotherapy. Recently, reduced intensity conditioning allogeneic transplants have been introduced with acceptably low toxicity and some success.

Lymphocyte predominant Hodgkin disease

Lymphocyte predominant Hodgkin disease (LPHD) is no longer regarded a subtype of HD, as it can now be distinguished as a very low grade B cell lymphoma. It usually presents as early stage disease in adolescent males and can be treated surgically. Using MRI and CT/PET, the completeness of surgical excision can be monitored, and a 'wait and watch' policy followed. If excision is impossible, inadequate or if the disease progresses, it appears to be very sensitive to short courses of low dose chemotherapy. Occasionally, the disease is more aggressive and requires classical HD type therapy. Interestingly, late relapses may occur with a diffuse large cell lymphoma (DLCL) picture suggesting a stem cell link between these two types of lymphoma.

Lymphoblastic lymphoma

As discussed above (Classification 🕮 p.448), LL is essentially ALL outwith the bone marrow and therefore carries the risk and treatment implications of central nervous system (CNS) involvement. Staging by lymph node group involvement does not influence therapy and LL protocols are similar to those used for ALL. However, T cell disease with mediastinal involvement is regarded as 'high stage' disease and is treated more intensively. B cell disease responds well and, interestingly, boys do not appear to need longer maintenance than girls (unlike ALL in general). Relapse on treatment carries an ominous prognosis, but late relapses can be salvaged using leukaemia type protocols including allogeneic stem cell transplant.

Burkitt's lymphoma

For treatment purposes this disease is divided into three groups:

- Very localized disease which appears to have been completely surgically removed. Only two cycles of moderately intensive chemotherapy needed.
- Clear residual disease post-laparotomy or post-superficial lymph node biopsy. Because of the risk of tumour lysis, in often already very sick children, chemotherapy is started at a very low dose for the first 1–2 weeks and then continued with four cycles of extremely dose-intensive systemic and intrathecal therapy.
- Bone marrow (BM) or CNS involvement at diagnosis. These are initially similarly treated to the second group, but go on to receive intensive chemotherapy for twice as long. As described above (Classification 📖 p.448), ALL (L3) (Burkitt's type) should be treated in this group.

Generally, cure rates are now high, even for the third group of patients. Relapse almost always occurs within the first 6 months of stopping therapy and successful salvage is unusual. Whilst the CD20 monoclonal antibody rituximab is as yet of unproven benefit in standard paediatric protocols, it can be useful as an interim therapy in progressive disease or patients too unwell to receive chemotherapy.

Anaplastic large cell lymphoma

ALCL is a very variable disease. Strong expression of T cell antigens and involvement of skin, mediastinum, lungs, liver, or spleen generally indicate a more aggressive form of the disease. Chemotherapy is cyclical and dose intensive with between 3 and 6 courses. Intrathecal CNS prophylaxis is given. Interestingly, some cases, which relapse even after intensive second line treatment will remain responsive to single agent vinblastine therapy. Some cases have been salvaged with autologous and allogeneic stem cell procedures.

Diffuse large cell lymphoma

The incidence of this type of lymphoma increases with age and is therefore mostly seen in adolescents. Unlike adult patients who are now treated with CHOP-R [cyclophosphamide, doxorubicin, vincristine, prednisolone and rituximab (anti-CD 20)], children are treated using the same strategies outlined for BL above, although marrow and CNS involvement are unusual. The results for children treated in this way are very good.

Other lymphomas

The lymphomas above account for more than 90% of those found in children. Treatment of the 10% of individually rarely seen subtypes requires expert involvement, often from adult colleagues who may see such diseases commonly in their more mature population.

Post-transplant lymphoproliferative disorders

With the increase in allogeneic transplantation, there is a rising incidence of PTLDs. A similar problem is also arising among the increasing population of genetically immuno-incompetent children awaiting stem cell transplant. Initially, this is a reactive polyclonal response to EBV reactivation. Unfortunately, this provides a lymphoproliferative background that predisposes to the chance of oncogene translocation and the emergence of malignant clonal disease. These lymphomas are responsive to treatment, but subsequent long-term survival probably depends on restoring, as much normal overall immune function as possible.

Section 9

Solid tumours

Neuroblastoma

Neuroblastoma is one of the embryonal malignancies of childhood (the others include Wilms' tumour, hepatoblastoma, retinoblastoma, and the embryonal subtype of rhabdomyosarcoma).

The neuroblastic tumours include:
- Neuroblastoma (NB).
- Ganglioneuroblastoma (GNB).
- Ganglioneuroma (GN).

They are derived from primordial neural crest cells, which subsequently develop into sympathetic ganglia and the adrenal medulla.

The variety of locations of neuroblastic tumours and the differing degree of histopathological differentiation results in an array of enigmatic tumours demonstrating diverse clinical and biological characteristics, and behaviour:
- May undergo spontaneous regression, especially stage 4s and localized tumours.
- May undergo spontaneous differentiation to benign GN.
- Often demonstrate initial response to treatment and then relapse later with chemoresistant disease, but may rarely undergo relentless progression.

Incidence
- Commonest extracranial malignant solid tumour.
- Incidence in childhood is ~8 per million person years in UK.
- 8% of childhood malignancy.

Age
- Median age of onset = 2 years.
- Peak age = 18 months.
- Commonest cancer of infancy (age <12 months).
- 2% diagnosed >10 years age.

Sex
Slight male predominance (1.2:1).

Geography
- Highest incidence in white children in industrialized nations.
- Lower incidence in India.

Predisposing factors
- Possible links with drugs in pregnancy, e.g. phenytoin, or illicit drugs and alcohol.
- Possible protective effect of folic acid in preventing NB.
- Most NB sporadic, ~1% familial associated with multiple primary tumours, usually occurring <18 months age.
- Linked with NF1, central hypoventilation syndrome (Ondine's curse) and Hirschprung disease.

Clinical features

- Initial features may be protean – around 50% of NB is misdiagnosed initially. NB is the 'great mimic' in paediatrics.
- Clinical presentation may reflect location of primary, regional, and metastatic disease.

Primary tumour

- Can occur anywhere along the sympathetic nervous system (SNS).
- Frequency of adrenal tumours is higher in children (40%) compared with infants (25%).
- Infants more likely to have thoracic and cervical 1° tumours.
- In order of decreasing frequency, 1° tumours occur in:
  - adrenal;
  - paravertebral retroperitoneum;
  - posterior mediastinum;
  - pelvis;
  - neck.
- 1° unknown in 1%.
- Abdominal tumours usually present with palpable mass.
- In head and neck region, Horner's syndrome may occur – ipsilateral:
  - miosis;
  - enopthalmos;
  - partial ptosis;
  - heterochromia (if <2 years at diagnosis) –
- pelvic tumours (organ of Zückerkandl) may alter bowel and bladder habit;
- paravertebral tumours may compress the spinal cord
  - ⚠ ' dumb-bell tumours' → flaccid leg paralysis and spinal cord compression with bladder and bowel dysfunction.

Secondary tumours

Distant lymphadenopathy

For example, supraclavicular (Virchow's node).

- Subcutaneous nodules, non-tender, bluish and blanching 'blueberry muffin' appearance. Classical of stage 4s disease.
- Rapidly enlarging liver ('Pepper syndrome') – also stage 4s.
- Proptosis and periorbital bruising from retro-orbital infiltraton.
- Metastatic spread to bone and bone marrow → fever, limp and bone marrow failure (anaemia, thrombocyteopenia) ('Hutchinson syndrome').
- CNS and meningeal involvement may occur in the late stages of the disease.

Paraneoplastic syndromes

Opsoclonus myoclonus ataxia ('Dancing Eyes') syndrome.

- 2–3% NB, median age 18–22 months.
- **Opsoclonus:** conjugate, non-phasic, fast and multidirectional eye movements occurring in bursts.
- Myoclonus/ataxia.
- Behavioural change and/or sleep disturbance.

- Usually localized, differentiated, good biology tumour.
- Neuropsychological sequelae common, particularly language, motor and cognitive deficit.
- Intractable secretory diarrhoea ('Kerner-Morrison') syndrome.

Failure to thrive

Hypertension

- From secretion of catecholamine metabolites (which may → flushing, sweating, ↑ heart rate).
- Stimulation of renin-angiotensin system.

Biochemical features

- ↑ Urinary catecholamines in >90% NB:
  - homovanillic acid (HVA) and vanillylmandelic acid (VMA) usually measured, but dopamine also recommended;
  - ↑ = HVA/Cr and/or VMA/Cr >3.0 standard deviations (SD) above mean for age;
  - no prognostic significance.
- ↑ LDH – may be prognostic, particularly in localized tumours.
- ↑ ferritin, only useful at diagnosis.
- ↑ neurone specific enolase (NSpE).

Imaging

- Plain abdominal or chest radiographs show calcification in ~50% of tumours.
- Ultrasound (US) initial imaging modality of choice for an infant or child with an abdominal mass, also provides baseline for follow up.
- CT scan recommended for abdominal tumours to demonstrate internal structure and relationship to important vessels.
- MRI recommended for paravertebral and pelvic tumours.
- ^{131}I or ^{123}I (preferred) meta-iodo benzyl guanidine (mIBG) scintigraphy highly sensitive and specific:
  - Useful for resolving differential diagnosis as well as evaluating metastases and assessing response;
  - Taken up specifically by neural crest tumours (90% of NB, phaeochromocytoma, paraganglioma, retinoblastoma and medullary thyroid carcinoma);
  - ^{131}I mIBG also used for therapy.
- Tc^{99m} MDP bone scanning now recommended to detect bone metastases only in cases where mIBG not taken up by the primary tumour.
- Positron emission tomography (PET) scanning using ^{18}F-FDG now being used to detect soft tissue and skeletal neuroblastoma:
  - FDG uptake correlates with tumour burden;
  - Improved accuracy with PET-CT.

Histopathology

Macroscopic

- NB are lobulated masses intimately related to the adrenal gland or sympathetic chain.
- Delicate, membranous capsules cover soft, fleshy, grey partially haemorrhagic tumours.
- Nodular GNB have grey haemorrhagic nodules in a firm, white-grey tumour mass.
- Intermixed GNB or GN have tan-yellow homogeneous cut surfaces.

Microscopic

- Neuroblastic tumours comprise 2 main cell populations:
  - neuroblastic/ganglion cells;
  - Schwannian stroma cells.
- Neuroblasts are tumour cells, whilst the majority of evidence to date suggests that Schwannian stroma cells are reactive, non-tumour cells.
- The International Neuroblastoma Pathology Classification (INPC) is now widely used to classify neuroblastic tumours into 4 groups:
  - neuroblastoma (Schwannian stroma-poor) – these can be undifferentiated, poorly differentiated (neuropil present, e.g. as rosettes) or differentiating;
  - ganglioneuroblastoma, intermixed (Schwannian stroma-rich);
  - ganglioneuroma (Schwannian stroma-dominant);
  - ganglioneuroblastoma, nodular (composite Schwannian stroma-rich/ stroma-dominant and stroma-poor).
- Using a combination of the above groups, patient age and assessment of proliferation and apoptosis (the mitosis-karyorrhexis index), a tumour is classified as having:
  - INPC unfavourable histology (UH);
  - INPC favourable histology (FH).
- This histopathological classification now forms part of the International Neuroblastoma Risk Group Classification (see Table 32.1).

Genetics

MYCN amplification

- Amplification of the *MYCN* oncogene at 2p24 occurs in around 25% of all NB (Fig. 32.1).
- Occurs more frequently in rapidly progressive tumours with advanced stage.
- Associated with poor prognosis in (a) infants <18 months age with localized and metastatic disease, and (b) older patients with localized disease.
- In these 2 groups treatment is intensified if *MYCN* is amplified (Neuroblastoma, Principles of treatment according to risk group in Europe 📖 p.462).

Allelic loss of 1p
- Loss of heterozygosity of 1p occurs in up to 35% NB.
- Predicts for recurrence in localized tumours without *MYCN* amplification, but not survival.

Unbalanced 17q gain
- Most frequent genetic abnormality in NB, occurring in up to 70% tumours.
- Independently associated with poor prognosis in retrospective studies.
- Very rarely a tumour is either *MYCN* amplified or 1p deleted without 17q gain.

Allelic loss/imbalance of 11q
- Occurs in 40% NB.
- Inversely associated with *MYCN* amplification.
- Predicts for recurrence in localized tumours without *MYCN* amplification, but not survival.

Genetic tests used
- Fluorescent *in-situ* hybridization (FISH) is method of choice for detecting *MYCN* amplification.
- Multiplex ligation-dependent probe amplification (MLPA), a multiplex PCR method, will identify all the above genetic abnormalities in a single experiment and is now being increasingly used for the diagnosis of molecular abnormalities in NB.
- Other methods: array comparative genomic hybridisation (📖 p.21)

Ploidy
- Hyperdiploid and near-triploid tumours in infants have whole chromosome gains with few structural rearrangements, good prognosis.
- Near-diploid tumours of any age, and hyperdiploid or tetraploid tumours in older patients usually have structural rearrangements such as deletions and unbalanced translocations.

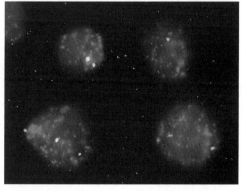

Fig. 32.1 *MYCN* amplification by FISH. Red signals = MYCN, green/yellow signals = 2p centromeric probe. Courtesy of N. Bown, Institute of Human Genetics, Newcastle.

Diagnosis

According to International Neuroblastoma Staging System (INSS) guidelines (Brodeur et al., 1993), diagnosis of NB established if:
- Unequivocal pathological diagnosis is made from tumour tissue ± immunohistology, ↑ urine catecholamines. If histology equivocal, genetics may help.
- Bone marrow aspirate or trephine biopsy contains unequivocal tumour cells, e.g. syncytia or immunocytological clumps of cells, *and* ↑ urine catecholamines.

Further information

Brodeur, G.M., Pritchard, J., Berthold, F. *et al.* (1993) Revisions of the international criteria for neuroblastoma diagnosis, staging and response to treatment. *J Clin Oncol 11*, 1466–1477.

Staging

- International Neuroblastoma Staging System.
- International Neuroblastoma Risk Group classification
  - New stratification based on:
    - age < or ≥18 months;
    - staging based on surgical resectability;
    - *MYCN* status (*MYCN* amp = *MYCNA*); ploidy;
    - histological features.
  - Staging –
    - L1 = localized, resectable;
    - L2 = localized, unresectable;
    - M = metastatic;
    - Ms = metastatic, special(s) – liver, skin and bone marrow.

Table 32.1 International Neuroblastoma Risk groups

Risk group Incidence	Stage	Age	Genetics	Histology
Very low 10%	L1/L2		Non-*MNA*	GN maturing GNB intermixed
	L1		Non-*MNA*	Any
	Ms	<18 months	Non-*MNA* 11q normal	Any
Low 20%	L2	<18 months	Non-*MNA* 11q normal	Any except GN maturing GNB intermixed
	L2	≥18 months	Non-*MNA* 11q normal	GNB nodular or differentiating NB
	Ms	<12 months	Non-*MNA*	Any
	M	<18 months	Non-*MNA* Hyperdiploid	Any
Intermediate 20%	L2	<18 months	Non-*MNA* 11q aberration	Any except GN maturing GNB intermixed
	L2	≥18 months	Non-*MNA* 11q aberration	GNB nodular or differentiating NB
	L2	≥18 months	Non-*MNA*	Poorly differentiated or undifferentiated
	M	<18 months	Non-*MNA* Diploid	Any
High 50%	Any	Any	*MNA*	Any
	Ms	<18 months	Non-*MNA* 11q aberration	Any
	M	≥18 months	Non-*MNA*	Any

Adapted from Cohn, S.L. et al. (2009) *J Clin Oncol* 27, 289–297.

Current principles of treatment according to risk group in Europe

Some current risk groups differ from those shown in Table 32.1.

Risk

Low risk
- Surgery alone for all L1 patients.
- L2:
  - if symptoms, etoposide and carboplatin (VP16/carbo);
  - if asymptomatic, proposed study of randomization between treatment and observation.
- M/Ms – treatment if symptomatic, usually VP16/carbo 1-4 courses.

Intermediate risk
- M, <12 months, (bone/lung/CNS metastases):
  - 4–8 courses VP/carbo and CADO (cyclophosphamide, doxorubicin, vincristine);
  - surgery to primary tumour if feasible.
- L2:
  - treatment dependent on histology;
  - if GN or GNB intermixed – observation;
  - FH, 2-4 courses of chemotherapy (VP16/carbo ± CADO);
  - surgery.
- L2, UH:
  - 3 courses VP16/carbo + 3 courses CADO;
  - surgery if feasible;
  - local radiotherapy if age >18 months;
  - possibly 13-*cis* retinoic acid.

High risk
- European HR-NBL-1 trial, opened 2002, including infants with *MYCNA* NB <12 months age (from 2006).
- 5 phases of treatment:
  - *Induction chemotherapy* – rapid COJEC (cyclophosphamide, vincristine, carboplatin, etoposide, cisplatin)
    - + 2 courses TVD (topotecan, vincristine, doxorubicin) if inadequate response;
    - + prophylactic granulocyte colony stimulating factor (G-CSF).
  - Surgical resection of primary tumour.
  - Myeloablative therapy and autologous stem cell rescue – busulfan and melphalan versus carboplatin, etoposide and melphalan.
  - Radiotherapy to primary tumour (21Gy).
  - 13-*cis* retinoic acid ± anti-GD$_2$ therapy.

Prognosis

Low risk
Excellent: 95–100% 5-year survival in last European infant study (NB99.1 and 2) and LNESG1.

Intermediate risk
Very good: 85–95% 5-year survival in most studies including European infant NB99 study. However, event-free survival only 60% in some groups hence selective addition of radiotherapy

High risk
Poor: 30–40% 5-year survival. Last European *MYCN* amplified infant study (NB99.4) – 28% overall survival.

Treatment for relapsed neuroblastoma

- **Low risk:** usually salvageable with conventional chemotherapy.
- **Intermediate risk:** often salvageable with conventional and high dose chemotherapy.

High risk
- At least 50% of patients with high risk NB will relapse.
- Relapsed high risk NB is rarely, if ever, curable, but lengthy responses may be seen particularly if non-*MNA* with:
  - TVD or topotecan and cyclophosphamide;
  - temozolamide;
  - oral etoposide;
  - ^{131}I mIBG ± topotecan;
  - palliative radiotherapy 2–8Gy.

Treatment of special conditions

Spinal cord compression
- ▶▶Neurological and oncological emergency.
- Begin dexamethasone whilst awaiting MRI imaging. 0.5mg/kg/day IV bolus then 0.2mg/kg/day in 3 divided doses.
- **Chemotherapy:** VP/carbo preferable to neurosurgery:
  - fewer late adverse effects, e.g. scoliosis;
  - tumour and spinal cord compression respond rapidly;
  - reassess after 1 course and plan 2–4 courses dependent on response and whether on a clinical trial.
- Continue dexamethasone until radiological evidence of improvement, then wean gradually.
- Complete neurological recovery is possible and is not necessarily related to duration of symptoms.
- Worse prognosis if present at birth.

Opsoclonus-myoclonus-ataxia syndrome
- Aetiology relates to cross-reactivity between neuroblastoma and CNS antibodies, e.g. anti-Purkinje cell.
- Surgical resection recommended for L1 tumours, may improve symptoms.
- Early treatment improves acute symptoms and may reduce the severity of neuropsychological sequelae.

- Therefore, immunosuppressive treatment used. European guidelines suggest:
  - **1st line:** dexamethasone 20mg/m^2/day for 3 days per month for 1 year;
  - **2nd line:** intravenous immunoglobulin (IVIg) 2g/kg monthly for 7 months and then bimonthly for 1 year;
  - **3rd line:** cyclophosphamide 750mg/m^2/month for 6 months and then 3 doses 2 months apart.

Antenatally/perinatally diagnosed adrenal masses
- European guidelines currently under construction.
- US evaluation and urinary catecholamines recommended at birth and at regular intervals thereafter.
- mIBG and MRI if mass persists beyond 3 months.
- Consider biopsy if evidence of progression or >5 cm in length.

Investigations of patients with Horner's syndrome
- Up to 25% of patients with non-surgical Horner's syndrome have an underlying mass lesion – the differential diagnosis includes NB.
- All such patients require investigations to exclude NB including:
  - urine catecholamines;
  - CXR;
  - brain, head, neck and chest MRI;
  - mIBG scan.

New treatments under investigation
Undergoing clinical trials
- **Gemox:** gemcitabine and oxaloplatin.
- **CEP-701:** tyrosine kinase inhibitor.
- Arsenic trioxide.
- Cox2 inhibitors.

Undergoing pre-clinical evaluation
- Proteosome inhibitors (e.g. bortezomib).
- DNA damage repair inhibitors, e.g. PARP inhibitors in combination with DNA damaging agents.

Conclusions
- NB remains one of the most fascinating and challenging childhood cancers to treat.
- Progress in the biological understanding of this tumour has led us to:
  - reduce treatment for low and intermediate risk tumours;
  - identify high risk tumours and treat them intensively.
- Improving cure rates of high risk patients will depend on identification of novel therapies that target the genetic abnormalities of this elusive tumour.

Retinoblastoma

Introduction

Retinoblastoma is a malignant tumour of the retina usually occurring in children under 5 years of age. It represents around 3% of childhood cancers with a frequency of 1 in 20–25,000 live births. Retinoblastoma is due to a mutation within the *RB* gene, located on the long arm of chromosome 13, and may be divided into:

- A heritable form in which there is a germline mutation within the RB gene. All bilateral cases and up to 15% of unilateral cases have heritable retinoblastoma. Around 15% of children with this form of retinoblastoma will have inherited the mutation from a parent and are likely to have a positive family history. In the remainder, the mutation will have arisen *de novo*.
- A non-heritable form that is unilateral and where the mutation within the *RB* gene is somatic.

About 60% of all cases are non-heritable and 40% heritable.

Presentation

Presenting signs include:
- Leukocoria, sometimes noted as absent red reflex on a flash photograph.
- Strabismus.
- Painful, red eye.
- Some cases will have no symptoms and will be picked up by screening.

Classification

The International Classification of Retinoblastoma grades the intraocular appearances as in Table 33.1.

Table 33.1 The International Classification of Retinoblastoma grades

Group	Features
A	Retinoblastoma <3mm
B	Retinoblastoma >3mm *or* Macular location (<3mm to foveola) *or* Located near the optic disc (<1.5mm to disc) *or* Subretinal fluid <3mm from margin
C	Retinoblastoma with subretinal seeds <3mm from tumour *or* Vitreous seeds <3mm from tumour *or* Both subretinal and vitreous seeds <3mm from tumour
D	Retinoblastoma with subretinal seeds >3mm from tumour *or* Vitreous seed >3mm from tumour *or* Both subretinal and vitreous >3mm from tumour
E	Extensive retinoblastoma occupying >50% of globe *or* Neovascular glaucoma *or* Anterior chamber involvement

In the developed world >95% of children diagnosed with retinoblastoma survive. By contrast, only about 50% of children survive retinoblastoma worldwide, mainly due to late detection of the disease in developing countries where children often present with locally invasive or metastatic disease.

Management

Treatment for retinoblastoma depends on the laterality of the disease, number, size, and location of the tumour(s), and likely visual prognosis. Treatment methods include:

- **Local therapy:** cryotherapy, laser photocoagulation, and plaque brachytherapy are used to treat smaller tumours or following primary chemoreduction.
- **Chemotherapy:** the indications for intravenous chemotherapy in retinoblastoma include:
  - intraocular retinoblastoma to chemoreduce larger tumours and render them amenable to local therapy;
  - post-enucleation where there is evidence of adverse histological features (deep choroidal invasion, retrolaminar nerve invasion, disease in the anterior chamber);
  - *metastatic retinoblastoma* – if there is evidence of either local or distant spread of RB, the prognosis is poor and aggressive multimodality treatment is required if cure is to be achieved.

Carboplatin, vincristine, and etoposide are the first line agents, administered intravenously on a 3-weekly basis for up to 6 courses (although more may be given in exceptional circumstances). Second-line chemotherapy may be required in situations of relapsed or progressive disease or to treat adverse histological features in an eye enucleated at the end of first line therapy. Currently, second line therapy in the UK consists of doxorubicin, ifosfamide, and vincristine. Carboplatin may also be administered in to the subconjunctiva in cases with vitreous involvement.

- **Enucleation:** surgical removal of the eye plays an important part in the management of retinoblastoma. Around 75–80% of unilateral tumours present with more advanced (grade D or E) disease, and for the majority of these patients, primary enucleation is the most appropriate treatment. In addition, around 60% of patients with bilateral disease will require secondary enucleation of the more advanced eye after chemoreduction.
- **Radiotherapy:** external beam radiotherapy is generally reserved as second-line treatment in an attempt to salvage some visual function in patients with bilateral disease.

In bilateral disease, treatment is planned according to the worst eye. Although the management is dependent upon each individual case, in general:

- Patients with group A disease can be managed with local therapy alone.
- Group B–D patients are likely to receive chemotherapy +/– local therapy.
- Group E eyes tend to require enucleation at diagnosis or following chemotherapy.

The success of chemotherapy in globe salvage (avoiding enucleation or external beam radiotherapy) is around 100% for group A, 93% for group B, 90% for group C, and 50% for group D.

Genetics

Offspring of patients with the heritable form of retinoblastoma have a 50% chance of inheriting the mutation from their parent. 90% of these children who have inherited the mutation will develop the disease. Unless it is known that the child has *not* inherited the mutation, a screening programme of regular fundal examinations is recommended for all children of affected parents, from birth, in order to detect the disease at the earliest opportunity.

Renal tumours

Wilms' tumour

Wilms' tumour is an embryonal neoplasm arising in the kidney. It is the most common renal malignancy in childhood. It was first described by Max Wilms in 1899. As with many other childhood cancers, the prognosis has improved significantly over the last 20–30 years with the development of multinational clinical trials combining surgery, chemotherapy, and radiotherapy.

Epidemiology
- Wilms' tumours account for about 8% of all childhood neoplasms.
- Annual incidence of 8 per million children under the age of 15 years.
- Peak age at diagnosis is 3rd and 4th years of life.
- Very rare in neonates and in children over 10 years of age
- No difference in incidence between genders.

Differential diagnosis
There are a number of other renal tumours of childhood from which Wilms' tumours must be differentiated on the basis of pathology:
- Abdominal neuroblastoma.
- Clear cell sarcoma.
- Malignant rhabdoid tumour.

Associated conditions
Several conditions are known to be associated with Wilms' tumours. However, associations such as those listed here form only a very small proportion of the total numbers of children with Wilms' tumour. Most cases are sporadic and not associated with any other abnormalities:
- **WAGR syndrome:** a rare genetic syndrome comprising a predisposition to the development of Wilms' tumour, in addition to Aniridia, genitourinary anomalies and mental retardation.
- **Aniridia:** a rare congenital condition characterized by the under development of the iris. It is associated with poor development of the retina.
- **Hemihypertrophy:** overgrowth of one side of the body and associated organs.
- **Beckwith-Wiedemann syndrome:** an overgrowth disorder present at birth and characterized by macroglossia, macrosomia, midline abdominal defects, ear creases/pits, and neonatal hypoglycaemia.
- **Denys-Drash syndrome:** characterized by gonadal dysgenesis, nephropathy, and Wilms' tumour.
- **Perlman syndrome:** polyhydramnios, foetal overgrowth, neonatal macrosomia, macrocephaly, dysmorphic facial features, visceromegaly, and high neonatal mortality.
- **Simpson-Golabi-Behmel syndrome:** X-linked recessive disorder. Males affected, females are carriers. Overgrowth syndrome with distinctive facial features often described as 'coarse'. The expression of the genetic defect is very variable and can affect a variety of organs.
- The incidence of familial Wilms' tumour is extremely low.

Genetics

The precise genetic mechanism in Wilms' tumour is unclear. There are a number of associated genetic abnormalities, particularly mutations in the WT1 and WT2 genes.

- WT1 gene on 11p - transcription factor. Deletion in one copy is found in WAGR syndrome. A germline mutation is found in Denys-Drash syndrome.
- WT2 gene 11p15 locus.
- Chromosome abnormalities in 16q, 1p and 7p.

Clinical features

- **Abdominal/flank mass:** 74% of patients.
- **Abdominal pain:** 44% of patients.
- Haematuria.
- Hypertension.
- Fever.

Pulmonary metastases may be present at diagnosis, but are rarely detected on clinical examination.

Investigations (Figs 34.1, 34.2, 34.3, 34.4)

- **Abdominal US:** confirms organ of origin, determines extent of any intra-abdominal spread and confirms patency of the inferior vena cava.
- **Chest X-ray** (PA and lateral): detects pulmonary metastases.
- **Urinary catecholamines:** excludes intrarenal neuroblastoma.
- **CT chest and abdomen:** to detect pulmonary metastases and define more clearly the anatomy of the tumour and surrounding organs.
- Full blood count to detect anaemia secondary to haemorrhage into tumour.
- **APTT/PT:** an acquired form of Von Willebrand disease (due to formation of an inhibitor to von Willebrand factor) may be associated with Wilms' tumour.
- U&Es and urinalysis to detect any gross abnormality in renal function.

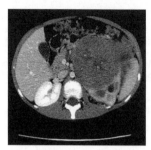

Fig 34.1 CT scan of abdomen showing a large Wilms' Tumour.

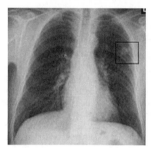

Fig 34.2 Chest X-ray showing pulmonary metastases.

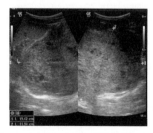

Fig. 34.3 A renal ultrasound showing the classical 'claw' sign and measurement of the tumour.

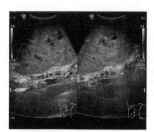

Fig 34.4 A Doppler flow study showing flow in renal vessels that can become blocked with tumour.

Treatment

There is overwhelming evidence from outcome data that Wilms' tumours should be treated in recognized paediatric oncology centres. Surgeons, radiotherapists, and paediatric oncologists need to work together to ensure that the children receive appropriate treatment. The development of Wilms' tumour treatment is often cited as a paradigm for multicentre clinical trials in childhood cancer.

Surgery

Surgical excision of the tumour if possible is and will almost certainly remain fundamental to the treatment of Wilms' tumour. There is debate about the timing of surgery, the place of percutaneous needle biopsy and the use of preoperative chemotherapy.

In North America the practice is immediate surgery followed by adjuvant chemotherapy and radiotherapy. In contrast in Europe, patients standard practice is treatment with preoperative chemotherapy and delayed surgery. Between 1991 and 2001 the UKCCSG conducted a prospective randomized trial (UKW3) comparing immediate surgery with 6 weeks of preoperative chemotherapy and delayed surgery. The trial showed that there was a significant reduction in the stage of the tumours in those having preoperative chemotherapy. As a consequence these patients received less chemotherapy, in particular anthracycline treatment, and also fewer patients received radiotherapy. Both the immediate surgery and the delayed surgery groups had equivalent event-free and overall survival rates.

Contraindications to surgery

- Bilateral disease.
- Hepatic invasion.
- Tumour invading inferiorly into the abdominal wall.

Biopsy

In Europe the majority of patients with suspected Wilms' tumour will have preoperative chemotherapy for 6 weeks with deferred surgery. Current UK practice is to biopsy the tumour using a Trucut needle. Data from the UKW3 trial demonstrated that biopsy was able to detect the 10% of cases with unfavourable histology or non-Wilms' pathology. There is, however, considerable debate as to the place that biopsy plays in management as it may give an unrepresentative sample of the tumour and, therefore, misleading histology, and there is also a risk of spillage of tumour cells along the biopsy track.

Pathology

Two broad groups of tumour can be recognized by their histological appearances:

- **Favourable histology:** the most common pathology. Classical triphasic histology – epithelial, blastemal, and stromal elements.
- **Unfavourable histology:** anaplasia.

Staging

In Europe the staging of a tumour is based on radiology and biopsy at diagnosis in conjunction with pathology post-surgery.

Chemotherapy

The use of chemotherapy as an adjuvant to surgery is now an essential part of Wilms' tumour treatment. The major advances in treatment have come as a result of the multicentre trials performed in North America, Europe and the UK. An essential determinant of adjuvant therapy is the surgical stage of the tumour. Consecutive studies have confirmed the role of chemotherapy as adjuvant agents in the treatment of Wilms' tumour. The intensity and length of post-operative treatment is directly related to the tumour stage.

Radiotherapy

The use of radiotherapy in low risk Wilms' tumour has decreased as trials have shown equivalent outcomes for patients treated with intensive chemotherapy with and without radiotherapy. Growing tissue, such as muscles, are damaged by radiotherapy, with consequent long-term sequelae. In low stage disease with excellent survival rates with chemotherapy alone, this morbidity has become unacceptable. Radiotherapy does, however, still have a significant role in high stage/unfavourable histology and relapsed Wilms' tumour treatment.

Follow-up

Pulmonary relapse is more common that local relapse. PA and lateral CXRs should be obtained regularly during and after treatment. Typically patients have CXRs every 2 months during treatment and for the first year post-treatment. Thereafter, CXRs should be performed every 3 months for 2 years, then 6-monthly for a year, and then at annual review.

It is sufficient to screen for local relapse with an abdominal US at the end of treatment and then 6-monthly for the next 2 years. Patients should also be monitored for hypertension and proteinuria.

Prognosis

The great majority of patients with Wilms' tumour will be cured as shown in Table 34.1 (SIOP9/UKW3 results).

Table 34.1 Cures for Wilms' tumour

Stage	Histology	5-year survival	Post-operative chemotherapy
I – Tumour completely within the renal capsule	Favourable	100%	None
	Unfavourable	93%	Actinomycin D, vincristine, doxorubicin
II – Extension of tumour outside renal capsule but still complete resection	Favourable – node negative	88%	Actinomycin D, vincristine, doxorubicin
	Unfavourable	85%	Etoposide, carboplatin, cyclophosphamide, doxorubicin plus radiotherapy
III – Incomplete excision of tumour but confined to abdomen	Favourable	85%	Actinomycin D, vincristine, doxorubicin
	Unfavourable	71%	Etoposide, carboplatin, cyclophosphamide, doxorubicin plus radiotherapy
IV – Metastatic spread to lung, liver, brain		70%	Actinomycin D, vincristine, doxorubicin plus radiotherapy
V bilateral renal disease		80%	

Late effects of treatment

Potential late adverse sequelae of treatment may include:
- Cardiotoxicity (due to anthracyclines).
- Restrictive pulmonary disease (due to radiotherapy to a field including lung tissue).
- Growth impairment and/or spinal asymmetry (due to radiotherapy to a field involving the spine).
- Risk of second malignancies (due to radiotherapy or etoposide).
- Hypertension.

Bone tumours

Introduction

Malignant, borderline and benign tumours can all arise in childhood.

The principal malignant bone tumours of childhood are *osteosarcoma* and *Ewing's sarcoma*, which comprise 8% of childhood tumours, occurring mainly in adolescence and early adulthood. Both tumours require systemic and local therapy, and a multidisciplinary approach is mandatory for optimal management

- *Chondrosarcomas* are rare in childhood, and surgery forms mainstay of treatment.
- *Giant cell tumours* can usually be managed with non-radical surgery, although they may very rarely metastasize.
- *Simple* and *aneurysmal* bone cysts do not have malignant potential and require orthopaedic management.
- *Osteoid osteomas* can be painful and may be treated surgically or with radiofrequency ablation.

Osteosarcoma

See Figs. 35.1 and 35.2.

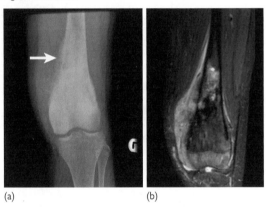

(a) (b)

Fig 35.1 Plain X-ray (a) and MRI (b) of osteosarcoma of distal femur. Note on (a) the raised periosteum with new bone formation leading to Codman's triangle (arrow). In this case the bone is sclerotic, rather than lytic.

- Commonest primary bone tumour of childhood.
- Rare under age of 10 years.
- Vast majority occur in long bones. Most are high grade tumours.
- Parosteal and low-grade osteosarcomas sub-types have low metastatic potential and can be treated with surgery alone.

Aetiology

Osteosarcoma in later adulthood may be associated with radiation exposure and genetic predisposition syndromes (retinoblastoma gene mutation and *Li-Fraumeni syndrome*). Rare predisposing syndromes, such as Rothmund-Thomson, exist, but account for only a small proportion of cases. Tumours occur most often at or towards the end of the pubertal growth spurt. Tumours are also more likely in tall individuals. In dogs, osteosarcoma is much more frequent in large breeds.

Presentation

- Pain is usual initial symptom.
- Vast majority of primary tumours occur in long bones, particularly the distal femur.
- Frequently dismissed as a sports injury or minor trauma.
- Persistent pain, especially at night and neuropathic in nature, mandates imaging.
- Subsequent symptoms include swelling and deformity.
- Many patients have symptoms for 6 months to 1 year before diagnosis.
- Pathological fractures are not uncommon.
- Clinical suspicion is aroused by plain X-ray in most cases, although X-ray abnormalities may be missed, giving false reassurance.

Diagnosis

- Initial take plain X-ray, if not already done.
- MRI of affected region to cover sufficient area to detect 'skip lesions' – lesions distinct from primary tumour in the same bone.
- All patients suspected of osteosarcoma must be referred to an oncological orthopaedic surgeon and preferably an appropriate multidisciplinary meeting for planning of biopsy and imaging. It is crucial that biopsy is carried out, bearing in mind eventual definitive surgery. Adequacy of imaging is also vital, since not all MRI scans are the same.
- Assessment of biopsy material also requires specific expertise and may require central referral. Key pathological feature is the formation of bone or osteoid in the tumour.

Staging

- CT chest and liver.
- Bone scan.
- MRI of any suspicious bone lesions.

Treatment

- All aggressive osteosarcomas need to be considered as metastatic, even when no metastases seen.
- High proportion of tumours recur where adequate surgery alone is used.
- Substantial cure rate only where chemotherapy and surgery used.
- Active drugs are cisplatin, doxorubicin, methotrexate, ifosfamide, and etoposide.
- Standard international regimen is cisplatin, doxorubicin, and high dose methotrexate.

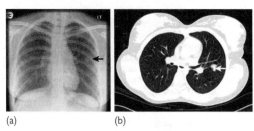

(a)   (b)

Fig. 35.2 Metastatic osteosarcoma arrowed on plain X-ray (a) and CT (b).

- There has been little change in survival rates over last 30 years.
- Neo-adjuvant chemotherapy (prior to definitive surgery) permits higher rate of limb salvage with endoprosthetic replacement, but does not improve survival.
- Response after neo-adjuvant chemotherapy is strongly prognostic.
- Tumours either show good response (≥90% necrosis) or poor response (<90% necrosis).
- Chemotherapy continues post-surgery (adjuvant).
- Current global trials randomize poor risk patients to treatment with additional ifosfamide and etoposide.
- Good risk patients are randomized either to added interferon treatment or not.

Primary surgery
- Crucial for cure.
- Needs to be *en bloc* with surrounding margin of normal tissue.
- Margins need to be wide or have anatomical boundary.
- Limb preservation is secondary to wide resection of tumour.
- Usually limb preservation depends on the ability to completely resect tumour and leave a functional limb. The proximity of tumour to neurovascular structures is crucial in this decision.
- Endoprostheses have improved greatly:
  - usually tailor-made for individuals based on careful measurement of bone using X-ray and MRI;
  - can be lengthened to match the growth of the patient.
- Endoprosthetic replacement does not recapitulate full limb function.
- Results are sometimes disappointing to patients who may choose to progress to amputation.

Metastastectomy
- Where possible demonstrated metastatic disease (usually lung) should be resected at or following primary surgery.
- During thoracotomy, careful palpation of lung parenchyma should be performed and will often identify further lesions.
- Even multiple and bilateral lesions should be resected where possible.

Toxicity

- Substantial toxicity associated with this treatment.
- Highly emetogenic chemotherapy regimen.
- Adequate nutrition is often hard to maintain.
- Long-term nephrotoxicity, cardiomyopathy, and hearing loss are all possible.
- Endoprostheses are at risk of infection, fracture, or loosening.
- Most will require revision within 10 years.

Prognosis

For 5- and 10-year survival rate see Table 35.1.

Table 35.1 5- and 10-year survival rate

	5-year overall survival	10-year overall survival
Localized tumours	70%	60%
Metastatic	30%	20%

The usual pattern of recurrence is metastatic in the lungs. Isolated lung recurrence should be treated with metastastectomy. Long-term survival has occurred even in the face of recurrent lung metastases.

- Rarely, isolated distant bone osteosarcomas occur in patients previously treated. These metachronous tumours may represent a new tumour, rather than recurrence. Where these tumours are treated as primary tumours, they can be associated with up to 50% survival.
- Multiple site recurrence is associated with a dismal prognosis.
- Death from cardiomyopathy may occur in cured patients.

Ewing's sarcoma

- Usually bone-associated, but can occur elsewhere – particularly soft tissue and renal.
- Majority appear localized on staging but need to be considered as occultly metastatic, if not overtly so.
- 95% have characteristic chromosomal translocation.
- Ewing's, peripheral primitive neuroectodermal tumours (pPNET), extra-osseous Ewing's sarcomas and Askin tumours all share the same translocation and form the Ewing's sarcoma family of tumours (ESFT; Fig. 35.3).

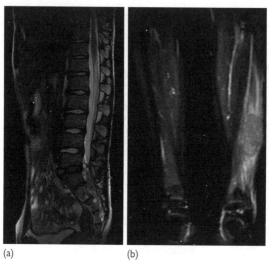

(a)   (b)

Fig. 35.3 (a) Ewing's sarcoma arising in sacral vertebra vertical arrow with infiltration of spinal canal horizontal arrow. (b) Ewing's sarcoma of fibula.

Aetiology

- Sporadic and unknown.
- Chromosomal translocation of Ewing's sarcoma gene *EWS* on chromosome 22 to an *ETS* family gene.
- *Ews-Fli1* transcript most common, associated with classical t(11;22) translocation.
- Combinations with other partner chromosomes/genes may occur.
- Translocation combines a potent transcriptional activator (*EWS*) and DNA binding domain (*ETS* e.g. *Fli1*).
- Fusion transcript seems important in malignant phenotype.

Presentation
- Pain is usual presenting symptom.
- An enlarging mass lesion will be evident except in internal sites (e.g. pelvis).
- Many sites of origin especially long bones, pelvic, and chest wall tumours.
- More rarely, can arise in soft tissues, especially kidney and subcutaneous.
- The majority are present in the 2nd decade of life.
- Very rare in young children or those over 30 years old.
- Diagnosis is often delayed.

Diagnosis
- Plain X-ray initially.
- Cross-sectional imaging MRI ± CT.
- All patients suspected of Ewing's sarcoma must be referred to an oncological orthopaedic surgeon and preferably an appropriate multidisciplinary meeting for planning of biopsy and imaging. It is crucial that biopsy is carried out bearing in mind eventual definitive surgery.
- Biopsy essential. Usually, small round blue cell tumour on haematoxylin & eosin (H&E) staining. Usually stains positive with CD99 on immunocytochemistry. Rearrangement of chromosome 22 and fusion gene formation demonstrated either by FISH or RT-PCR is diagnostic.

Staging
- Chest CT.
- Bone marrow examination.
- Bone scan.

Treatment
- All Ewing's family tumours need to be considered as metastatic even when no metastases seen.
- Require combination of effective systemic therapy and good local therapy.

Systemic therapy
- Active agents include vincristine, ifosfamide, cyclophosphamide, etoposide, doxorubicin, actinomycin D, melphalan, and busulfan.
- Euro-Ewing 99 induction: vincristine, ifosfamide, etoposide, and doxorubicin.
- Megatherapy with stem cell rescue is one option.
- Continuation of lower dose chemotherapy is another option.

Local therapy
- Options include surgery or radiotherapy.
- Surgery preferred, where it can be complete, wide, and non-mutilating.
- Radiotherapy may be used alone or in addition to surgery.
- Local therapy decision may change depending on response.

Toxicity
- High level of toxicity.
- Risk of cardiomyopathy.
- Risk of nephrotoxicity: glomerular and tubular.
- Risk of infertility.
- Long-term toxicity associated with radiotherapy.
- Surgical morbidity.

Prognostic indicators
For 3-year event-free survival see Table 35.2.

Table 35.2 3-year event-free survival

	3-year event-free survival
Localized tumours	66%
Metastatic lung only	42%
Metastatic other	29%

- **Site:** extremity tumours better than axial.
- **Size:** larger tumour volume worse.
- **Age:** younger patients fare better.
- **Metastases:** any detectable metastases markedly affects prognosis. Bone or bone marrow metastases are particularly grave.
- Early response to treatment predicts prognosis.
- Recurrence most frequently occurs in lung, bone, bone marrow, or primary site.
- Recurrence is a very grave situation. Prognosis of <10% is particularly serious for early recurrence and recurrence at sites other than the lung.

Extracranial germ cell tumours

Germ cell tumours (GCTs) are a rare and heterogeneous group of tumours, encompassing both benign and malignant subtypes, often with more than one subtype being present in any one tumour. They are unique in that their age of occurrence ranges from the neonatal period through to adulthood, and they may occur at both intracranial and extracranial sites.

Epidemiology

- Incidence of malignant germ cell tumours (MGCTs) is 3–5 per million children under 15 per year (3% of childhood malignancies).
- Incidence has a bimodal distribution with a peak in infancy/early childhood, rising again in late adolescence (15–19 years).
- In late adolescence (15–19 years), incidence increases:
  - *males* – 35/million;
  - *females* – 25/million.
- Incidence by gender varies according to site:
  - *sacrococcygeal* – females > males;
  - *thorax and CNS* – males > females;
  - *testicular GCTs* > ovarian GCTs.
- Incidence rose by around 25% from 1975 to 1995, largely accounted for by CNS tumours and testicular tumours in adolescents.
- There is racial variation with higher incidence of intracranial GCTs in Japan and lower incidence of testicular GCTs in African Americans.

Aetiology

- Evidence supports origin from primordial germ cells with either normal (gonadal) or aberrant (extragonadal) midline migration:
  - embryonal carcinoma and teratoma show some evidence of embryonal differentiation;
  - yolk sac tumour and choriocarcinoma show evidence of extra-embryonal differentiation;
  - germinoma remains undifferentiated (totipotent).
- **Associations:**
  - **Klinefelter's syndrome** (47, XXY): thoracic GCT.
  - XY gonadal dysgenesis, androgen insensitivity, Turner's syndrome (45, X) gonadoblastoma/germinoma.
  - Down syndrome.

Pathology

- GCTs comprise a variety of histological subtypes. Teratomas are composed of elements from all 3 embryonic germinal layers:
  - *mature teratoma* – all elements are well differentiated;
  - *immature teratoma* – contain some blastemal or undifferentiated neuroectodermal elements in addition, graded 1–3 according to amount of undifferentiated tissue.
- **Gonadoblastoma:** benign GCT exclusively associated with intersex disorders. Tendency to give rise to germinoma.

- **Malignant germ cell subtypes:**
  - yolk sac tumour (endodermal sinus tumour);
  - choriocarcinoma;
  - embryonal carcinoma;
  - germinoma (seminoma in testis, dysgerminoma in ovary).
- GCTs are frequently mixed:
  - *neonates/early childhood* – yolk sac tumour with mature/immature teratoma;
  - *peri- and post-puberty* – germinoma, embryonal carcinoma, choriocarcinoma, yolk sac tumour with mature/immature teratoma.
- A non-germ cell malignancy may rarely arise within mature/immature teratoma, e.g, neuroblastoma, peripheral neuroectodermal tumour, squamous cell carcinoma.

Tumour markers

- Secretion of tumour markers is a common feature of GCTs.
- α-fetoprotein (AFP) – an α-globulin, foetal serum binding protein:
  - half-life 5–7 days;
  - elevated in normal neonates, falling to adult normal values (<10ng/mL) by 12–18 months;
  - produced by yolk sac tumours and to lesser extent by embryonal carcinoma and immature endothelium in immature teratoma.
- Human chorionic gonadotrophin (β-HCG) – a glycoprotein, α subunit common to FSH, LH , TSH and melatonin, β subunit unique to β-HCG
  - half-life 24–36h;
  - produced by choriocarcinoma and (at low levels) by some germinomas;
  - high levels can cross react with LH receptor and trigger precocious puberty.

Biology

- The biology of GCTs continues to be unravelled.
- There is emerging evidence of differences between adult and paediatric GCTs, and between different histologies
  - *early childhood* – tumours are usually diploid or tetraploid, invariably yolk sac sub-type. Losses on 1p, 4, and 6q, and gain on 3p. Gain of 12p11 also seen, but less frequently than in adults;
  - *adolescence and adult* – tumours often aneuploid. Frequent gain of 12p (50–80% cases). Variable loss on 11, 13 and 18, and gain on 1, 7, 8, 21 and X.

Clinical presentation

Varies by site
- **Sacrococcygeal tumours** (40%): in neonates present as visible mass (often detected by antenatal scans). In children mass may be less prominent or not visible, and bladder, bowel, or lower limb dysfunction may be only sign.
- **Testis** (10%): painless scrotal mass.
- **Ovary** (25%): abdominal distension and pain. 7% are bilateral and 10% associated with intersex condition.

- **Mediastinum** (7%): respiratory symptoms, cardiac failure, associated Klinefelter's syndrome in adolescence.
- **Other extragonadal** (12%): include retroperitoneum, vagina, head and neck, liver. Vaginal tumours present with bleeding and are an important differential in suspected foreign body or sexual abuse in early childhood.

Investigation

- Suspect GCT in midline or gonadal mass.
- Measure AFP and β-HCG pre-operatively.
- Image primary site (CT or MRI). Heterogeneity and calcification suggest mature/immature teratoma.
- Malignant GCTs also need staging scans of lungs, liver, bones (include brain if HCG >10,000IU/L).
- Staging:
  - historically different staging systems have been used for tumours at different sites e.g. FIGO staging for ovarian tumours;
  - national groups are now using a TNM staging system in order to facilitate comparison of outcomes.

Management

GCTs are treated with surgery, with or without chemotherapy. Radiotherapy rarely has a role in treatment of extracranial GCTs.

Surgery

- Resectable tumours should have initial surgery. This is usually confined to gonadal primaries. However, tumours at other sites that have negative markers and have imaging consistent with pure teratoma should also have initial surgery.
- Testicular tumours should be resected via an inguinal route.
- The role of laparoscopic resection of ovarian tumours is not defined.
- Unresectable or metastatic tumours should be biopsied.
- If tumour markers are unequivocally raised and biopsy felt to be hazardous, diagnosis can be made on markers and imaging alone.

Chemotherapy

- Pure mature/immature teratoma does not require chemotherapy.
- Stage 1 malignant GCTs are managed with surgery only initially and close surveillance. About 20% overall and about 40% with AFP >10,000 at diagnosis will relapse. Chemotherapy is given at relapse.
- All stage 2–4 malignant GCTs require adjuvant chemotherapy. Chemotherapy should be platinum-based. Different strategies are used by different international groups.
- The most commonly used chemotherapy is bleomycin, etoposide, and cisplatin. In children one dose of bleomycin per cycle is used. The number of courses is determined by stage and site of the tumour and is either 3 or 4 courses.
- In the UK, carboplatin is used instead of cisplatin, with the aim of minimizing long-term toxicity. It is used in a dose intense manner, aiming for an AUC of 6.9. Although there has been no randomized study, the results appear to be as good as those using cisplatin in children.

Prognosis
- Germ cell tumours are generally highly curable tumours.
- Mature and immature teratomas have a survival close to 100%, the main risk being death from surgical complications in neonates.
- Up to 10% of neonatal sacrococcygeal teratomas will have a malignant recurrence.
- Overall outcome for malignant GCTs in the most recent UK paediatric germ cell study (GC 8901) is 5-year event-free survival (EFS) of 88% and overall survival (OS) 91%. Equivalent figures for the most recent North American study are 5-year EFS 86% and OS 92%.
- International groups are currently trying to clarify prognostic factors to define the small number of high-risk paediatric GCTs.

Chapter 37

Soft tissue sarcomas

Introduction

Sarcomas are malignancies arising from connective tissue. They may arise from skeletal tissue (Bone tumours 📖 pp.477–484) or in non-bony sites (soft tissue). In children and young people, the most common soft tissue sarcoma (STS) is rhabdomyosarcoma (RMS).

A range of non-rhabdomyosarcomatous soft tissue sarcomas also occur. Some are specific to childhood and some are tumours more commonly seen in adults.

Rhabdomyosarcoma (Fig. 37.1)

Commonest soft tissue sarcoma of childhood

- Wide range of age at presentation, including infants and continuing into young adult life.
- Variable phenotype with age. Younger children predominantly have more biologically favourable disease.

Aetiology

Most cases are sporadic. However, RMS may be associated with genetic predisposition syndromes (retinoblastoma gene mutation and *Li-Fraumeni syndrome*). Neurofibromatosis type 1 (NF1) often associated with bladder/prostate RMS.

Pathological characterization

- Histological appearance 'small round blue cell tumour'.
- Shows expression of a range of muscle markers.
- Pathological sub-types have strong prognostic significance.
- Botyroid, spindle cell and embryonal sub-types are favourable.
- Alveolar and solid variant of alveolar sub-types are unfavourable.
- Older patients and unfavourable sites are more likely to show unfavourable histology, but also are independent predictors of outcome.
- Any area of alveolar morphology makes a tumour alveolar.

Cytogenetics

- No characteristic abnormalities for favourable sub-types.
- Alveolar forms characteristically have translocation of *FKHR* gene on chromosome 13 and either *Pax3* (from chromosome 2 → t(2;13) translocation) or *Pax7* (from chromosome 1 → t(1;13) translocation):
  - these fusion genes appear to be crucial in determining poor prognostic of these tumours;
  - presence of these translocations make the tumour alveolar irrespective of morphology.

Presentation
- Most commonly presents as a mass.
- May be painful or cause site specific symptoms.
- Sites of original disease is an important prognostic indicator:
  - favourable sites include orbital, non-parameningeal head and neck, and non-bladder prostate/genitourinary (e.g. paratesticular);
  - these sites present early with obvious aberrant masses;
  - other sites are unfavourable, including extremity tumours, para-meningeal and bladder/prostate tumours;
  - these sites present with more advanced disease and have site-associated symptoms at presentation more frequently.
- Bladder/prostate tumours usually present with urinary tract obstruction and renal failure.
- Parameningeal tumours present with cranial nerve palsies and upper airways obstruction.

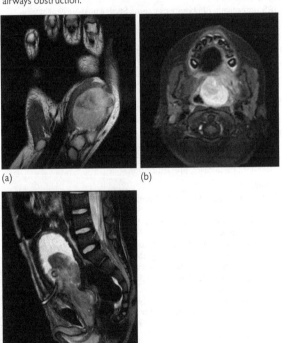

(a) (b)

(c)

Fig. 37.1 MRI showing (a) rhabdomyosarcoma of thenar eminence, (b) parameningeal rhabdomyosarcoma, and (c) bladder/prostate rhabdomyosarcoma.

Diagnosis
- Cross-sectional imaging is mandatory. CT or preferably MRI of primary lesion.
- Biopsy also mandatory for diagnosis.
- Consideration needed regarding definitive therapy prior to biopsy. Biopsy track requires subsequent local treatment.
- Specimen requires expert pathology review and cytogenetic analysis.

Staging
- CT chest.
- Bone scan.
- Bone marrow aspirate and trephine.
- CSF examination for parameningeal tumours.
- Scrotal US for paratesticular tumours.

Staging systems
- **IRS** (Intergroup Rhabdomyosarcoma Study): post-surgical staging.
- **TNM** (tumour, nodes, metasases): pre- or post-surgical staging system.

IRS
- **Group I:** localized disease, completely resected.
- **Group II:** total gross resection with evidence of regional spread.
- **Group IIa:** grossly resected tumour with microscopic residual disease.
- **Group IIB:** involved nodes grossly resected, but with microscopic residual disease in nodes.
- **Group III:** incomplete resection or biopsy.
- **Group IV:** distant metastases.

TNM
- **T:** primary tumour site, size, degree of invasion.
- **N:** regional lymph nodes, involved or not.
- **M:** distant metastases, present or not.

Treatment
- RMS need to be considered as metastatic even when no metastases seen.
- High proportion of tumours recur where adequate local therapy alone has been used.
- Much higher recurrence rate without local therapy.
- Not all these patients are salvageable.
- Optimal therapy for most patients requires local and systemic therapy.
- Active drugs include vincristine, actinomycin D, cyclophosphamide, ifosfamide, doxorubicin, topotecan.
- Prognosis is dependent on phenotype, site, size, age, and stage.
- Currently open EpSSG study in Europe.
- Therapy stratified in intensity according to prognosis.
- Neo-adjuvant chemotherapy (prior to definitive surgery) is the most common strategy, with subsequent reassessment and decision about local therapy.
- Adjuvant chemotherapy continues post-local therapy.

Local therapy
- Unavoidable for most tumours.
- Surgery or radiotherapy (or both).
- Surgery preferred where it can be non-mutilating and have a wide excision margin.
- Radiotherapy preferred in difficult surgical sites.

Metastatic disease
- <20% overtly metastatic at presentation.
- Overt metastases are the worst prognostic indicator.
- Prognosis worsens with number of sites, and involvement of bone and bone marrow.

Toxicity
- Toxicity proportional to intensity of treatment.
- Substantial morbidity from local therapy.

Prognosis
- Very wide range despite increasing intensity of treatment.
- **Low risk tumours:** >90% 5-year EFS.
- **Moderate risk:** 80% 5-year EFS.
- **High risk localized tumours:** 60% 5-year EFS.
- **Lower risk metastatic:** 30% 5-year EFS.
- **Higher risk metastatic:** 7.5% 5-year EFS.

Other soft tissue sarcomas

Synovial sarcoma
- Most common non-RMS STS.
- Most tumours occur in extremity sites.
- Occur in adolescence to young adulthood.

Aetiology
- Sporadic and unknown.
- Chromosomal translocation t(X;18) seen in >90% of tumours.

Presentation
- Pain present in up to 50% of cases.
- An enlarging mass lesion will be evident except in internal sites (e.g. pelvis).
- May be slow-growing.
- May be slow to present and diagnosis is often delayed.

Diagnosis
- Plain X-ray initially.
- Cross sectional imaging MRI +/– CT.
- All patients with an extremity mass lesion must be referred to an oncological orthopaedic surgeon, and preferably an appropriate multidisciplinary team meeting for planning of biopsy and imaging. It is crucial that biopsy is carried out bearing in mind eventual definitive surgery.
- Biopsy is essential. Classically, may contain spindle cell or epithelial cell morphologies. Hence, may be monophasic or biphasic.
- Fusion gene formation from SYT gene on chromosome 18q11 and a SSX gene from chromosome Xp11 demonstrated either by FISH or RT-PCR is diagnostic.

Staging
- Chest CT.
- Bone scan.
- IRS staging system applies (Rhabdomyosarcoma 🕮 p.494).

Treatment
- Metastatic disease is rare in tumours <5cm dimension.
- Local therapy is mainstay of treatment.
- Current open EpSSg study.

Local therapy
- Wide surgical excision is curative in most small tumours.
- Consideration should be given to radical surgery for all tumours.
- Combined orthopaedic and plastic surgery may be necessary for optimal results.
- Other surgical specialties: retroperitoneal, thoracic, spinal or neurosurgical may also have a role depending on site.
- Radiotherapy is added where tumours >5cm or margins are close.
- Radiotherapy may be given pre-operatively.

Systemic therapy
- Controversial in adults, but usual in children.
- Based on ifosfamide/doxorubicin.
- May be adjuvant or neo-adjuvant (pre-operative).
- Currently reserved for larger or harder to resect tumours.

Prognostic indicators
Prognostic indicators are shown in Table 37.1

Table 37.1 Prognostic indicators

	5-year EFS	5-year overall survival
IRS Group 1	79%	90%
IRS Group 2	75%	98%
< 5 cm dimension	92%	98%
> 5 cm dimension	56%	78%

- Failure to achieve local control carries a dire prognosis.
- Metastatic disease is associated with poor survival.

'Adult type' soft tissue sarcomas

Sarcomas more classically presenting in adult life can also present in children and young people. These tumours include fibrosarcomas, malignant peripheral nerve sheath tumours (especially in patients with NF1), liposarcomas and malignant fibrous histiocytomas. These tumours are individually very rare.

Where possible wide excision is the most effective treatment. In large tumours or where surgical margins are difficult, radiotherapy has a clearly beneficial role. In adults there has not been any demonstrable benefit from chemotherapy in this group of tumours. In children and young people unpredictable chemotherapy responses do occur.

The management of these tumours in young people should not be undertaken outside a specialist multidisciplinary team, but may involve chemotherapy in addition to surgery and radiotherapy, and is similar to the therapeutic approach to synovial sarcoma.

Infantile fibrosarcoma
- Most common soft tissue sarcoma of infancy.
- Classical t(12;15) translocation.
- Range of behaviours from rapid growth, through involution, to spontaneous resolution.
- Generally good prognosis for survival: 80–100%.
- Surgical treatment is mainstay.
- Chemosensitive tumour.
- Recommended strategy for unresectable tumours is initial low toxicity chemotherapy with vincristine and actinomycin D.
- Tumours not responding well may be managed by the addition of ifosfamide and/or doxorubicin.

Liver tumours

Introduction

- All types of liver tumours are found in children, both primary and secondary, benign and malignant.
- The most common primary malignant tumours of the liver are hepatoblastoma (HB) and hepatocellular carcinoma (HCC). These are epithelial liver tumours.
- The most common secondary malignant liver tumour in children is neuroblastoma.
- The age of the child, a history of travel abroad, or a history of underlying liver disease can help in the differential diagnosis.
- The most frequent benign tumours, haemangiomas, are more likely to occur in infancy. Young children are more likely to have HB. Older children or those with underlying liver disease are more likely to have HCC.
- The highest incidence of HCC comes in countries where hepatitis B is widespread.
- Non-neoplastic cysts do occur in the liver, but benign teratomas, malignant embryonal sarcomas and malignant germ cell tumours are rare.
- The cure rate for HB has considerably improved over the last three decades in the developed world, due to international collaboration in clinical trials. The incidence of HCC has decreased in the wider world due to active vaccination campaigns against hepatitis B, most notably in Asia, and particularly in Taiwan.

Presentation and history

- Most children present with an abdominal mass.
- Occasionally, they may have fever or show signs of malnutrition or bleeding. Only children with underlying liver disease will be jaundiced.
- Even a large hepatic mass, encompassing most of the liver, will not affect liver function.
- The history should include a full perinatal and maternal history, including vaccinations administered.
- Any travel abroad should be detailed (may suggest increased risk of hepatitis).

Investigations and screening

- Providing that the child is clinically stable, the most useful initial diagnostic investigation is an abdominal ultrasound (US). This should be able to clarify the localization of the tumour to the liver or, if pedunculated, as lying under the liver. During the US, it is important to watch the movement of the mass through a respiratory cycle to visualize the interface with the more stationary kidney. This helps differentiate between a mass arising from the upper pole of the kidney or adrenal gland and one from an inferior sector of the liver.

- A full blood count may show a raised platelet count. In the rare case of bleeding or rupture of the tumour, the haemoglobin may be low. If there is a large haemangioma and the Kasabach-Merritt syndrome is present (with platelet consumption within the haemangioma), then severe thrombocytopenia may be present.
- Liver function tests including AST, APT, ALP, GGT, bilirubin, and a coagulation screen will give a clear idea of underlying liver disease.
- A full viral screen for hepatitis should also be carried out. Urinalysis should be performed, looking for haematuria suggestive of Wilms' tumour.
- If a malignant tumour is suspected then serum α-fetoprotein (AFP) and human chorionic gonadotrophin (ß-HCG) should be taken and the results compared with the normal levels for age. Serum AFP levels are very high at birth and reach normal adult levels around the age of 8 months.
- CXR will reveal any significant metastatic disease. Malignant liver tumours metastasize preferentially to the lungs.
- If a haemangioma or malignant lesion remains the first differential diagnosis, then further cross sectional imaging with IV contrast should be obtained. MRI is preferable to CT in the abdomen for defining liver disease. However, spiral CT scan is the optimal imaging for staging the lungs. Young children may need two general anaesthetics to obtain adequate imaging.
- To confirm the diagnosis of a benign or malignant tumour, a biopsy is advisable. There are only a few exceptions:
  - An infant with a haemangioma diagnosed on US and MRI.
  - A cystic lesion that is likely to be non-neoplastic and can easily be removed surgically.
  - A child between the ages of 6 months and 3 years with a raised AFP above 1000ng/mL and a liver mass which is likely to be HB on imaging.
  - In the past, this latter group has been treated without a biopsy. In recent years, however, more is being understood about the different histopathological subtypes of HB as a result of the increasing number of children with the disease safely undergoing diagnostic biopsy and the central review of this tissue. Tissue can also then be analysed for biological features. To date, treatment is not stratified according to biology as it is in some malignancies; however, in the future this may become possible.
- Screening children with overgrowth syndromes for benign tumours and HB, with US 3-monthly up to the age of 7 years, allows for early diagnosis and treatment. Screening of children with predisposition syndromes to HCC is also of benefit. This screening, however, needs to be life-long.

Staging and prognosis

- In the case of malignant disease staging is essential prior to treatment. HB and HCC metastasize almost exclusively to the lungs.
- It is the extent of the locoregional disease, outside of the liver, which defines the potential for complete surgical excision. The presence of metastatic disease and incomplete macroscopic surgical excision remain the key prognostic factors in malignant liver tumours.
- If necessary total hepatectomy, followed by liver transplant, is indicated. However, for liver transplant to be successful there should be no extra-hepatic disease at the time of transplant. Whether transplant is technically possible or not will also depend on the extent of peri-hepatic vascular invasion. This should be assessed at diagnosis by a combination of cross-sectional imaging and Doppler US.
- In the case of embryonal sarcoma of the liver, staging should be completed with bilateral bone marrow aspirates and trephines, and a technetium bone scan.
- Staging of malignant epithelial tumours differs in North America and Europe:
  - The North American system takes into account the potential of primary surgery, as well as the extent of metastatic disease, and defines disease in a traditional way as being stage I, II, III, or IV.
  - The European system relies on image-defined risk factors at diagnosis and is based on the pretreatment extent of disease or PRETEXT system specifically designed for the liver.
  - This system divides the liver into four surgical sectors, and defines PRETEXT I, II, III, and IV as image defined potential surgical groups. A PRETEXT I tumour could potentially be removed by a right or left lobectomy, a PRETEXT II tumour could be excised by hemihepatectomy, a PRETEXT III tumour by an extended right or left hemihepatectomy, and a PRETEXT IV tumour by total hepatectomy (see Fig. 38.1 and Table 38.1).

Table 38.1 The PRETEXT system

PRETEXT I	Three adjoining sections free, one section involved
PRETEXT II	Two adjoining sections free, two sections involved
PRETEXT III	Two non-adjoining sections free, or just one section free, in the latter case three sections are involved
PRETEXT IV	No free section, all four sections involved

- Additional letters are used for disease outside of the liver: M for metastatic disease, E for extra-hepatic regional disease, V for hepatic venous disease, and P for portal vein disease.

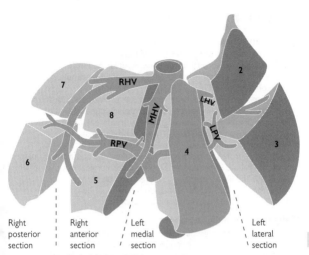

Fig. 38.1 Diagram showing schematic representation of hepatic anatomy as used in the staging of liver tumours under the PRETEXT system. Reproduced with permission from Roebuck DJ, Aronson D, Clapuyt P, *et al.* International Childhood Liver Tumor Strategy Group. 2005 PRETEXT: a revised staging system for primary malignant liver tumours of childhood developed by the SIOPEL group. Pediatr Radiol. 2007 Feb; 37(2):123–32, with kind permission of Springer Science and Business Media.

Further information

Roebuck, D.J., Aronson, D., Clapuyt, P., Czauderna, P., de Ville de Goyet, J., Gauthier, F., Mackinlay, G., Maibach, R., McHugh, K., Olsen, O.E., Otte, J.B., Pariente, D., Plaschkes, J., Childs, M., Perilongo, G., and the International Childhood Liver Tumor Strategy Group (2007) PRETEXT: a revised staging system for primary malignant liver tumours of childhood developed by the SIOPEL group. International Childhood Liver Tumor Strategy, 2005 Group. *Pediat Radiol 37*, 123–132.

Treatment

Benign tumours

- The most frequent benign tumours of the liver are haemangiomas, and can be diagnosed through a combination of US and MRI.
- These may regress spontaneously, but may need treatment if they are symptomatic.
- Initial treatment is usually with steroids or a combination of steroids and vincristine. If they become life-threatening due to congestive heart failure and/or consumptive coagulopathy, treatment with resection, embolization, or arterial ligation may become necessary.
- Other benign tumours such as mesenchymal hamartoma or focal nodular hyperplasia require a diagnostic biopsy to confirm their nature, as imaging alone is inadequate. Depending on surgical risk they may be left *in situ* and intermittently monitored with US or resected.
- In the rare case of liver teratoma, excision should be undertaken to reduce the risk of malignant transformation.

Malignant epithelial tumours

- There are four main groups designing treatment protocols for paediatric epithelial liver tumours, the North American Clinical Oncology Group (COG), the International Society of Paediatric Oncology Epithelial Liver Tumour Strategy Group (SIOPEL), the Japanese Liver Tumour Group (JPLT) and the German Liver Tumour Group (GPOG). The main difference between treatment approaches has been that of primary surgical excision versus pre-operative chemotherapy, rather like in Wilms' tumour.
- COG use primary surgery where possible in both HB and HCC, and SIOPEL use pre-operative chemotherapy in all cases of HB and primary surgery where possible in HCC. The Germans and Japanese are currently moving towards pre-operative chemotherapy for HB. HB is known to be more chemosensitive than HCC.

Hepatoblastoma

- The cure rate for HB has increased considerably since the introduction of cisplatin chemotherapy in the early 1980s.
- Cisplatin was shown to be the most active agent in xenograft models and new agents continue to be compared to this gold standard.
- Carboplatin is not as effective and attempts to increase the intensity of platinum by alternating cisplatin and carboplatin therapy have failed. Alternating platinum regimens which have increased the cure rate in high-risk disease have combined carboplatin with another active agent e.g. doxorubicin.
- The definition of standard and high risk disease differs across the Atlantic. However, inoperable tumours, defined either as PRETEXT IV, or stage III and metastatic disease are HR. More recently, tumour rupture at diagnosis (rare) and a serum AFP <100ng/mL is considered HR as well.

- Treatment depends on achieving complete remission (CR) with no evidence of disease on imaging, either in the lungs or the liver, and a normal serum AFP level.
- If necessary this needs to include surgical resection of lung metastases remaining after induction chemotherapy, prior to surgical resection of the liver mass.
- Liver surgery, whether it is a lobectomy or a total hepatectomy followed by liver transplant, induces a process of liver regeneration in the weeks following surgery.
- If lung metastases remain, they are likely to be stimulated during this regenerating phase.
- Combining aggressive surgery with multi-agent chemotherapy has increased the cure rate of high risk HB to 75%. Cisplatin monotherapy and surgical resection is sufficient to cure over 90% of standard risk HB. The current challenge in standard risk HB is to reduce the long-term renal and ototoxicity of the cisplatin without compromising the cure rate.
- The use of the chemoprotectant amifostine failed to reduce toxicity. The current SIOPEL 6 trial aims to reduce cisplatin ototoxicity by using sodium thiosulphate as a chemoprotectant.

Hepatocellular carcinoma

- HCC often presents as a large inoperable tumour. It is known to be highly angiogenic and has a propensity to metastasize.
- It is less chemosensitive than HB. Cisplatin and doxorubicin remain the most active chemotherapeutic agents, but surgical resection is the mainstay of cure.
- Primary resection should be carried out where possible.
- In inoperable tumours, the addition of anti-angiogenic agents to standard chemotherapy may increase the resection rate. Trans-arterial chemoembolization (TACE) may also be of benefit by enabling an unresectable tumour to become resectable.

Embryonal sarcoma and malignant germ cell tumours

- Embryonal sarcoma of the liver is a discrete tumour of the liver that is not synonymous with rhabdomyosarcoma occurring in the liver. However, due to its rarity, it has not been specifically studied in clinical trials in children.
- It is currently advised to treat embryonal sarcoma of the liver according to the most available rhabdomyosarcoma protocol (e.g. the EPSSG treatment protocol) and not as might be expected under the non-rhabdomyosarcoma soft tissue sarcoma protocol.
- Malignant germ cell tumours should be treated according to the current available malignant germ cell tumour protocol.

Conclusion

- Most liver tumours in children are curable.
- Cisplatin-based chemotherapy and surgery are the mainstay of cure in standard risk HB.
- The rare cases of high-risk HB require more aggressive treatment and where necessary additional surgery to clear lung metastases prior to liver surgery.
- The incidence of HCC, related to hepatitis B infection, is reducing worldwide thanks to national immunization programmes.
- Treatment of HCC, which is highly angiogenic, remains a challenge.
- Serial US screening of children with predisposition syndromes for HB or HCC is helpful.

Central nervous system tumours

Central nervous system tumours

Initial management of brain tumours

- Children and young people with brain tumours present with a variety of symptoms including raised intracranial pressure, focal seizures, neurological signs, and endocrinopathies.
- Children with brain tumours should be treated in an institution which is used to treating such children.
- If the child is to be transferred, dexamethasone should be given to reduce tumour swelling prior to transfer (recommended dose = 0.1mg/kg per dose bd, although often an initial loading dose of 0.2mg/kg is given).
- A multidisciplinary team approach is essential for the complex management of such children.

Raised intracranial pressure headaches

- Typically, but not exclusively, present on waking.
- Vomiting may occur in isolation and an index of suspicion must be maintained.
- The headaches typically get worse over time and last for longer each day.
- Papilloedema is a relatively late sign.
- *In extremis*, the child will show signs of coning (drowsiness and even loss of consciousness, hypertension, bradycardia, neck in extension) and become obtunded.
- Children with raised intracranial pressure should be seen immediately by a medical professional.

Focal seizures

All *unexplained focal seizures* in children require CNS imaging, as do unexplained neurological signs.

Biopsy

If a *biopsy* is performed, results should be seen initially or reviewed by a neuropathologist with significant experience with paediatric brain tumours before further treatment is started. It is preferable to discuss the case with a neuropathologist prior to surgery. Neurosurgical procedures in children with brain tumours should be performed only by surgeons with experience of such patients. Occasionally, life-saving surgery (usually in the form of a CSF diversion procedure) may need to be performed by surgeons without this experience, but this should be limited to urgent essential procedures.

Endocrine deficiencies

Children with suspected *endocrine deficiencies or excesses* should be seen by an endocrinologist prior to surgery (unless the surgery is urgent and life-saving).

General comments

- *Detailed clinical examination* should be performed whenever possible in order to establish any baseline neurological deficits:
- A *neuroradiologist* with expertise in paediatric brain tumours should review the imaging.
- Ideally, the *multidisciplinary team* should meet to discuss management options prior to surgery, but this is not always possible. However, a minimum of the neuroradiologist, neurosurgeon, and oncologist should meet to discuss the case prior to surgery.
- *A doctor and member of the nursing staff should give detailed explanations to the patient and parents.* Parents and children are understandably very scared by the mention of a brain tumour, and since major neurosurgery often follows shortly after the initial consultation the patients and parents need to be fully informed and supported.
- Initial serum investigations should include viral serology:
  - *VZV, measles* – to guide post-exposure prophylaxis in susceptible patients) (Other aspects of supportive care, Immunization 📖 pp.270–274);
  - *HSV* – to assist differential diagnosis and management of mouth ulcers;
  - CMV ± EBV are performed routinely in some units;
  - in high risk areas, hepatitis B/C and HIV screening will usually be performed;
  - the blood sample should be taken *before* any blood product transfusion to avoid passive transfer of antibodies giving a false positive result.

Children and young people with brain tumours have high morbidity and, as such, need a lot of input from all healthcare professionals, including psychologists, social workers, nurses, teachers, physiotherapists, and occupational therapists, in addition to those healthcare professionals mentioned above.

Low grade glioma

Introduction

Low grade glioma (LGG) are frequently underestimated due to their perceived benign nature, but often have significant morbidity and even mortality. Site is important in terms of treatment and outlook. Comprise 30–40% of childhood CNS tumours. Can occur at any age, mean 6–11 years.

Genetic factors

Certain genetic conditions predispose to these tumours:

- **Neurofibromatosis type 1 (NF1)**: due to mutation in neurofibromin gene (17g11.2), which is thought to be a tumour suppressor gene. NF1 predisposes children to visual pathway astrocytomas, which arise in 5–15% of NF1 children. Conversely, half of all children with visual pathway tumours have NF1.
- **Tuberous sclerosis (TSC):** condition characterized by multiple hamartomas. Sub-ependymal giant cell astrocytomas (SEGA) are one of the diagnostic criteria. Approx 15% of TS children have a SEGA at some point during childhood/adolescence.
- **Li-Fraumeni syndrome:** due to mutation in p53 tumour suppressor gene. More commonly develop medulloblastomas, but can develop LGG although usually in 3rd and 4th decade.

Presentation

Very dependent on site and can have a myriad of presentations. History is usually, but not inevitably, longstanding.

- **Eye signs:** including nystagmus, loss of vision in visual pathway tumours.
- **Endocrine presentation:** may include delayed puberty, precocious puberty, diencephalic syndrome, hypothalamic-pituitary axis dysfunction, growth failure.
- **Headaches**: either due to hydrocephalus, particularly for posterior fossa tumours, or as a result of mass effect.
- **Raised intracranial pressure**: signs and symptoms of raised intracranial pressure may be present especially in posterior fossa tumours.
- **Seizures, particularly focal ones:** all children who suffer a focal seizure should have a scan. MRI if possible or CT scan as a screening scan.
- **Cranial nerve signs:** may be present in pilocytic tumours of the brain stem.
- **Long tract signs:** these may be present depending on the site of the tumour.
- Spinal cord compression with motor and/or sensory signs and/or loss of bladder/bowel function.
- Cerebellar tumours may present with ataxia.
- Hypotonia and developmental delay more often present in those with extensive tumours, and especially in NF1 patients.
- Rarely may have disseminated disease at presentation or at relapse (usually hypothalamic chiasmatic tumours).

Diagnosis

- MRI is the imaging of choice. CT scan may be used as screening test.
- If child has stigmata of NF1 and the lesion is typical on neuroimaging then a biopsy may not be necessary. This may also be the case for other typical visual pathways tumours, as well as tectal plate tumours (see Figs 39.1–39.6).
- For all other patients a biopsy or resection should be performed. This depends on ease of proposed resection and possible morbidity. If possible a resection is the best treatment.

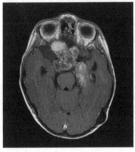

Fig. 39.1 Visual pathway astrocytoma. Non NF-1.

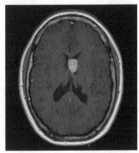

Fig. 39.2 Subependymal giant cell astrocytoma (SEGA) in patient with TS.

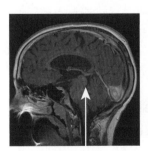

Fig. 39.3 Tectal plate glioma with hydrocephalus (arrowed).

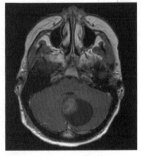

Fig. 39.4 Pilocytic astrocytoma of cerebellum. There is a small solid and large cystic component.

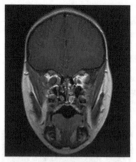

Fig. 39.5 Optic pathway glioma with large optic nerves (NF1).

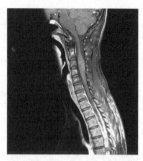

Fig. 39.6 Intrinsic spinal cord tumour.

Pathology

WHO grading system

WHO grade 1
- Pilocytic astrocytoma.
- Subependymal giant cell astrocytoma.

WHO grade 2
- Fibrillary astrocytoma.
- Protoplasmic.
- Gemistocytic.
- Mixed.

Other
- Pilomyxoid glioma.
- Ganglioglioma.
- Gangliocytoma.
- Dysembryoplastic neuroepithelial tumour (DNET).

Oligoastrocytoma

Treatment
- Surgical resection is treatment of choice if possible without significant morbidity.
- Chemotherapy used generally for patients younger than 8 years old and radiotherapy for those older.
- Some children who have tumours that are not progressing, or are not expected to, may be observed with serial MRI scans. Generally, these are children with either NF1 (and no progressive visual deterioration) or tectal plate gliomas.
- Often managed as a chronic disorder and multiple strategies may be used at different time points in the same patient.
- Supportive care in terms of nutrition may be necessary especially for those children presenting with diencephalic syndrome.
- Treatment for those presenting with disseminated disease needs to be planned on an individual basis.

Surgery
- Patients with posterior fossa tumours may need CSF diversion in form of 3rd ventriculostomy or ventriculo-peritoneal shunt.
- Surgical resection is usually possible for posterior fossa tumours and many hemispheric lesions.
- Not usually possible for hypothalamic tumours, visual pathway tumours, brainstem including tectal plate tumours, or intrinsic spinal cord tumours.
- If incomplete resection is possible with a small residuum (especially for non-hypothalamic tumours), a watch and wait policy is advisable as often these tumours do not regrow.

Chemotherapy
- Usually given if surgery not possible, and a watch and wait strategy inappropriate.
- Usually prolonged therapy (1 year or greater). Number of agents have been used but usually includes one or more of the following:
  - vincristine and carboplatin (occasionally cisplatin) most common;
  - cyclophosphamide and etoposide;
  - single agent vinblastine and more recently temozolomide have been used.
- Multiple therapies may be used in an attempt to delay radiotherapy.
- Many children treated on chemotherapy eventually require radiotherapy.

Radiotherapy
- Radiotherapy usually reserved for those over 8 years of age.
- Generally given as focal radiotherapy. Radiosurgery is unsuitable for most children with low grade gliomas.
- Dose usually in region of 54Gy.
- Intellectual long-term effects dependant on site and age of patients.
- Central midline tumours have risk of hypopituitarism.

Prognosis
See Table 39.1.

Table 39.1 Treatment and 5- and 10-year overall survival rates

Treatment	5-year overall survival	10-year overall survival
Complete resection	76–100%	69–100%
Incomplete resection	62–87%	62–87%
Incomplete resection + radiotherapy	80%	67–94%

- Morbidity can be high and a multidisciplinary team approach is usually necessary, often including other specialists, such as ophthalmologists, developmental paediatricians, endocrinologists, and neurologists.
- Usually a chronic disease and relapse is not uncommon, particularly for midline tumours.
- Relapse or progression should be treated on an individual basis – consider surgery first, but if not possible either chemotherapy or radiotherapy.
- Progression of Grade II tumours to Grade III or IV tumours is unusual in children, but may occur in older adolescents.

High grade glioma

High grade glioma (WHO Grade III and IV), which account for 15% of brain tumours in children, are tumours arising from glial tissue (supporting structure of brain). Can occur at any age, but more common in teenagers. Male to female ratio 1:2. Usually supratentorial, but occasionally occur in posterior fossa. Half in cerebral cortex and half in thalamus, hypothalamus, 3rd ventricle and basal ganglia. Transformation from low grade glioma is unusual in children.

Presentation

- Dependant on location.
- Duration of symptoms vary, but may be up to a year in length
- Headaches, seizures (often focal), and motor deficits most common in supratentorial tumours.
- Basal ganglia tumours may present with abnormal movements, such as choreiform movements.
- Hydrocephalus may be present, but total obstruction of CSF flow due to the tumour is unusual.
- History of NF1 or NF2 should be sought.

Diagnosis

- Clinical suspicion followed by imaging, preferably MRI, but may use CT as a screen.
- High grade gliomas seen usually as non-homogenous, infiltrating, space-occupying lesion, which is diffuse with poorly defined margins. Haemorrhagic and cystic areas common, but calcification uncommon. Usually take up contrast (see Fig. 39.7).
- Surrounding oedema common.
- Hydrocephalus may be present depending on site.
- Distant spread within the CNS is uncommon, but does occur.

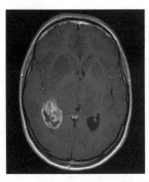

Fig. 39.7 Right-sided supratentorial high grade glioma (T1 axial post-contrast view) showing contrast enhancement and central necrosis.

Pathology

WHO grading system

WHO grade III
- Anaplastic astrocytoma.
- Anaplastic oligodendroglioma.
- Malignant oligoastrocytoma.
- Gliomatosis cerebri.

WHO grade IV
- Glioblastoma multiforme.
- Giant-cell glioblastoma.
- Gliosarcoma.
- Glioblastoma with sarcomatous elements.

- Features include cellular anaplasia, mitotic figures, angiogenesis and necrosis.
- Usually glial fibrillary acid protein (GFAP) and S100-protein positive. MIB-1 proliferation usually high.
- Diagnosis can be difficult. Disagreement between pathologists on central review can be as high as 20%.

Treatment

- Dexamethasone should be given prior to surgery to reduce oedema.
- **Surgery** is first line and is necessary for diagnosis. Extent of surgical resection is dependant on site. A biopsy may be only procedure that is possible. Maximum amount of safe resection should be aimed for. Children who have >90% resection have a better prognosis, unlike adults.
- **Radiotherapy** is mainstay of treatment. 54Gy focal radiotherapy is considered standard.
- **Chemotherapy** has a less clear role. A number of studies have been done, none of which show definitive effect. Adult studies showing benefit with temozolomide not reproduced in children. However, various combinations are still in use – temozolomide with radiotherapy (concomitant) and subsequent adjuvant use of temozolomide probably the commonest strategy. Studies with small numbers of paediatric patients and with differing degrees of resection are difficult to interpret.
- **Immunotherapy:** much research is in progress in this area, but has to overcome immunosuppressive mechanisms.
- **Small molecules:** these are being tried at the current time.
- **Anti-angiogenic** treatments have been tried with little success thus far, but there is hope that a new generation of these agents may be more effective.

Prognosis
- Grade III have better survival (28% 5-year) than grade IV (16% 5-year). This is in contrast to adults where histology has no significant effect.
- Oligodendrogliomas with 1p and 19q loss have a more favourable outlook than those without. The prognosis of oligoastrocytomas and other variants as separate entities is not clear.
- Children under 3 years old (90%) have worse outlook.
- Extent of resection is related to better survival in children, but often such extensive surgery is not feasible.

Medulloblastoma and PNET

Primitive neuroectodermal tumours (PNET) are embryonic tumours accounting for 25% of paediatric CNS tumours. Medulloblastomas are those with the primary in the posterior fossa (85%), whilst the term PNET refers to those found elsewhere in the CNS (usually supratentorial) and outside the CNS. Peak age at presentation 5-7 years old.

Presentation
- Signs of raised intracranial pressure (ICP), esp. in medulloblastomas:
  - headaches particularly early morning (lying down eliminates any CSF flow due to gravity, hence pressure builds up if obstructive hydrocephalus), initially headaches improve during day;
  - vomiting with or without headaches usually early morning;
  - papilloedema, but often not recognized;
  - head tilt;
  - occasionally pre-terminal with lowering of conscious level, bradycardia and hypertension.
- Ataxic gait.
- Cranial nerve deficits especially VI.
- Supratentorial PNET may present with seizures, headaches, loss of motor function.
- Nystagmus and diplopia may occur.

Diagnosis
- Clinical suspicion followed by imaging. CT can be used as screen. MRI necessary if a mass is seen and must include spine (pre-operatively) as drop metastases occur in up to 20%.
- **Medulloblastoma:** usually vermal mass, usually enhances strongly, relatively homogeneous (Fig. 39.8).
- Metastatic spread outside the CNS occurs (rare, but if present, usually bone and bone marrow).
- **PNET:** similar characteristics, but in other site.
- Histology should differentiate subtypes; classic most common, anaplastic, desmoplastic, large cell.
- Early post-operative MRI essential (within 48 h).

Staging: Chang staging
- **M0:** no evidence of metastasic disease.
- **M1:** positive CSF cytology.
- **M2:** meningeal metastasis within the cranial vault.
- **M3:** MRI visible spinal metastatic disease.
- **M4:** metastasis outside the CNS (usually bone).

Risk groups
- **Standard risk:**
  - <1.5cm^2 residuum on early post-operative MRI;
  - M0 staging.
- **High risk:**
  - >1.5cm^2 residuum on early post-operative MRI;

- M1–4 staging;
- large cell or anaplastic histology believed to have worse outlook.

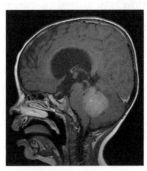

Fig. 39.8 Homogeneous midline vermal mass with contrast enhancement (saggital T1 post-contrast) resulting in hydrocephalus from compression of IV ventricle typical of a medulloblastoma.

Biology

Playing a more important role. Future stratification using biology is likely. Current factors conferring a better prognosis include β–catenin, Trk C, desmoplastic histology. Poorer outlook in presence of *c-myc*, or anaplastic or large cell histology.

Treatment and side effects

- **Surgery:** initial treatment with maximum resection (usually only for primary lesion and not metastases if they are present).
- MRI scan for residuum within 48h.
- For over 3-year-olds, craniospinal radiotherapy (24Gy) with boost of up to 54Gy to site of primary tumour for standard risk. For high risk patients, 36Gy to primary site, with boost up to 54–59Gy.
- Followed by chemotherapy depending on national or local protocol. Common protocols include the use of agents in varying combinations of carboplatin, cisplatin, vincristine, CCNU, and cyclophosphamide.
- For under 3-year-olds, primarily chemotherapy based strategy, but an increasing number of groups are using focal radiotherapy.
- Side effects may be varied but usually of moderate severity. Include nausea, vomiting, hair loss, neutropenia (all acute), hearing loss, moderate ataxia, intellectual deterioration, panhypopituitarism including growth failure and infertility (usually chronic).

Outcome

- For standard risk disease (medulloblastomas) over the age of 3 years, 5-year survival approximately 80%.
- For high risk disease, 5-year survival approximately 50%, but many variables may influence outcome.

- Non metastatic supratentorial disease: 5-year survival about 50%, but lower if M1–4.
- Pinealoblastomas have better outcome than other supratentorial PNETs.
- Under 3-year-olds have a worse prognosis (better if desmoplastic or have extensive nodularity).

Ependymoma

Derived from ependymal cells that line the ventricles. Usually arise in brain but can arise rarely in spinal cord. Account for 6–10% of CNS tumours in children. Peak age at presentation 3–8 years with no apparent gender bias. Two thirds of cases arise in posterior fossa.

Presentation

- Signs and symptoms of raised intracranial pressure most common presentation (Haematological and oncological emergencies, Raised intracranial pressure 📖 pp.98–100).
- Signs and symptoms may be present for days to months before diagnosis established.
- May have specific cerebellar signs or cranial nerve dysfunction.
- If supratentorial, may present with seizures, loss of function, or headaches.
- Nystagmus and diplopia may occur.

Diagnosis

- Clinical suspicion followed by imaging. CT can be used as screen. MRI necessary if a mass is seen and must include spine (pre-operatively) as drop metastases occur in up to 22%.
- MRI usually shows contrast enhancement and can have signal heterogeneity (haemorrhage, necrosis, calcification, with the latter shown best on CT scan). Often midline and intra-ventricular. Spread into foramen magnum or cerebellopontine angle more characteristic of ependymoma than the main differential diagnosis of medulloblastoma (see Fig. 39.9).

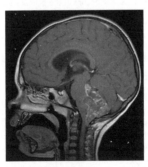

Fig.39.9 Midline posterior fossa tumour arising within the IV ventricle (saggital T1 post contrast) with resulting hydrocephalus. The tumour is heterogeneous with contrast enhancement.

Pathology

WHO grading system

- **Grade 1:** subependymoma and myxopapillary.
- **Grade 2:** low grade (includes cellular, papillary, clear-cell and tancytic).
- **Grade 3:** anaplastic.
- Histology: can be difficult to grade accurately (high degree of discordance in studies – in region of 70%).

Treatment

- Steroids should be started at initial diagnosis.
- Surgery is mainstay of treatment.
- May need urgent relief of raised ICP prior to definitive surgery that needs to be performed by experienced paediatric neurosurgeon. An external ventricular drain may be used to relieve the pressure prior to transfer to distant neurosurgical centre, although steroids alone are often adequate.
- Intra-operative frozen section should be performed. If diagnosis of ependymoma established intra-operatively, maximal surgical resection should be attempted even at cost of increased neurological deficit.
- If residuum visible on 48h scan, then second look surgery should be contemplated (53% have some residuum).
- If metastatic disease then gross total resection (GTR) is not as important.
- In over 3-year-olds, focal radiotherapy to tumour site should be given (tumour recurrence usually occurs in the primary site). Recurrence can be treated with chemotherapy to try and reduce tumour volume, and make the lesion resectable.
- In under 3-year-olds, chemotherapy has been employed due to the reluctance to use radiotherapy. This can delay use of radiotherapy. Ependymomas not particularly chemosensitive in majority of cases.

Prognostic factors

- Have been difficult to analyse accurately.
- As yet, no definitive evidence that anaplastic ependymoma has a worse outlook than Grade II.
- No definitive biological prognostic markers yet proven.
- Under 3-year-olds (at diagnosis) have a worse outlook.
- No major difference associated with site (supratentorial versus posterior fossa).
- Tumour resection is most powerful prognostic factor (approx 70% survival after total resection vs. 30% for incomplete resection). MRI within 48h used as an assessment measure, since the surgeon's intra-operative assessment is incorrect in 32% of cases.

Outcome

- 5-year survival ranges from 39 to 64%, while 10-year survival is approximately 45%. Complete surgical resection has higher rate of long-term survival.
- Often left with moderate to severe neurocognitive outcome.

Choroid plexus tumours

- These are rare tumours (1–4% of childhood CNS tumours). Half occur in children less than 1 year of age.
- Lateral ventricles are the commonest site (75%), other sites include 4th ventricle and cerebello-pontine angle (15%) and 3rd ventricle (10%).
- Choroid plexus tumours are either:
  - papillomas (CPP) (grade I) (80%) (Fig. 39.10);
  - carcinomas (CPC) (grade 3) (20%).

Presentation

- Hydrocephalus, increasing head size and bulging fontanelle if young enough. Choroid plexus papillomas may secrete cerebrospinal fluid.
- Other signs of raised intracranial pressure, e.g. vomiting and headache (in older children who are able to verbalize).
- May present with an intracranial bleed.

Diagnosis

- Clinical suspicion followed by imaging. As most of these patients are young, remember not to sedate a child with possible raised ICP.
- MRI scan is the investigation of choice. These tumours are intraventricular. Papillomas resemble florets of cauliflower and a stalk is often seen (Fig. 39.10). Carcinomas are usually large very vascular lesions within the ventricles.
- Magnetic resonance angiograms (MRA) or formal angiograms may be necessary prior to definitive treatment (Fig. 39.11).

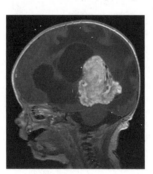

Fig. 39.10 Saggital T1 post-contrast MRI scan showing a large intraventricular choroid plexus papilloma.

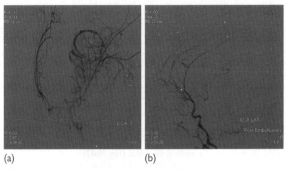

(a)   (b)

Fig. 39.11 (a) Pre- and (b) post-embolization of a CPP.

Pathology

- **Classic CPP (WHO grade I):** rest on basement membrane as simple layer of cuboid/columnar cells, may have the occasional mitosis. Often very vascular.
- **Carcinoma (CPC) (WHO grade III):** anaplasia, mitoses and invasion of adjoining brain often seen.
- **Atypical CPP:** increased mitotic activity and some invasiveness, may transform if not resected.

Treatment

- Surgery is the treatment of choice. Only experienced paediatric neurosurgeons should attempt to resect these tumours. CPP usually need surgery alone. CSF diversion needed in 60% (usually VP shunt) for persisting communicating hydrocephalus. As with most CNS tumours, dexamethasone should be given prior to surgery.
- Pre operative embolization should be considered, since risk of significant bleeding during surgery is high. High intraoperative mortality, particularly for CPC, has made some clinicians suggest preoperative chemotherapy.
- If incomplete resection, then second look surgery should be considered.
- CPC should have a combination therapy approach using chemotherapy (usually multi-agent containing platinum/cyclophosphamide) and possibly radiotherapy.

Prognosis

- Excellent survival for CPP (approaching 100%).
- CPC cure rate is poor (about 25%). Complete resection is difficult due to tumour invasiveness, but if achieved it improves the outcome.

Infant central nervous system tumours

Infants have often been considered to be a separate group in terms of CNS tumours. The reason for this is mainly the different disease patterns seen, as well as differing outcomes from older children. The lack of willingness to give radiotherapy due to long-term effects on a developing brain has also distinguished this age group. Approximately one-third of all CNS tumours in children occur in the under 3-year-old age group. Congenital tumours tend to occur in first 6 months of life.

Specific tumour types

PNET and medulloblastoma

- A third of medulloblastomas/primitive neuroectodermal tumours (PNET) occur in the under 3-year-olds (Fig. 39.12).
- Usually have a worse prognosis, probably due to unfavourable biology, as well as the inability to give optimal radiotherapy (due to long-term side effects).
- One subcategory is thought to have more favourable outcome – medulloblastoma with extensive nodularity (MBEN), although it is additionally suggested that desmoplastic medulloblastoma in this age group is also more favourable.
- Supratentorial PNETs have a very poor prognosis.
- Treatment usually involves intensive chemotherapy. Recently, more groups are using focal radiotherapy especially for medulloblastoma.

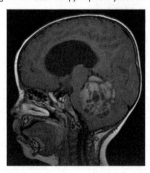

Fig. 39.12 Infant medulloblastoma.

Ependymoma

- A third of all ependymomas occur in the under 3 years age group.
- Surgery, as with older children, is the treatment of choice, followed up with chemotherapy in first instance.
- Radiotherapy should be reserved for progressive disease.
- Outcome dependent on resection (as with older children), but overall survival lower.

Ependymoblastoma

- Rare, distinguished by multilayered rosettes.
- More commonly found in lateral ventricles.

- Characterized by rapid growth and leptomeningeal dissemination.
- High dose treatment should be considered.
- Usually fatal within a year.

Astrocytoma

Low grade
- 21% of CNS tumours in children under 3 years.
- Most commonly midline supratentorial tumours (25% have NF1).
- NF1 children have better prognosis.
- Chemotherapy is usually given unless resectable and radiotherapy is reserved for older children (in Europe currently those >8 years old).

High grade.
- Surgery and chemotherapy usually used as initial treatment.
- Anaplastic astrocytomas do better than glioblastoma multiforme (GBM).
- Believed by some that there is better outlook than in older children (?chemotherapy inducing some maturation of tumour).

Infantile desmoplastic ganglioglioma

- WHO grade 1. Usually supratentorial in children under 2 years of age.
- Often involves extension to more than one lobe.
- Histological appearance often more aggressive than clinical behaviour.
- Surgery is treatment of choice.
- Prognosis excellent, but high incidence of neurocognitive and neuromotor late adverse effects.

Teratoma

- 4% of brain tumours in infancy.
- Surgery alone is preferable, but if residual immature elements are left post-operatively, then chemotherapy is usually given.

Choroid plexus tumours

- Choroid plexus tumours.
- Either papillomas or carcinomas.
- Usually vascular.
- Surgery often difficult.
- Carcinomas need further therapy, but outcome is poor.

Atypical teratoid rhabdoid tumour (ATRT)

- Highest incidence in first 2 years of life.
- Usually arises in posterior fossa, but is often metatstatic..
- Particular genetic abnormalities include chromosome 22 deletion and absence of *INI 1* gene (on 11q22).
- Chemotherapy usually used after initial surgery, but with little success. Vast majority of patients, especially in infancy, die of their disease.

Outcome

In general outcome is worse in infants probably due to a combination of the biological characteristics as well as the increased difficult of neurosurgery in a small brain and the unwillingness to give radiotherapy due to adverse late neurocognitive outcome. Trials are more difficult to run due to the relatively small numbers. Multinational trials are the obvious way forward.

Craniopharyngioma

Craniopharyngiomas occur as a result of maldevelopment (thought to be from Rathke's pouch remnants) and account for about 7–10% of childhood CNS tumours. Although benign by nature, they often require repeated treatment and have considerable morbidity. Peak incidence is at 5–10 years of age with no gender predilection.

Presentation

- Can present in a myriad of ways usually as a result of compression of adjacent suprasellar structures.
- Most common presenting features include headache and vomiting due to hydrocephalus as a result of compression of 3rd ventricle, diabetes insipidus, TSH insufficiency, LH/FSH insufficiency, ACTH insufficiency and raised serum prolactin.
- Precocious or delayed puberty may also be presenting features. Weight gain is a common finding, the short over weight child being a classic presentation.
- Other rarer presenting features may include unsteadiness, developmental delay, and seizures.

Diagnosis

- Clinical suspicion followed by neuroimaging, preferably MRI scan.
- Calcification may be seen on CT scan.
- Tumour usually has cystic and solid components, which usually enhance on imaging (Fig. 39.13). These suprasellar tumours are often extensive and compress adjacent structures. Hydrocephalus is commonly seen. Hypothalamic invasion may be seen which makes total removal difficult.
- An endocrine workup is essential prior to definitive treatment, but more extensive investigation may be left until after treatment, as surgery may result in further endocrinopathies. It is preferable to involve an endocrinologist from the outset.
- Germ cells markers should be checked if there is any suspicion this may be a germ cell tumour (AFP and βHCG).

Suggested initial endocrine work-up

- Height, weight (plotted on centile charts).
- Pubertal staging and bone age.
- Electrolytes (paired plasma and urine).
- Urine and serum osmolalities.
- TSH/T$_4$, LH/FSH, IGF1, prolactin, testosterone (males), oestradiol (females) if age 8 years and above.
- Synacthen test.

- Ophthalmological assessment is also essential. This should include visual acuity, visual fields, fundoscopy, and possibly electrophysiology.
- Differential diagnosis includes optic pathway glioma, germinomas, and rarely, Rathke's pouch cysts.

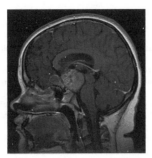

Fig. 39.13 MRI scan showing a typical craniopharyngioma with cystic and solid components.

Pathology

Histologically, craniopharyngiomas consist of squamous epithelium lining cystic cavities and solid components, which often contain calcium and/or keratin.

Treatment

There are a number of components to treatment.

Surgery
- **Direct tumour surgery**: as much of the tumour should be removed with as little morbidity as possible. If there is residual tumour on post-operative scan (performed at 3 months), then radiotherapy should be considered. Repeated surgery for control of cysts (over a long time period) may be necessary. Occasionally, Ommaya reservoirs are used to aspirate cysts on a repeated basis. Regular MRI scanning is necessary for follow-up.
- **Hydrocephalus**: direct surgery may clear a passage for CSF flow. An external ventricular drain may be necessary as a temporary measure, or a ventriculo-peritoneal shunt as a more permanent measure. A 3rd ventriculostomy is more difficult since this is the site of obstruction.

Radiotherapy
- Radiotherapy is often necessary if tumour residuum is present post-operatively or if subsequent progression occurs. Focal radiotherapy is usually used, but may have the long-term side effects of worsening pituitary function and increasing visual impairment.
- Intracavity radiotherapy may be used especially if a single discrete cavity is seen.

Endocrinopathies
- Lifelong endocrine follow-up is required.
- Hormone replacement is usually necessary for one or more of the following – growth hormone, hydrocortisone, thyroid hormone, DDAVP, sex hormones.

Long-term effects

There is a high degree of morbidity associated with this benign tumour. This may include:

- Endocrinopathies and their associated problems. Lifelong hormone replacement is usual.
- Neuropsychological effects from both the tumour and the treatment including radiotherapy. Educational difficulties of some degree occur in 75% of patients.
- Repeated surgery can also produce increased morbidity.
- Weight gain and increased appetite is a constant problem in a large number of patients and psychological input is often necessary. Excess weight, in turn, leads to an increase in morbidity and even mortality.
- Significant visual loss also impinges on quality of life.

Prognosis

- Overall survival at 10 and 20 years is around 80–90%, but progression-free survival is lower (65–70%). This is, however, dependent on the type of treatment, with those having received radiotherapy having lower rates of progression.
- The main cost of this tumour relates to frequent morbidity (Long-term effects 📖 p.532).

Intracranial germ cell tumours

Intracranial germ cell tumours are rare (10% of paediatric GCTs). Like their extracranial counterparts, they are a heterogeneous group of tumours comprising benign and malignant subtypes with single tumours often containing more than one subtype. Whilst they are histologically similar to their extracranial counterparts, their position dictates a different approach in terms of surgery, chemotherapy, and the use of radiotherapy.

Epidemiology

- 0.4–3.4% of primary paediatric CNS tumours in Western countries.
- 5–8 times more common in Japan and Far East (11% of CNS tumours).
- Overall male:female ratio is 2:1:
  - male predominance higher for non-germinoma;
  - in germinoma, male predominance confined to pineal tumours, whilst suprasellar germinoma is commoner in females.
- Peak incidence around puberty (10–12 years old):
  - mature and immature teratomas are usually seen in neonates and infants;
  - malignant germ cell tumours exceptional under 5 years age;
  - 90% diagnosed before 20 years age.

Presentation

Germ cell tumours should always be suspected in cases of midline intracranial tumours, particularly at suprasellar or pineal sites. Germ cell tumours may present in a number of ways, with signs and symptoms being determined by the site and histology of the tumour.

- The length of the symptoms is determined by the tumour histology, non-germinoma having a shorter history. Germinoma can be very indolent with an endocrine history of many months.
- Pineal tumours usually present as neurosurgical emergencies with raised intracranial pressure and Parinaud syndrome (paralysis of upward gaze). This is due to invasion of the tectal plate and involvement of the superior colliculus.
- Suprasellar germ cell tumours present with endocrine symptoms (often diabetes insipidus over months or short stature secondary to growth hormone deficiency), visual field loss and occasionally with significant weight loss (diencephalic syndrome).
- Secretion of human chorionic gonadotrophin (β-HCG) may stimulate the LH receptor and result in precocious puberty.
- Other rarer sites (basal ganglia) may present with seizures or focal neurological signs
- Spinal metastases may present with symptoms of spinal cord dysfunction.
- 5–10% of tumours are bifocal (pineal and suprasellar) at diagnosis.

Histology of germ cell tumours

Germ cell tumours comprise several histological sub-types including teratomas and malignant histiotypes. Several components may be mixed in one tumour.

- Teratomas are either mature (grade 0) or immature (grades 1–3).
- Malignant germ cell tumours include germinoma, embryonal carcinoma, yolk sac tumour, and choriocarcinoma. They are often grouped as germinoma and non-germinoma for treatment purposes in CNS tumours.
- Approximately 50% of CNS germ cell tumours are germinomas.
- Tumour markers – it is a characteristic of GCTs that several sub-types secrete tumour markers which may aid diagnosis (Extracranial germ cell tumours 📖 pp.485–489).
  - α-fetoprotein (AFP) is secreted by yolk sac tumour, in small amounts by some embryonal carcinomas and occasionally by immature teratoma;
  - β-HCG is secreted by choriocarcinoma and to a lesser extent by some germinomas;
  - the implications of β-HCG secretion by germinomas is unclear – some groups suggest it may imply a less good prognosis;
  - in current European protocols, a level of AFP >25ng/mL and/or HCG >50IU/L is used to define non-germinomatous tumours, where biopsy is not required for diagnosis;
  - in CNS germ cell tumours, markers should be measured in serum and CSF at diagnosis. A small percentage of non-germinomatous tumours only have positive markers in the CSF.

Biology

- The biology of GCTs continues to be researched.
- Emerging evidence of differences between adult and paediatric GCTs and different histologies:
  - *early childhood* – tumours usually diploid or tetraploid, invariably yolk sac sub-type, losses on 1p, 4 and 6q and gain on 3p, gain of 12p11 also seen, but less frequently than in adults;
  - *adolescence and adult* – tumours often aneuploid, frequent gain of 12p (50–80% cases), variable loss on 11, 13 and 18, and gain on 1, 7, 8, 21 and X.

Diagnosis

For an initial approach to a child thought to have a newly diagnosed brain tumour see Initial diagnosis of brain tumours, Pineal, suprasellar, and atypical tumours 📖 pp.60–61; see Fig. 39.14)

- If a germ cell tumour is suspected on neuroimaging, due to a midline site or a heterogeneous appearance, then germ cell markers must be checked prior to any biopsy.
- CSF diversion may be necessary urgently. Third ventriculostomy is often appropriate. This can often be combined with CSF sampling for cytology and measurement of CSF markers. If serum markers are negative a biopsy can be done at the same time.
- If tumour markers show β-HCG >50IU/L or AFP >25ng/mL, the diagnosis of a non-germinomatous germ cell tumour can be made and biopsy should not be performed.
- Prior to biopsy it is important to image the whole CNS to exclude metastatic disease.
- Initial resection is never indicated for either germinoma or non-germinoma.
- Teratomas (mature and immature) do not secrete markers, have a typical MRI appearance and do need excision, or biopsy followed by excision.
- Endocrine consultation should be arranged at diagnosis to assess possible endocrinopathies, and to advise on hormone replacement and fluid/electrolyte management in the presence of diabetes insipidus.

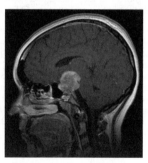

Fig. 39.14 Suprasellar secreting germ cell tumour.

Treatment

- Treatment is dependent on the type of germ cell tumour.
    - Teratomas should be resected if possible. Immature teratomas may be more likely to regrow. The role of chemotherapy and radiotherapy is unclear.
    - Germinomas are very sensitive to therapy. These tumours can be treated with craniospinal radiotherapy (24Gy) and a tumour boost (40Gy), with whole ventricular radiotherapy and a tumour boost, or with a combined chemotherapy and radiotherapy approach. All seem equally effective for localized tumours and depend on the treatment protocol used. Resection of the tumour does not improve the outcome and should be avoided.
    - For non-germinomatous germ cell tumours, a combination of chemotherapy followed by surgical resection of any residual lesion and then involved field radiotherapy is used (craniospinal radiotherapy for metastatic disease).
    - Tumour response can be monitored by following tumour marker levels.
    - Chemotherapy for germinoma and non-germinoma should include a platinum drug.
- Hormonal deficiencies usually predate the diagnosis and there is a high risk of pituitary hormone deficiencies developing subsequently.
- Late adverse effects of chemotherapy may occur, especially ototoxicity and nephrotoxicty in those receiving cisplatin and/or ifosfamide.

Outcome

- After the neonatal period, mature teratoma has an excellent outcome if total resection is possible. In newborns these tumours are often massive and fatal.
- Immature teratoma does well if completely resected, but grade 3 (higher grade) or incompletely resected tumours have at least a 20% risk of relapse.
- Germinomas (localized and metastatic) have a survival of 95% if treated with radiotherapy and 86% treated with combination therapy in the recent SIOP CNS GCT 96 protocol. These outcomes were not statistically different.
- Non-germinomatous germ cell tumours have a survival rate of approximately 70% provided that residual disease can be resected. Those with metastatic disease have an equivalent outcome, but require craniospinal radiotherapy.

Brainstem glioma

Brainstem gliomas constitute 8–15% of CNS tumours. Occur more commonly in mid/late childhood and have no gender predominance. The brain stem is taken to include the thalamus, midbrain, pons, and medulla.

Presentation

- Cranial nerve dysfunction dependant on level of tumour, e.g. facial weakness (VII), diplopia (III and/or IV and/or VI), facial sensory loss (V), dysphagia, dysarthria, drooling.
- Other eyes signs, e.g. dysconjugate gaze.
- Pyramidal signs, i.e. limb weakness.
- Raised intracranial pressure is rare, but headache and vomiting may occur.
- Length of history gives a clue about whether the tumour is fast or slow growing
- Can be relatively insidious and difficult to diagnose.
- Patients with NF1 are predisposed to astrocytic tumours and, although these usually occur in the optic chiasm/hypothalamus, they may be seen in the brainstem.

Diagnosis

- High index of suspicion required.
- MRI scan is the preferred option since CT does not give a good view of the brainstem. However, CT is a reasonable screening tool. IV contrast should always be given.
- **Thalamic tumours:** High grade gliomas, low grade gliomas.
- **Midbrain tumours:** usually tectal plate gliomas. Usually small low grade astrocytomas, often present with hydrocephalus. No need for biopsy unless clinical behaviour unusual. Occasionally germ cell tumours occur in midbrain – if clinical behaviour atypical of glioma, check AFP and HCG (may be raised in a germ cell tumour).
- **Diffuse intrinsic pontine gliomas** (DPG): diagnosis can be made on MRI alone (Fig. 39.15a), but increasingly a biopsy is performed to understand the biology and clinical behaviour. Usually behave in a high grade manner with rapid progression. Resection is not possible. Occasionally, hydrocephalus may require CSF diversion.
- Focal medullary or pontine tumours are often low grade gliomas and more amenable to treatment.
- Cervicomedullary tumours are usually focal and low grade gliomas (Fig. 39.15b).

Treatment

- **Tectal plate gliomas:** usually 'watch and wait' as the tumour is unlikely to increase in size. CSF diversion is often necessary. If progression occurs, biopsy is advisable. If treatment is necessary, either chemotherapy or radiotherapy is used, depending on the patient's age (currently in Europe children below 8 years of age receive chemotherapy and above this age radiotherapy).
- **Diffuse pontine glioma:** no effective curative treatment is possible. Radiotherapy is the best palliative treatment. Various chemotherapeutic

strategies have been tried, so far unsuccessfully. Hyperfractionated radiotherapy has not shown any advantage over conventional radiotherapy. Targeted biological therapies are being considered as best way forward.

- **Focal tumours**: may be amenable to resection. This depends on the risk of morbidity. Usually they are low grade, so it is feasible to follow a 'watch and wait' strategy. If further treatment is necessary (or if the tumour is unresectable), either chemotherapy or radiotherapy depending on age and NF1 status (age criteria as above, NF-1 patients receive chemotherapy as a preference). At a minimum, biopsy should be performed in all these tumours (to determine the grade and type).
- Steroids are often needed as an adjunct to treatment to reduce local swelling. Short courses are considered best as morbidity is then much lower. However, some patients, especially those with diffuse pontine gliomas, become steroid-dependant and require prolonged low dose use.

Outcome

- Tectal plate tumours and other low grade gliomas have a good outcome. The site and treatment determines long-term morbidity (mainly neurological and intellectual). Those treated with surgery alone usually have best outcome.
- High grade pontine and other brainstem tumours have a very poor outlook. Diffuse pontine gliomas <1% survival, with mean duration of survival of approximately 9 months.

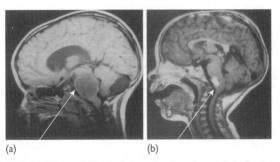

(a)   (b)

Fig. 39.15 (a) MRI scan of diffuse intrinsic pontine glioma (arrowed). (b). Focal tumour of cervico-medullary junction (arrowed).

Spinal cord tumours

Spinal cord tumours are rare in childhood, accounting for approximately 4% of childhood CNS tumours. Tumours are either intradural or extradural, whilst intradural tumours are either intra- or extramedullary. A high index of suspicion is needed, remembering that back pain in children is rare and almost always warrants imaging.

Site of spinal tumours

Intradural

Intramedullary

- *Astrocytoma*:
- *ependymoma* – classic or myxopapillary;
- *lipoma*.

Extramedullary:

- *primitive neuroectodermal tumour* (PNET) – usually a metastasis from medulloblastoma or supratentorial PNET;
- *ependymoma* – metastasis;
- *germ cell tumour* – germinomas or secreting germ cell tumours;
- *meningioma*;
- *benign tumour* – dermoid or vascular abnormality.

Extradural

- *Neuroblastoma*.
- *Sarcoma*.
- *Metastasic disease*.
- *Lymphoma*.
- *Other*.

Clinical presentation

- Pain is the major presenting symptom, often waking the child at night. Children with persistent back pain should always have MRI imaging.
- Neck stiffness and torticollis may be presenting symptom in upper spinal cord tumours.
- Problems in walking and stiffness predominate in lower spinal cord lesions.
- Scoliosis or kyphoscoliosis may be present (especially in NF1). All children with scoliosis should have a spinal MRI. CT imaging or plain X-rays are not adequate.
- Clinical evaluation should include a careful search for neurological symptoms (including bowel and bladder dysfunction) and signs.

Diagnosis

- Diagnosis is made by clinical suspicion and MRI scan (Fig. 39.16) followed by biopsy if appropriate.
- Further investigation is determined by appearance of the lesion and the likely diagnosis (e.g. stage IV neuroblastoma diagnosed by raised catecholamines and bone marrow infiltration and a typical MRI scan may be treated with chemotherapy and dexamethasone without an initial biopsy).
- Biopsy is usually required and, if possible, resection in primary tumours.

Treatment and outcome

Treatment and outcome vary with the diagnosis (covered under individual tumour types elsewhere in this book).

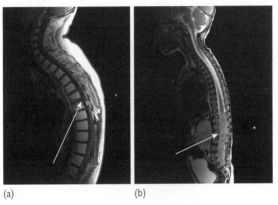

(a)　　　　　　　　　　(b)

Fig. 39.16 (a) Glioma of upper spinal cord (arrowed). (b) Neuroblastoma with intraspinal extension compressing spinal cord (arrowed).

Rare central nervous system tumours

The tumours mentioned below are unlikely to be seen outside paediatric neuro-oncology centres. Most present in the same way as other CNS tumours. The list below is not exhaustive, but covers the most common of the rare tumours.

Ganglioglioma

Gangliogliomas and ganglioneuromas account for about 4–5% of paediatric CNS tumours and occur at a median age of 10 years, although they may occur at any age. These tumours are differentiated, and have both neuronal and glial elements.

Presentation
- Slow growing from nerve cells.
- Temporal region most common, but may occur almost anywhere else in CNS.
- Presentation depends on site, but focal seizures predominate in supratentorial tumours. These may be longstanding and difficult to control.
- May have learning disability and behaviour problems.

Diagnosis
- Usually well circumscribed cystic lesions on MRI and CT (Fig. 39.17).
- Calcification seen in about 25% (seen best on CT).
- Midline and hemispheric gangliogliomas may appear histologically different. Variation in histological features does not correlate with outcome.

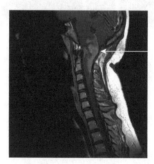

Fig. 39.17 Ganglioglioma of brainstem and upper cervical cord (arrowed).

Treatment
- Complete excision is best treatment.
- Second look surgery should be contemplated as outlook is better with complete excision.
- Brain stem gangliogliomas have a worse prognosis due to inability to resect the tumour.
- Radiotherapy is usually used for recurrent or progressive disease.
- No evidence of benefit from chemotherapy.

Outcome
The outlook is usually good, but worse for those with unresectable tumours.

Dysembryoplastic neuroepithelial tumours

Usually occur in 2nd and 3rd decades of life. Incidence unclear, but probably around 1–3% of childhood (CNS) tumours. They are also mixed neuroglial tumours.

Presentation
- Usually supratentorial.
- Classically present with epilepsy (usually focal and often intractable).
- Affect males more commonly than females.

Diagnosis
- Usually temporal lobe, well circumscribed lesions with no mass effect.
- Usually don't enhance.
- Histologically have a multi-nodular architecture often with elements of cortical dysplasia.

Treatment
- Can usually be completely resected.
- Even if unable to perform complete resection, a 'watch and wait' strategy is usually best due to their benign nature.
- Resection often cures the epilepsy, but not always.

Outcome
Generally excellent.

Oligodendroglioma

These tumours are more common in adults, but do occur in children (about 1% of childhood CNS tumours). Usually occur supratentorially. Infiltrative, but well differentiated.

Presentation
- Seizures are most common presentation.
- Raised intracranial pressure is the other common presenting feature.
- History often prolonged before diagnosis.

Diagnosis
- About 50% lesions are calcified.
- Usually low-density infiltrative lesions found supratentorially, but may be found anywhere in CNS.
- Posterior fossa tumours are more likely to have leptomeningeal dissemination.
- Either well differentiated WHO grade 2 lesions or anaplastic grade 3.
- OLIG2 marker may help in diagnosis of these tumours.
- 1p or 19q loss of heterozygosity is felt to imply improved treatment outcome as they render tumours more sensitive to chemotherapy.

Treatment.
- Complete resection is best treatment.
- Chemotherapy is useful in adults with 1p or 19q loss (procarbazine, lomustine, vincristine), but its benefit is not as clear in children as in adults.
- Radiotherapy is often used even in Grade II tumours. Some advocate craniospinal radiotherapy for posterior fossa tumours as they often have leptomeningeal spread.

Outcome.
- Grade 3 tumours have a considerably worse outcome in children.
- Posterior fossa tumours also have a worse outcome.

Pleomorphic xanthoastrocytoma

Rare tumour of childhood that usually occurs in young people in 2nd decade of life. Exact incidence unknown, but thought to be <1% of CNS tumours of childhood

Presentation
- Usually present with fits, raised intracranial pressure, or focal neurological deficits.
- Most common site is temporoparietal region, often superficial.

Diagnosis
- Mixed neuroglial tumours.
- MRI usually demonstrates superficial supratentorial tumour, which strongly enhances with contrast.
- Histologically resemble glial tumours (GFAP +ve), also contain a lot of lipid, hence yellow appearance. Usually have features of desmoplasia and neuronal differentiation.

Treatment
- Best treatment is complete surgical resection.
- May use pre-operative chemotherapy to reduce size first.
- If there is recurrence or inability to remove the tumour, then low grade glioma treatment should be offered (see Low grade glioma 📖 pp.512–515).

Outcome.
Long-term outcome thought to be very good (about 90% survival), but occasionally these tumours behave aggressively.

Gliomatosis cerebri

This refers to a separate disease entity that consists of proliferation of glial cells diffusely through the central nervous system, but particularly the cerebrum. There are two types of this disease:

- Type I is not associated with an obvious tumour mass (classic type).
- Type II is associated with a tumour mass.

Usually occurs in adults (median 40–50 years), but can occur at any age.

Presentation

- The presentation varies widely and may include many symptoms, including seizures, headache, nausea, vomiting, and focal neurological signs.
- Less common symptoms include sensory and visual changes, and pain.

Diagnosis

- Diagnosis is often delayed.
- MRI is the best way to detect suspected gliomatosis cerebri. Shows high signal intensity on T2 imaging.
- Biopsy should be performed (often performed stereotactically) to confirm the diagnosis.
- Histologically neoplastic glial cells that infiltrate brain with very little destruction of other structures are seen. Ki67 stationing is variable and does not seem to be related to prognosis.

Treatment

- CSF diversion may be necessary for associated hydrocephalus.
- Whole brain radiotherapy is thought to have some survival advantage.
- Chemotherapy has not yet been shown to be of any value.

Outcome

The prognosis is poor with most patients dying of their disease within the first year.

Hypothalmic hamartomas

- These are not tumours, although often referred as such (Fig. 39.18). They are congenital malformations of ectopic neurones and may present in a number of ways.
- The most common presenting features are gelastic seizures and/or precocious puberty.
- Although medical control of symptoms is possible, deterioration often occurs over time. Surgical removal may be attempted, often with good results.

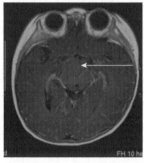

Fig. 39.18 Hypothalamic hamartoma in axial T1 view (arrowed).

Meningiomas

These account for about 1–2% of childhood CNS tumours. They tend to occur either in the first few years of life, when they are usually malignant, or in the over 10-year age group, when they tend to behave more like adult meningiomas.

Presentation

- There is no gender preponderance in children unlike adults, where females are more likely (70%) to have a meningioma.
- Presentation is varied, with the most common symptoms including headache, vomiting, and focal neurological deficits. Other symptoms include deafness and ataxia.
- Optic nerve sheath meningiomas may present with proptosis and visual disturbances (Fig. 39.19).
- Meningiomas are most commonly supratentorial.
- May be associated with NF1 and NF2.

Diagnosis

- MRI is the best imaging modality.
- Meningiomas are usually superficial (cerebral hemispheres), appear attached to the dura, enhance strongly, and may be calcified (best seen on CT scan).
- There are many histological subtypes, but their relation to prognosis is not well established.
- Malignant meningiomas are not well classified at the current time.

Treatment
- Complete surgical resection is the treatment of choice. If possible second look surgery should be contemplated.
- Intraoperative bleeding is the major complication.
- For recurrent tumours, radiotherapy should be considered.
- Chemotherapy should be considered for infants where radiotherapy is contraindicated.

Outcome
- Prognosis is poor for infant tumours.
- Prognosis is good (about 75% at 5 years) for tumours in older children.

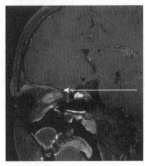

Fig. 39.19 Meningioma of optic nerve (arrowed).

Chordoma

These are mainly skull base or lower spinal cord tumours that arise from the developmental notochord. These are more common in adults and in males. Tend to be slow growing.

Presentation

- Depends on site of tumour. Brainstem signs (cranial nerves, especially VI) and hydrocephalus are most common for skull base tumours and lower spinal cord neurological signs for spinal cord lesions.
- They can also occur in vertebral and extra-axial sites and may metastasize (to lung and bones).
- History often prolonged, related to invasion of tumour or pressure on adjoining structures.

Diagnosis and treatment

- CT and preferably MRI scans suggest the diagnosis, but histological confirmation is necessary (Fig. 39.20).
- Surgery is the treatment of choice. Total removal is usually not possible, but is associated with a better outcome.
- Radiotherapy plays a useful role. Proton beam radiotherapy is thought to give the best local control.
- Chemotherapy has also been used, mainly anthracyclines and ifosfamide. This has also been used for pre-operative treatment in order to maximize the resection as long as there is no risk of further neurological deterioration.
- Histologically, classical and atypical (more sarcomatoid in appearance) variants seen.

Outcome

About half of patients are still alive with some control of the tumour at 10 years. The tumour is very slow growing and difficult to remove so often only local control is possible.

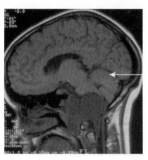

Fig. 39.20 Large clival chordoma (arrowed).

Pituitary tumours

Pituitary adenomas are the most common pituitary tumour in childhood accounting for about 3% of childhood CNS tumours. Majority of these tumours are hormone-secreting, whilst chromophobe adenomas (non-secreting) account for only 5% in children. The vast majority of pituitary tumours present after the age of 12 years. Prolactimomas (Fig. 39.21) account for 50% of childhood pituitary tumours.

Presentation

- Symptoms related to pressure on surrounding structures or secretion (or deficiency) of excess (or lack) of hormone.
- Headaches, visual disturbances (including field defects) are most common.
- Prolactin-secreting tumours may result in galactorrhorea.
- Adrenal insufficiency, thyroid insufficiency, and growth hormone insufficiency may be presenting features due to compression of pituitary and subsequent lack of hormone production.
- Prolactinomas are associated with McCune–Albright syndrome (*café-au-lait* spots, precocious puberty, polcystic ovaries), as well as MEN-1 (multiple endocrine neoplasia – pituitary, parathyroid and pancreatic islet cell neoplasms). Excess hormone production resulting in syndromes such as gigantism is very rare.

Diagnosis

- Diagnosis is best made by MRI scanning after clinical suspicion is raised.
- Serum prolactin levels should always be measured prior to surgery since surgery is not essential for prolactinomas.
- A full endocrine work-up should be considered prior to surgery.

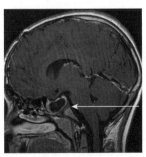

Fig. 39.21 Prolactinoma (arrowed).

Treatment

- Surgery for non-prolactinomas is considered the treatment of choice. Usually a trans-sphenoidal route is chosen, but sometimes this approach is not advised, especially for tumours that extend superiorly or are large in size.
- Prolactinomas are usually treated with ergot-dopamine agonist analogues (such as cabergoline, 1–2 doses per week orally), but

occasionally surgery is required for decompression, especially if there is an acute threat to vision.

- Growth hormone secreting tumours may also be treated with somatostatin analogues.
- With all pituitary tumours in childhood and adolescence, urgent evaluation by a paediatric endocrinologist is required.
- Radiotherapy may be used for recurrent tumours.

Outcome

- Outcome is good in terms of survival, although there is often morbidity associated with endocrine dysfunction.
- Microadenomas have a operative cure rate of about 70%, whereas macroadenomas have an operative cure rate of about 33%.

Section 11

Other conditions

Histiocytosis

Histiocytes are tissue cells of monocyte/macrophage lineage that can have both antigen-presenting (dendritic) and phagocytic phenotypes. Dysregulated histiocytic function results in a clinically heterogeneous group of diseases that is difficult to put into a single comprehensive classification. However, for practical purposes they can be grouped as:

- **Langerhans cell histiocytosis** [LCH; multisystem (MS), or single system (SS)].
- Non-Langerhans cell histiocytoses (JXG family or non-JXG family).
- Haemophagocytic lymphohistiocytosis (congenital or acquired).
- Malignant histiocytoses (leukaemia or sarcoma).

Langerhans cell histiocytosis

Including all presentations of LCH, there are around 5 per million affected children in the UK annually. Normal Langerhans cells are part of the wider dendritic cell family and sit in the epidermis, where they monitor and ingest invading organisms. Whilst digesting these foreign proteins they migrate to lymph nodes where they present this processed antigen to other immune cells. The various manifestations of LCH are due to a clonal, but essentially reactive, possibly T cell driven, expansion of Langerhans-like dendritic cell precursors (LCH cells) affecting a diverse variety of organs.

Table 40.1 Disease systems, manifestations, and investigations required

System	Manifestation	Investigations
Skin	Recalcitrant eczema	Biopsy
Bone	Eosinophilic granuloma	Biopsy, age-appropriate, skeletal survey, CT ± MRI, craniofacial bones
Lymph nodes	Lymphadenopathy	Biopsy
Intestine	Malabsorption	Biopsy
Posterior pituitary	Diabetes insipidus	MRI
Lung	Honeycomb lung	CXR, high resolution CT (HRCT), bronchoalveolar lavage, (BAL) or biopsy
Liver	Sclerosing cholangitis	LFTs, clotting, US, MRI, biopsy
Bone marrow	Cytopenias	Biopsy
Spleen	Splenomegaly	Ultrasound

Presentation

The disease manifests in one or more of the systems above (Table 40.1).

MS disease that includes involvement of the lungs, liver, spleen, or bone marrow (described as risk organ positive, RO+) usually occurs in infancy and carries a potentially grave prognosis. Fortunately, it is rare with an annual incidence in UK children of less than 0.5 per million. This group commonly present with a history of unusual 'eczema' and failure to thrive and can rapidly progress to multisystem failure.

MS disease not involving a risk organ (risk organ negative, RO–) is rarely fatal, but like single system (SS) disease, requires treatment to reverse the acute problem and limit late sequelae, especially those resulting from multiple chronic reactivations of bony disease.

SS bony lesions tend to present with musculoskeletal pain or visible lumps. Typical presentations in skin include cradle cap and chronic aural discharge.

A characteristic late and severe neurodegenerative syndrome has been recognized in some patients. Its aetiology is unknown, and preventive strategies and treatment have not been systematically evaluated. It is fortunately rare.

Diagnosis

A careful history and examination often gives clues about which systems are, or have been, involved with LCH. Ideally, affected tissue is biopsied and the typical morphological appearance found. Electron microscopy for Birbeck granules is now rarely performed. Definitive confirmation relies on the immunohistochemical demonstration of CD1a or the Birbeck granule-associated protein langerin (CD207) on the LCH cells. LCH affecting the odontoid peg or the posterior pituitary gland may not be amenable to biopsy requiring the diagnosis to be made on suspicion of LCH and exclusion of alternative diagnoses.

Investigations

- Affected skin is generally easy to biopsy and will establish the diagnosis.
- The presence of a bony lesion suggestive of LCH should lead to an age-appropriate skeletal survey. A bone scan may not identify early lesions. There is exciting early data regarding the value of positron emission tomography (PET) scanning at diagnosis and for response evaluation.
  If the only manifestation is an isolated and typical lytic lesion, and there is no suspicion of a malignant bone tumour, biopsy with curettage as a definitive therapy is appropriate. For involvement of craniofacial bones, CT and MRI are useful to look at areas of bony involvement and the degree of soft tissue extension.
- SS disease involving lymph nodes or the intestine is rare. In the context of MS disease, it is generally not necessary to perform a biopsy, except to exclude opportunistic infection in a node or confirm severe protein losing enteropathy.
- The MRI appearance of LCH involvement of the posterior pituitary is characteristic with thickening of the stalk and absence of the vasopressin bright spot. With careful exclusion of other differential diagnoses and close follow up with regular MRI, biopsy can be avoided.

- SS disease affecting the lungs is rare and the diagnosis will normally require biopsy. In MS disease the presence of typical HRCT changes is generally enough to establish pulmonary disease, but opportunistic infection may need exclusion by BAL. As a screening test in recently diagnosed cases of LCH, a normal CXR is adequate to exclude pulmonary involvement.
- At diagnosis the liver may be directly involved by LCH cells causing sclerosing cholangitis, which may eventually progress to biliary cirrhosis. Normal clotting and LFTs (especially γGT) are adequate to exclude hepatic involvement.
- Bone marrow involvement can be assumed in recently diagnosed cases with significant, otherwise unexplained cytopenias, even if an aspirate and biopsy fail to show infiltration with CD1a + LCH cells.
- Splenic dysfunction is difficult to demonstrate and involvement can be assumed if there is significant enlargement in the absence of any other possible causes.

Treatment

Approximately half the cases occurring in UK children have a SS unifocal bony lesion, previously known as an eosinophilic granuloma. Commonly, these will resolve after biopsy and of those that do not, many respond to further curettage and intra-lesional steroids.

For MS disease, International Histiocyte Society protocols (LCH I–III completed, IV in preparation) provide detailed information on diagnostic criteria, staging, first line of treatment (in the context of randomized studies), and response evaluation. The strategies are described in outline below:

- **MS RO+ disease:** intensive induction therapy with vinblastine/prednisolone (VBL/Pred) for up to 12 weeks is recommended. If the patient's disease progresses despite this, intensive acute myeloid leukaemia (AML)-type chemotherapy, with the option of allogeneic haemopoieic stem cell transplantation (HSCT), is recommended. For responders, maintenance to one year with VBL/Pred and 6-mercaptopurine (6MP) is currently recommended.
- **MS RO– disease:** induction therapy with VBL/Pred for 6 weeks followed to a total of 1 year's maintenance treatment with VBL/Pred is currently recommended. SS multifocal bone (MFB) and some special site disease (e.g. odontoid peg) can also be treated with this approach.
- Reactivation of bony lesions is a major problem that causes acute dysfunction and may result in chronic deformity. Unlike malignancy, however, the disease does not become resistant to therapy and will eventually burn out. It appears that the longer maintenance therapy is continued the lower the reactivation rate becomes.

Progression with involvement of new organs in LCH is unpredictable. In general, patients with DI do not regain any useful function with systemic therapy, so in cases where this is the only site of involvement there is no clear rationale for LCH treatment. There is continued discussion concerning whether using local treatment alone for base of skull and orbital lesions may predispose to subsequent pituitary problems, supporting an argument for systemic therapy.

Non-Langerhans cell histiocytosis (JXG family or non-JXG family)

'Non-LCH' is similar to other 'non'-based classifications in that it includes a wide diversity of histiocytic disorders that have different presentations, treatment requirements and outcomes. Broadly speaking, they fall into a group with biology resembling JXG and those that do not!

Haemophagocytic lymphohistiocytosis (congenital or acquired)

Haemophagocytic lymphohistiocytosis (HLH) is a process in which phago-cytic histiocytes inappropriately engulf and destroy normal peripheral blood, bone marrow precursor, and immune system cells. The process results from a failure of down-regulatory killer lymphocytes to turn off normal immune responses. This failure can be due to a single gene defect or occur as part of an acquired paraneoplastic or infection-associated dysregulation.

A defect in the gene coding the CD8 T cell and NK lymphocyte cyto-toxic pore-forming protein (perforin) has been recognized as an auto-somal recessive cause of congenital HLH. This deficiency leads to impairment of the cellular down-regulatory arm of the immune response. The uncontrolled proliferation of immune cells and cytokine production results in the pathological picture of extensive haemophagocytosis. This presents in early infancy as a systemically very unwell child with fever, hepatosplenomegaly with abnormal liver function, variable cytopenias and often severe cental nervous system (CNS) disturbance. The diagnosis is supported by the finding of haemophagocytosis in bone marrow, nodes or CSF, and a series of other laboratory abnormalities, including decreased NK function, raised soluble IL2 receptor (sCD25), hypertriglyceridaemia, hypofibrinogenaemia, and raised ferritin levels. Therapy is aimed at damping down the immune response with chemotherapy (etoposide) and ciclosporin or immunotherapy (ATG) until HSCT can be performed to replace the defective gene.

A superficially similar immune disorder can be acquired by older patients in the context of malignancy or infection. In these cases, immune suppression can be used, depending on the severity of the haemophagocy-tosis, whilst urgently treating the underlying cause.

Malignant histiocytoses (leukaemia or sarcoma)

Histiocyte lineage-related malignancies include chronic myelomonocytic leukaemia (CMML), some acute myeloid leukaemias (M4 and M5), and a variety of extremely rare dendritic, monocytic, and histiocytic sarcomas. Treatment of the leukaemias is along standard AML lines, although CMML is almost universally fatal without HSCT. Therapy for the sarcomas generally involves surgery with adjuvant chemo and radiotherapy.

Rare tumours

Rare tumours

Cancer is rare in childhood, compared to older age groups, affecting approximately 1 in 600 children during the first 15 years of life. However, some paediatric malignancies are so rare that even paediatric oncologists only encounter them once in their lifetime practice.

For this chapter, rare tumours in childhood are arbitrarily defined as those that have an age-standardized annual incidence (ASR) of less than one per million children in Great Britain. This chapter cannot cover all rare tumours in childhood, but will focus on those that only occur in children outside the central nervous system and currently have a poor prognosis. Also included is nasopharyngeal carcinoma, which more recently has had an improved prognosis, but still poses treatment challenges.

Nasopharyngeal carcinoma

- Most nasopharyngeal carcinomas (NPCs) in children and teenagers are of the undifferentiated type. Incidence of childhood NPC in western populations is generally low, but in parts of North Africa and the Middle East it can be as high as 2 per million.
- Epstein-Barr virus appears to be implicated in the aetiology of NPC.
- Survival is up to 90% in non-stage IV disease.

Presentation and staging

- Commonly presents with enlarged cervical lymph nodes, whilst symptoms related to the primary tumour (trismus, pain, nasal regurgitation) may occur, but are less common.
- Staging requires cross-sectional imaging of primary tumour – assessing local nodal spread, and the presence or not of skull base erosion, which is a poor prognostic factor.
- Metastatic spread is a poor prognostic factor. It requires assessment with CT scan of chest and skull base. Other poor prognostic factors include cranial nerve involvement.

Treatment

- Neoadjuvant chemotherapy with cisplatin and 5-fluourocil has improved significantly the survival of NPC in children, but most series have relatively small numbers.
- This is followed by radiotherapy to the primary and nodal disease with doses up to 60Gy.
- Some groups now routinely use immunotherapy with interferon after radiotherapy.
- Surgery other than biopsy has a very limited role.

Pleuropulmonary blastoma

- Occurs in the thorax almost exclusively in children younger than 5 years.
- 25% of cases occur in constitutional/familial settings in which the PPB patient themselves or younger family members have other dysplastic or neoplastic features.
- 3 main histopathological subtypes:
  - *Type I* – cystic tumours typically in infant;
  - *Type II* – solid and cystic areas;
  - *Type III* – purely solid.
- There may be progression from lung cysts through from Type I to II to III.

Presentation and staging

- Usually with respiratory symptoms.
- Cerebral metastases are more frequent than in other childhood sarcomas, hence CT head should be part of routine staging along with CT chest and bone scan.

Treatment

- PPB is commonly treated with soft tissue sarcoma protocols.
- Total surgical resection if possible is important and leads to an improved relapse-free survival.
- Chemotherapy may have a role in aiding surgical resection and as an adjuvant in preventing recurrence.
- The role of chemotherapy is more clearly defined in Type II and III disease.
- In small series from various national groups, sarcoma regimens seem to be useful including vincristine, actinomycin, ifosfamide, and anthracyclines.
- The International PPB registry continues to collect data to improve the understanding of its clinical behaviour and management.

Pancreatoblastoma

- Similarities to hepatoblastoma, often found in identical age group with similar morphology.
- Associated with Beckwith-Wiedemann syndrome.
- Plasma α-fetoprotein (AFP) often elevated.
- Overall, there is at least an 80% survival with a completely resected tumour
- Skeletal, hepatic and chest metastases herald a very poor prognosis.
- ASR 0.04.

Presentation and staging

- Usually present late with upper abdominal pain and mass.
- CT/MRI of abdomen and AFP.
- Full metastatic workup: CT chest, bone scan and bone marrow assessment.

Treatment

- Complete surgical excision with neo- or adjuvant chemotherapy leads to a good outcome.
- Chemotherapy regimens as for hepatoblastoma: cisplatinum and doxorubicin (PLADO) are most commonly used.

Extracranial malignant rhabdoid tumour

- Although less than 1% of childhood malignancies with an ASR 0.56 their poor prognosis results in a significant number of relapses and hence death.
- Reported at most anatomical sites, most commonly in the kidney.
- Most have a mutation of *INI1* gene (a tumour suppressor gene).

Presentation and staging

- Commonest site is kidney. Classic presentation of mass, haematuria, fever, and hypercalcaemia.
- Next most common site is liver.
- CT and MRI of primary site, including assessment of nodal drainage.
- Full metastatic work up is important: high rate of metastases including brain.
- Renal rhabdoids are staged as in Wilms' tumour. Other sites with TNM system. Outcome is 50% survival at best for localized completely resected renal rhaboids, but most patients are metastatic with an outcome of less than 25% survival.

Treatment

- Total surgical resection including nodes is important. Up-front surgery may explain significantly better outcome for localized disease.
- Not always possible at diagnosis to perform surgery therefore an attempt should be made to do so after neo-adjuvant chemotherapy.
- Traditionally, renal rhabdoids are treated on the Wilms' tumour protocol, but the outcome is poor particularly in Stage IV patients.
- Several recent case reports of survivors of Stage IV disease who have been treated with ICE (ifosfamide, carboplatin, etoposide), alternating with vincristine, cyclophosphamide and doxorubicin chemotherapy.
- This regimen has been adopted by most groups as a treatment regimen, with surgery for metastases and radiation to all sites of disease.
- Overall, less than 25% of patients survive.

Adrenocortical carcinoma

- Bimodal age distribution curve with a peak incidence at 3.5 and 57 years.
- ASR 0.24, but an unusually high incidence in Brazil for unknown reasons.
- Increased incidence of ACC in patient with isolated hemihypertrophy, Beckwith-Wiedemann syndrome, and Li-Fraumeni syndrome.
- In Li-Fraumeni, ACC occurs 100 times more frequently than would be expected and, hence, most children with ACC have germline P53 mutations and.
- However, this is not the case in Brazilian patients.

Presentation and staging

- Most cases in children and adolescents are hormone secreting with signs and symptoms of virilization.
- CT/MRI scan of abdomen and full metastatic work-up with CT chest and bone scan.
- 24h urinary profile of sex steroids and corticosteroids.
- Distinction between benign and malignant tumours is purely on size:
  - *Stage I* – small tumours <200cm³ behave benignly; accounts for two-thirds of tumours and has an excellent outcome;
  - *Stages II – IV* – larger and/or metastatic tumours behave malignantly; account for one-third of tumours and have a very poor prognosis.

Treatment

- Complete radical surgery is the treatment of choice and may be curative in small tumours.
- Survival is dismal if complete resection is not obtained.
- Patients with incomplete resection or metastatic disease seem to benefit from chemotherapy and mitotane.
- The combination of mitotane, cisplatinum, etoposide, and doxorubicin has become a standard regimen in children with ACC.

New treatment strategies

New treatment strategies

New treatment strategies

The modern management of paediatric haematological and solid cancers has evolved from the study of successive new treatments by clinical trials. This process is relevant for all modalities of treatment, including the evaluation of surgery, radiotherapy, chemotherapy, or any combination of these. However, most new treatment strategies currently concentrate on the development of new anti-cancer drugs.

Newer treatment strategies can be categorized as:
- Improved use of current drugs.
- New drugs [including targeted therapy acting against either the tumour itself or angiogenesis (new vessel formation that is the basis of growth and survival of most solid tumours), New treatment strategies, Drug development 📖 p.568].
- Immunotherapy (including monoclonal antibodies and vaccines).
- Radiotherapeutic advances (e.g. proton beam therapy, radioablation using antibodies as carriers).
- Others.

Oncology has entered a new era of targeted anti-cancer drugs, which are designed to attack cancer cells more specifically and offer the hope of not only being more effective, but also being less toxic than conventional chemotherapy. Examples of such drugs include bevacizumab (a monoclonal antibody targeting the tumour blood vessels) and erlotonib (a small molecule targeting the epidermal growth factor receptor, which is over-expressed in malignant glioma).

Drug development

The process of drug development in paediatric oncology includes the following steps:
- Target identification and validation.
- Drug discovery.
- Pre-clinical testing.
- Clinical testing.

Target identification and validation

Most conventional chemotherapy agents are relatively untargeted in their mechanism of action, and exhibit their anti-cancer activity by inhibiting cell division or DNA synthesis. Modern molecular biology techniques have allowed the identification of new specific anti-cancer targets, such as the fusion product *bcr-abl* that results from the Philadelphia chromosome in chronic myeloid leukaemia. Inhibition of this protein in the laboratory effectively kills CML cells, validating this targeted approach. The increasing knowledge of the differences between the normal human and cancer genome has lead to an explosion in possible new targets to study.

Drug discovery

In the past, most drugs were discovered by screening natural compounds or adapting existing drugs. With the identification of new targets a more rational drug design process is required, which involves candidate identification, synthesis, characterization, screening, and therapeutic efficacy assays. This results in a *lead compound*, which is taken forward for further evaluation. Most current new oncology drugs are either small molecules or monoclonal antibodies.

Pre-clinical testing

This essential non-clinical step in drug development aims to establish important safety and pharmacological data. This will include both *in vitro* (cell line) and *in vivo* (animal) testing to establish the pharmacokinetics (how the body handles the drug) and pharmacodynamics (how the drug affects the body/tumour) and will help to estimate a safe starting dose of the drug for clinical trials in humans. This information is critical to the development of a drug and,. along with the clinical study and manufacturing of all medicines, is regulated by a competent authority in each country (MHRA in the UK, FDA in the US) according to agreed standards known as the ICH guidelines.

- **MHRA:** Medicines and Healthcare Products Regulatory Agency.
- **FDA:** Food and Drug Administration.
- **ICH:** International Conference on Harmonization.

Clinical testing

The clinical testing of a new drug in humans is usually conducted in three phases, each with a different aim, endpoint and design.

- **Phase I trial:** the aim is to test the safety of a new treatment. This will include characterizing any side effects, especially any serious *dose limiting toxicities*. A safe dose that can be used in further trials is defined and often termed the *maximum tolerated dose*. The pharmacokinetics and pharmacodynamics in humans are also studied by taking biological samples such as blood, urine, and tumour biopsy. Phase I clinical trials involve only a small number of people (possibly as few as 15–20). In oncology these patients usually will have no other curative options to treat their cancer. If the treatment is considered safe in a phase I trial, it will progress to a phase II clinical trial.
- **Phase II trial:** the aim in these trials is to test the effectiveness of the new treatment, at least in the short term. Effective in the case of cancer could mean that the treatment shrinks the size of a tumour or leads to longer survival. These studies are larger (30–200 people). Phase II clinical trials also collect information about safety in this larger group of people. The new treatment must meet a defined effectiveness to move to Phase III.

- **Phase III trial:** the aim of this clinical trial is to test the new treatment in comparison to the best treatment currently in use. Although this can be done by comparing outcomes with those from historical data, the preferred method is to allocate patients to either the standard or the trial treatment by randomization. As phase III trials are looking at long-term treatment effects, they usually last for many years, and often several hundreds or thousands of patients will be involved in many different hospitals and countries. If successful a drug will be registered and marketed after the phase III trial for use as a standard anti-cancer therapy.

Clinical trial conduct

All clinical trials are governed by 'Good clinical practice (GCP)', which is a set of internationally recognized ethical and scientific quality requirements that must be observed when designing, conducting, recording, and reporting clinical trials that involve the participation of human subjects. GCP covers the following areas of trial conduct:

- Ethical and regulatory review and approval.
- Consent (informed consent backed by appropriate information).
- Drug supply and administration.
- Safety monitoring and reporting (pharmacovigilance).
- Training and responsibilities.

Anyone involved in the conduct of a clinical trial should ensure that they are familiar with GCP requirements and receive appropriate training to ensure compliance with the relevant standards.

Immunotherapy

- Newer therapies that are being developed include the use of monclonal antibodies. The first such antibody to find an established role was rituximab (anti-CD20) in non-Hodgkin lymphoma. In theory, monoclonal antibodies can be made against any tumour antigen.
- Radio-labelling of antibodies is also being explored. This can deliver very focal radiation to tumour cells. However, so far, this has not resulted in total ablation of tumours.
- Tumour vaccines have been used in trials, but there are several problems that remain to be overcome before effective vaccines become available for widespread use. The main problem is that tumour vaccines generally require T cell help to enable a sustained response, but T-cell receptors are deficient in most tumour cells.

New treatment strategies continue to be developed, but it is likely to take many years for these to enter routine clinical use.

Appendix 1

Parameter	1st day	0–1 days	1–7 days	7–14 days	14–28 days	1–2 months	2–3 months	3–6 months	6–24 months	2–6 years	6–12 years M	6–12 years F	12–18 years M	12–18 years F
Haemoglobin (g/dL)	13.5 19.5	14.5 22.5	13.5 21.5	12.5 20.5	10.0 18.0	9.0 14.0	9.5 13.5	10.5 13.5	11.5 13.5	11.5 15.5	13.0 16.0	12.0 16.0	13.5 17.5	12.0 16.0
RBC × 10^{12}/L	3.90 5.50	4.00 6.60	3.90 6.30	3.60 6.20	3.00 5.40	2.70 4.90	3.10 4.50	3.70 5.30	3.90 5.30	4.00 5.30	4.50 5.30	4.10 5.10	4.50 5.90	4.00 5.20
Hct	0.42 0.60	0.45 0.67	0.42 0.66	0.39 0.63	0.31 0.55	0.30 0.42	0.29 0.41	0.33 0.39	0.34 0.40	0.35 0.45	0.37 0.49	0.36 0.46	0.41 0.53	0.36 0.46
MCV (fl)	98 118	95.0 121	88 126	86 124	85 123	77 115	74 108	70 86	75 87	77 87	78 98	78 102	83 101	83 101
MCH (pg)	31.0 37.0	31.0 37.0	28.0 40.0	28.0 40.0	28.0 40.0	26.0 34.0	25.0 35.0	23.0 31.0	24.0 30.0	25.0 33.0	25.0 35.0	25.0 35.0	27.0 34.0	27.0 34.0
MCHC (g/dL)	30.0 36.0	29.0 37.0	28.0 38.0	29.0 38.0	29.0 37.0	29.0 37.0	30.0 36.0	30.0 36.0	31.0 37.0	31.0 37.0	31.0 37.0	31.0 37.0	31.0 37.0	31.0 37.0

Parameter	Day 1 Full tem	1–7 days	7 days–1 month	1–6 months	6 months–1 year	1–2 years	2–4 years	4–6 years	6–8 years	8–10 years	10–16 years	16–21 years
WBC × 10⁹/L	9.0	5.0	5.0	6.0	6.0	6.0	5.5	5.0	4.5	4.5	4.5	4.5
	30.0	21.0	19.5	17.5	17.5	17.0	15.5	14.5	13.5	13.5	13.0	11.0
Neutrophils	6.0	1.5	1.0	1.0	1.5	1.5	1.5	1.5	1.5	1.8	1.8	1.8
	26.0	10.0	9.0	8.5	8.5	8.5	8.5	8.0	8.0	8.0	8.0	7.7
lymphocyte	2.0	2.0	2.5	4.0	4.0	3.0	2.0	1.5	1.5	1.5	1.2	1.0
	11.0	17.0	16.5	13.5	10.5	9.5	8.0	7.0	6.8	6.5	5.2	4.8
Monocytes	0.5	0.3	0.7	0.7	0.7	0.7	0.7	0.7	0.2	0.2	0.2	0.2
	1.5	1.1	1.5	1.5	1.5	1.5	1.5	1.5	0.8	0.8	0.8	0.8
Eosinophils	0.1	0.2	0.3	0.3	0.3	0.3	0.3	0.3	0.04	0.04	0.04	0.04
	1.25	2.0	0.8	0.8	0.8	0.8	0.8	0.8	0.4	0.4	0.4	0.4
Basophils	0.0	0.0	0.0	0.0	0.0	0.0	0.0	0.0	0.0	0.0	0.0	0.0
	0.1	0.1	0.1	0.1	0.1	0.1	0.1	0.1	0.1	0.1	0.1	0.1
Plts × 10⁹/L	150	150	150	150	150	150	150	150	150	150	150	150
	450	450	450	450	450	450	450	450	450	450	450	450
RDW (%)	10.0	10.0	10.0	10.0	10.0	10.0	10.0	10.0	10.0	10.0	10.0	10.0
	14.0	14.0	14.0	14.0	14.0	14.0	14.0	14.0	14.0	14.0	14.0	14.0

Values are lower and upper reference ranges. Reference ranges are those used in Newcastle Hospitals NHS Trust but may vary from laboratory to laboratory.

Appendix 2

Blood

Sodium, serum

- **0–4 weeks:** 130–145mmol/L.
- **5 weeks–12 months:** 132–142mmol/L.
- **≥13 months:** as adult.
- **Adult:** 135–145mmol/L.

Potassium, serum

- **0–4 weeks:** 3.8–7.0mmol/L.
- **5 weeks–12 months:** 4.0–6.0mmol/L.
- **13 months–4 years:** 3.5–5.0 mmol/L.
- **≥5 years:** as adult.
- **Adult:** 3.4–5.0mmol/L.

Creatinine, serum

Age range	Male (µmol/L)	Female (µmol/L)
1st week of life	35–85	35–85
2nd week	35–80	35–80
3rd week	35–75	35–75
4th week	30–65	30–65
1 month–2 years	25–55	25–55
3–5 years	30–65	30–65
6–9 years	35–70	35–70
10–12 years	40–80	40–80
13–14 years	45–90	45–90
15–16 years	55–105	50–95
17–55 years	70–110	55–95

Urea, serum

- **0–8 weeks:** 1.3–5.4mmol/L.
- **9 weeks–2 years:** 1.8–7.5mmol/L.
- **≥3 years:** as adult.
- **Adult:**
  - *male –* 3.1–7.9mmol/L;
  - *female –* 2.5–6.4mmol/L.

Bicarbonate (CO_2 content), serum

- **0–4 weeks:** 14–32mmol/L.
- **5 weeks–3 years:** 15–28mmol/L.
- **4–8 years:** 20–30mmol/L.
- **≥9 years:** as adult.
- **Adult:** 22–30mmol/L.

Chloride, serum

- **0–12 weeks:** 95–112mmol/L.
- **≥13 weeks:** as adult.
- **Adult:** 96–106mmol/L.

Calcium (total and adjusted), serum

- **0–4 weeks:** 1.80–2.85mmol/L.
- **5 weeks–2 years:** 2.25–2.80mmol/L.
- **3–16 years:** 2.18–2.63mmol/L.
- **≥17 years:** as adult.
- **Adult:** 2.12–2.60mmol/L.

Phosphate, serum

- **0–4 weeks:** 1.20–2.75mmol/L.
- **1–11 months:** 1.10–2.30mmol/L.
- **12–24 months:** 1.10–2.00mmol/L.
- **2–12 years:** 1.10–1.85mmol/L.
- **13–15 years:** 0.90–1.70mmol/L.
- **≥16 years:** as adult.
- **Adult:** 0.80–1.44mmol/L.

Glucose, plasma

- **≥2 weeks:** as adult.
- Adult.

Fasting glucose
- Levels ≥7.0mmol/L are consistent with a diagnosis of diabetes.
- Levels between 6.1 and 7.0mmol/L reflect impaired glucose handling.

Random glucose
- Levels ≥11.1mmol/L are consistent with a diagnosis of diabetes.
- Levels between 7.9 and 11.1mmol/L reflect impaired glucose handling.

Urate, serum

- **0–12 months:** 0.10–0.50mmol/L.
- **≥13 months:** as adult.
- **Adult:**
    - *male* – 0.16–0.43mmol/L;
    - *female* – 0.09–0.36mmol/L.

LDH (lactate dehydrogenase), serum

- 0–4 weeks: <1000U/L.
- 5 weeks–12 months: <450U/L.
- 1–6 years: <375U/L.
- 7–12 years: <325U/L.
- 13–16 years: <275U/L.
- Adult (≥17 years): ≤215U/L.

Magnesium, serum

- **0–7 days:** 0.40–0.90mmol/L.
- **1 week–23 months:** 0.74–1.10mmol/L.
- **≥2 years:** as adult.
- **Adult:** 0.70–1.00mmol/L.

Protein (total), serum

- **0–4 weeks:** 50–70g/L.
- **5 weeks–6 months:** 52–72g/L.
- **7–12 months:** 56–76g/L.
- **13 months–10 years:** 60–82g/L.
- **≥11 years:** as adult.
- **Adult:** 58–78g/L.

Albumin, serum

- **0–12 weeks:** 30–45g/L.
- **13 weeks–2 years:** 34–50g/L.
- **3–16 years:** 38–53g/L.
- **≥17 years:** as adult.
- **Adult:** 34–50g/L.

Bilirubin (total), serum

- **Day 1:** <110µmol/L.
- **Day 2:** <150µmol/L.
- **3–6 days:** <170µmol/L.
- **7–14 days:** <80µmol/L.
- **15–21 days:** <50µmol/L.
- **22–28 days:** <30µmol/L.
- **≥1 month:** as adult.
- **Adult:** <19µmol/L.

ALT (alanine aminotransferase), serum

- 0–23 months: 3–50U/L.
- ≥24 months: as adult.
- Adult:
  - *male* – ≤45U/L;
  - *female* – ≤40U/L.

Alkaline phosphatase, serum

Age range	Male (U/L)	Female (U/L)
0–4 weeks	150–300	150–300
1 month–9 years	150–375	150–375
10 years	120–375	120–420
12 years	100–420	100–375
13–14 years	80–500	80–280
15 years	60–450	60–200
16 years	40–375	40–150
17 years	40–280	40–150
18 years	40–200	40–150
19 years	40–150	40–120
20 years	As adult	As adult
Adult	35–120	35–120

AST (aspartate aminotransferase), serum

- 0–6 months: 15–90U/L.
- 7 months–3 years: 20–60U/L.
- 4–6 years: 15–50U/L.
- ≥7: as adult.
- Adult: ≤40U/L.

Gamma–GT (γ–glutamyl transpeptidase), serum

- **0–4 weeks:** 0–240U/L.
- **5 weeks–16 weeks:** 0–145U/L.
- **≥17 weeks:** as adult.
- **Adult:**
  - *male* – ≤70U/L;
  - *female* – ≤50U/L

Cholesterol, serum

LDL cholesterol, serum

- **0–1 year:** lower than adult.
- **≥2 years:** as adult.
- **Adult:** desirable: less than 3.0mmol/L.

HDL cholesterol, serum

- **Up to 14 years age:**
  - *male* – slightly above adult range;
  - *female* – slightly below adult range.
- **About 14 years**: as adult.
- **Adult:**
  - *male* –1.0–1.5mmol/L;
  - *female* – 1.2–1.8mmol/L.

Triglycerides, serum

- As young adult (difficult to get fasting samples from young children to set ranges)
- Adult: 0.5–1.8mmol/L.

HbA1$_c$ (glycosylated haemoglobin), blood

- **Paediatric:** as adult.
- **Adult:**
  - *non–diabetic* – <6.1%.
  - *inadequate control* – greater than 7.5.

Serum α–fetoprotein (AFP), serum

Age (days)	Mean AFP (ng/mL)	AFP range (ng/mL)
0	41,687	9120–190,546
1	36,391	7943–165,959
2	31,769	6950–144,544
3	27,733	6026–125,893
4	24,210	5297–109,648
5	21,135	4624–96,605
6	18,450	4037–84,334
7	16,107	3524–73,621
8–14	9333	1480–58,887
15–21	3631	575–22,910
22–28	1396	316–6310
29–45	417	30–5754
46–60	178	16–1995
61–90	80	6–1045
91–120	36	3–417
121–150	20	2–216
151–180	13	1.25–129
181–720	8	0.8–87
>720	Normal range 0–10	

Human chorionic gonadotrophin (β–HCG), blood
Normal: 0–10IU/L.

Urine

Creatinine, urine

NB. Paediatric ranges are approximate figures, calculated using tables of average body weight.

- **0–4 weeks:** 0.2–0.6mmol/24h.
- **1–12 months:** 0.3–1.7mmol/24h.
- **13 months–4 years:** 0.9–3.3mmol/24h.
- **5–17 years:** 1.7–16.8mmol/24h.
- **Adult:**
  - *male* – 9.0–17.7mmol/24h;
  - *female* – 7.0–15.9mmol/24h.

Protein (total), urine

24h urine (g/24h)

- 1/3 adult level at birth.
- Gradual rise thereafter.
- **≥4 years:** as adult.
- **Adult:** < 0.10g/24h.

Random urine (mg/mmol creatinine)

- **≤2 years:** <56mg/mmol creatinine.
- **>2 years:** <20mg/mmol creatinine.

Catecholamines (includes noradrenaline, adrenaline, dopamine, HMMA (4–hydroxy–3–methoxy–mandelate),VMA (vanillylmandelic acid), urine.

HVA/creatinine, HMAA creatinine

- **0–2 years:** 3.5–12.0μmol/mmol creatinine.
- **3–5 years:** 2.0–6.5μmol/mmol creatinine.
- **6–9 years:** 1.8–5.0μmol/mmol creatinine.
- **10–15 years:** 1.0–4.0μmol/mmol creatinine.

Adrenaline

Adult: 0–10nmol/mmol creatinine.

Noradrenaline

Adult: 0–48nmol/mmol creatinine.

Dopamine

Adult: 0–300nmol/mmol creatinine.

Phosphate (urine)

24h urine
- **Paediatric:** similar to adult – 0.33–1.28mmol/kg/24h.
- Varies widely depending on diet.
- **Adult:** 15–50mmol/24h.

Random urine (mmol/mmol creatinine):
- **6–12 months:** 1.2–19.0mmol/mmol creatinine.
- **1 year:** 1.2–14.0mmol/mmol creatinine.
- **2 years:** 1.2–12.0 mmol/mmol creatinine.
- **3–4 years:** 1.2–8.0mmol/mmol creatinine.
- **5–6 years:** 1.2–5.0mmol/mmol creatinine.
- **7–9 years:** 1.2–3.6mmol/mmol creatinine.
- **10–13 years:** 0.8–3.2mmol/mmol creatinine.
- **14–17 years:** 0.8–2.7mmol/mmol creatinine.
- **Adult:** < 2.9mmol/mmol creatinine.

All values are lower and upper reference ranges

Reference ranges are those used in Newcastle upon Tyne Hospitals NHS Foundation Trust but may vary from laboratory to laboratory.

Useful websites for children, young adults, and parents

The following websites may be useful for children and young people with cancer and their family members. The list is not exhaustive, but it includes many important support organizations and websites. Some are broad in scope, covering cancer or leukaemia in general, whilst others focus on childhood malignancies.

www.acor.org/ped-onc/
American site. Lots of links to various other information. Easy to use. It is designed and run by parents of children with cancer for parents of children with cancer.

www.brainandspine.org
Information and leaflets in relation to brain and spinal tumours. Glossary of neurological terms. Link to 'Headstrong' website, which is a site specifically for children and young people with brain and spinal tumours. Also link to the 'All About ABI' website, which is a website dedicated to information for children and young people with acquired brain injuries.

www.braintumourtrust.co.uk
Samantha Dickson Brain Tumour Trust. UK based charity for those with brain tumours. Information, advice, on-line support group in relation to low grade gliomas, stories.

www.cancerbackup.org.uk
Cancer Backup and Macmillan have joined forces for this website. Information on childhood cancers and their treatment, advice, and suggestions. Online discussions and forums for chatting with others.

www.cancercounselling.org.uk
Provides telephone counselling service for those who have cancer and their families.

www.cancer.gov/search/cancer_literature
American site. A lot of medical articles in relation to cancer and its treatment – use search facility to find exactly what you are looking for.

www.cancerguide.org
Guide to help research the child's diagnosis, treatment etc.

www.cancerhelp.org.uk
The patient information part of Cancer Research UK website. Provides information about cancer and cancer care for people with cancer and their families. Includes a list of cancer support organizations.

www.cancerimprovement.nhs.uk/patinfopath
Follows a path through different stages of treatment and links with further information.

www.cancerindex.org/ccw
Children's Cancer Web with links to other information in UK and USA, including supports.

www.cancerinyoungadults-throughparentseyes.org
Information for parents around the specific issues associated with being an adolescent/young adult diagnosed with cancer.

www.cancerresearch.org.uk
Information about cancer, its treatments, trials, side effects. Also has a discussion forum.

www.cbituk.org
Child Brain Injury Trust. A charity offering support, information, and training on acquired brain injury in children.

www.cbtrc.org
Children's Brain Tumour Research Centre. Information regarding treatments for brain tumours and a good glossary of terms (go through 'research' in menu on left hand side and it is down at the bottom).

www.cclg.org.uk
Childhood Cancer and Leukaemia Group (CCLG): the national professional body responsible for the organization and management of children with cancer in the UK. Information on clinical trials, support groups, resources and advice for the family, and a good glossary of terms.

www.chect.org.uk
Childhood Eye Cancer Trust: support and information for those whose child is diagnosed with a retinoblastoma.

www.childcancer.org.uk
Has a wide range of publications that can be downloaded or ordered (generally free of charge) – part of CCLG site.

www.childhoodbraintumour.org
American site. Information and personal stories.

www.click4tic.org.uk
Teen information on cancer. Has basic information about cancer, information concerning feelings, body changes, practical issues, and a message board for teenagers and young adults.

www.clicsargent.org.uk
CLIC Sargent's website. Basic information on childhood cancers, information on CLIC Sargent's current campaigns and resources, and publications that can be downloaded or ordered (generally free of charge).

www.clicsargent.org.uk/Aboutchildhoodcancer/youth
'U Need 2 Know' website by CLIC Sargent specifically for teenagers and young adults with cancer. Has helpful hints, information around feelings and worries, about what is happening/the changes during treatment, goal setting and an online discussion forum and message boards.

www.fanconi.org
Support for families and young people with Fanconi anaemia, based in the USA.

www.fanconi.org.uk
UK and Ireland Fanconi Anaemia Family and Clinical Network, supported by the Fanconi Hope Charity. A new and very useful website.

www.gapsline.org.uk
Support network site and helpline for parents. Online support network.

www.hawc-co-uk.com
Helping Adolescents with Cancer, a site run by adolescents and young adults for adolescents and young adults.

www.jimmyteenstv.com
Information sharing site for teenagers with news, blogs and videos.

www.leukaemiacare.org.uk
A site for those effected by leukaemia, lymphoma, and allied blood disorders. Has information and booklets, message boards, clinical trials, and welfare and benefits advice.

www.naccpo.org.uk
Site with information and support for those children diagnosed with cancer/leukaemia

www.ncbi.nlm.nih.gov/PubMed
PubMed a site with medical articles in relation to cancer and its treatment.

www.nhsdirect.nhs.uk
General information on cancer types and treatments.

www.pasic.org.uk
Parents Association of Seriously Ill children.

www.royalmarsden.org/captchemo
Website for children with clear and detailed information.

www.siblinks.org
A network for young people who have a family member affected by cancer.

www.squirreltales.com
American site. Practical tips, encouragement, and humour for parents and families.

www.supersibs.org
American site for siblings of children diagnosed with cancer.

www.support-oscar.org
For brain and spinal tumours. Information, resources and weblinks.

www.teenagecancertrust.org
The website of the Teenage Cancer Trust (TCT). Information following diagnosis, other people's stories and information about events TCT are running for teenagers and young adults with cancer.

www.theaat.org.uk
Support for families and young people with aplastic anaemia, based in UK.

www.virtualtrials.com
Information about trials for brain tumour treatments.

www.wilmsineurope.net
Information and support for children diagnosed with Wilms' tumour.

www.winstonswish.org.uk
Winston's Wish, a charity that aims to help grieving children and their families. Information for parents/carers, schools and other professionals and young people.

www.2bme.org
American site – non-medical information for teenagers and young adults.

Index